BIRTH DEFECTS
Risks and
Consequences

BIRTH DEFECTS INSTITUTE SYMPOSIA

Ernest B. Hook, Dwight T. Janerich, and Ian H. Porter, editors:
MONITORING, BIRTH DEFECTS AND ENVIRONMENT:
The Problem of Surveillance, 1971

Ian H. Porter and Richard G. Skalko, editors: HEREDITY AND
SOCIETY, 1972

Dwight T. Janerich, Richard G. Skalko, and Ian H. Porter, editors:
CONGENITAL DEFECTS: New Directions in Research, 1973

*Hilaire J. Meuwissen, Richard J. Pickering, Bernard Pollara, and
Ian H. Porter, editors:* COMBINED IMMUNODEFICIENCY
DISEASE AND ADENOSINE DEAMINASE DEFICIENCY: A
Molecular Defect, 1975

S. Kelly, E. B. Hook, D. T. Janerich, and I. H. Porter, editors:
BIRTH DEFECTS: RISKS AND CONSEQUENCES

ACADEMIC PRESS RAPID MANUSCRIPT REPRODUCTION

BIRTH DEFECTS
Risks and
Consequences

Edited by

Sally Kelly

Ernest B. Hook

Dwight T. Janerich

Ian H. Porter

Birth Defects Institute
New York State Department of Health
Albany, New York

Proceedings of a Symposium on Birth Defects: Risks and Consequences
Sponsored by the Birth Defects Institute of the
New York State Department of Health
Held in Albany, New York, November 7–8, 1974

Academic Press, Inc.
New York   San Francisco   London
A Subsidiary of Harcourt Brace Jovanovich, Publishers
1976

IK

ACADEMIC PRESS, INC.
111 Fifth Avenue, New York, New York 10003

United Kingdom Edition published by
ACADEMIC PRESS, INC. (LONDON) LTD.
24/28 Oval Road, London NW1

Library of Congress Cataloging in Publication Data

Symposium on Birth Defects: Risks and Consequences,
    Albany, 1974.
    Birth defects, risks and consequences.

    (Birth Defects Institute symposia)
    Bibliography: p.
    Includes index.
    1.   Deformities—Causes and theories of causation—
Congresses.   2.   Medical genetics—Congresses.
I.   Kelly, Sally.   II.   Birth Defects Institute.
III.   Title.   IV.   Series: Birth Defects Institute.
Symposia.
RG627.S89   1974   618.9'2'0043   76-7368
ISBN 0—12—403450—0

PRINTED IN THE UNITED STATES OF AMERICA

CONTENTS

CONTENTS

CONTENTS

PARTICIPANTS

Mary G. Ampola, Department of Pediatrics, Tufts University, Boston, Massachusetts

Corrado Baglioni, Department of Biological Sciences, State University of New York at Albany, Albany, New York

Arthur D. Bloom, Department of Pediatrics, College of Physicians and Surgeons of Columbia University, New York, New York

Helen C. Chase, Office of Research and Statistics, Social Security Administration, Washington, D.C.

Marilyn Cowger, Department of Pediatrics, Albany Medical College, Albany, New York

Betty Shannon Danes, New York Hospital-Cornell University Medical Center, New York, New York

Robert J. Desnick, Department of Pediatrics, and Dight Institute for Human Genetics, University of Minnesota, Minneapolis, Minnesota

J. Harold Elwood, Institute of Clinical Science, The Queen's University of Belfast, Belfast, Ireland

J. Mark Elwood, Department of Epidemiology and Community Medicine, University of Ottawa, Ottawa, Canada

Irvin Emanuel, Child Development and Rehabilitation Center, University of Washington, Seattle, Washington

Arthur E. Greene, Institute for Medical Research, Camden, New Jersey

PARTICIPANTS

Olli P. Heinonen, Boston University Medical Center, Boston, Massachusetts

Ernest B. Hook, Birth Defects Institute, New York State Department of Health, Albany, New York

Dwight T. Janerich, Birth Defects Institute, New York State Department of Health, Albany, New York

Sally Kelly, Birth Defects Institute, New York State Department of Health, Albany, New York

Jonathan T. Lanman, Department of Obstetrics and Gynecology, Downstate Medical Center, Brooklyn, New York

K. Michael Laurence, Department of Child Health, Welsh National School of Medicine, Cardiff, Wales

Charles E. Lawrence, Rensselaer Polytechnic Institute, Troy, New York

Harvey L. Levy, Department of Public Health, State Laboratory Institute, Jamaica Plain, Massachusetts

William J. Mellman, Department of Human Genetics, University of Pennsylvania, Philadelphia, Pennsylvania

Lechaim Naggan, Johns Hopkins School of Public Health, Batimore, Maryland

Ian H. Porter, Director, Birth Defects Institute, New York State Department of Health, Albany, New York

Godfrey P. Oakley, Jr., Center for Disease Control, Atlanta, Georgia

David Rush, School of Public Health, Columbia University, New York, New York

Richard G. Skalko, Birth Defects Institute, New York State Department of Health, Albany, New York

Dennis Slone, Boston University Medical Center, Boston, Massachusetts

Zena A. Stein, School of Public Health, Columbia University, New York, New York

PREFACE

This volume is the record of the 5th Birth Defects Institute Symposium held under the auspices of the New York State Department of Health in Albany, New York, November 7 and 8, 1974.

In general, the aim of these symposia is to review and discuss emerging problems and information for the purpose of evaluating them in a larger context and for the purpose of promoting investigation. Thus, for example, the problems of monitoring birth defects became a concern in the late 1960s *pari passu* with the evolution of the environmental movement and sparked the idea for the topic of our first symposium in 1970.

At our last symposium in 1973, geneticists, immunologists, and biochemists met to discuss adenosine deaminase deficiency, the first described inborn error of an immune deficiency disease and the second recognized inborn error of purine metabolism. The interaction of scientists from these disciplines enabled them to delineate a new syndrome and to chart future research, some results of which have already appeared in the literature.

The aim of this symposium has been to bring together new information about the factors which might adversely affect the outcome of pregnancies and the implications of some of these outcomes. The contributions concerning neural tube defects illustrate epidemiological and biochemical advances in pursuit of prevention of a single birth defect. The more general discussion of adverse pregnancy outcomes, such as fetal loss, low birth weight and infant mortality, deal with themes that are likely to be interrelated with congenital malformation, both in etiology and impact. Smoking, malnutrition, and drugs may be viewed as only a few of the environmental factors with which we must be concerned in seeking answers to the question of preventable causes of birth defects and other adverse outcomes. Inborn errors of metabolism may appear to raise different types of questions concerning screening, prevention, and treatment than for birth defects of unknown etiology, yet it is likely that, at least with regard to prevention, the problems will become similar in the near future. Our current incomplete knowledge of the etiology of most birth defects and other adverse outcomes, and the difficulties that arise in even investigating such issues in humans, raises vexing problems for public policy decisions.

It is difficult to embrace all such themes in a single title and we have taken the license of interpreting the term "Birth Defects" broadly, encompassing not only structural malformations but, simply, all defective births. Hence, this volume on "Birth Defects: Risks and Consequences."

SECTION I

ANENCEPHALUS AND SPINA BIFIDA IN NORTH AMERICA*

J. Mark Elwood

The prevalence at birth of anencephalus and spina bifida, referred to together as ASB, varies with impersonal factors, as geography, year and season and also with personal factors, as race, age, parity and socioeconomic status of the mother. My data relate to these variables and provide a framework for the "descriptive epidemiology" of ASB in the United States and Canada.

Natural History and Methods of Study

Since ASB is an abnormality which apparently develops in the 3—4 week old fetus,[1] differences in method of ascertainment make it difficult to compare estimates of frequency by different investigators. The possibility that a difference in prevalence at birth of ASB between persons, times or places may reflect different early abortion rates instead of, or as well as, different rates of occurrence of the malformation is brought to mind by the Japanese data[2] of high ASB prevalence in therapeutically aborted fetuses, suggesting that many fetuses die *in utero* and, as early spontaneous abortions, usually go unrecorded. The increased early abortion rates in mothers of ASB infants[3] are also suggestive. The problem of valid frequency estimates is compounded by the difference in gestation age at which stillbirths are reported, which will include the later *in utero* deaths. Since the legal requirements for stillbirth notification varies, usually from 20 to 28 weeks, the completeness of notification will increase with increasing gestational age.

Although referred to as incidence rates, my measurements are of prevalence at birth and are based on two sources of information: notification of abnormalities in births in hospitals or localized region and mortality data. Errors in figures from birth data will most likely include underreporting of early stillbirths and misdiagnosis. Errors in mortality figures (stillbirth and death certificates) will also include underreporting of early stillbirths, misdiagnosis and inadequate certification. In addition, affected children may be certified as

*Supported by Physician's Services Incorporated, Ontario and Grant 606-1038-29 from Health and Welfare, Canada

3

TABLE 1

Numbers of Stillbirths and of Infant Deaths from Anencephalus and Rates per 1,000 Total Births, Canada, by Time Period

	Stillbirths		Infant Deaths		% of Anencephalus as Stillbirths and S.E.
	No.	Rate	No.	Rate	
1943–49	3,092	1.30	393	0.17	88.7 $\pm$ 0.6
1950–54	2,684	1.31	613	0.31	81.9
1955–59	2,072	0.88	686	0.27	75.1
1960–64	1,612	0.67	892	0.39	64.4
1965–69	1,048	0.54	753	0.40	58.2 $\pm$ 1.2
1943–69	10,508	0.99	3,337	0.30	76.0

4

dying of some other cause, *e.g.,* meningitis; the error will increase in proportion to their length of survival.

By comparing numbers of cases of anencephalus in Canada reported by still-births and death certificates with those reported by studies of hospital records of mortality and birth since 1960, we found that ascertainment was about 90% based on mortality data alone.[4] Thus, mortality data of anencephalus may be used to estimate incidence. The compatibility would be expected from the nature of the disease, of which most cases are stillborn or survive only briefly. Conversely, the ratio of mortality of spina bifida to incidence is only from 30 to 50% and, furthermore, is variable. Thus, the interpretation of mortality data on spina bifida is more difficult than anencephalus.

Data based only on death (not stillbirth) certifications or on assessment of abnormalities in liveborn children may be misleading. We found, for example, by comparing total mortality rates and stillbirth and infant death rates from anencephalus in Canada since 1943 (Table 1), that the death rate based only on liveborn infants rose, due to a fall in the proportion of deaths certified as still-births, despite the fact that the total death rate had fallen by about 50%. Kurtze, Goldberg and Kurland,[5] furthermore, have shown that the anenceph-alus death rate per 100,000 population in the United States from 1950 to 1970 was stable and thus the rate per 1,000 births would have increased. As more detailed studies show a fall in anencephalus incidence, the same type of classification shift has probably occurred. The fall in the proportion of anen-cephalus cases certified as stillbirths seems more likely to reflect different interpretations of livebirth used by physicians than a biological change. In New York State from 1945–1959, for example, 85% of anencephalics were recorded as stillbirths[6] while in England and Wales most studies show that over 90% are so described, although the percentage has fallen from 90% in 1961 to 86% in 1967.[7] The greater use of resuscitative measures may increase the tendency to classify a severely deformed child as a livebirth and, conversely, the higher stillbirth proportion reported from Britain may reflect the greater number of deliveries performed by midwives than in the United States or Canada.

Stillbirth and death rates of spina bifida decreased over time. The percent-age classified as stillborn also fell, due perhaps to the same type of classification change and to the longer survival of liveborn children.[8]

Mortality data, therefore, may be used to estimate incidence of anenceph-alus if they include both stillbirths and livebirths. The interpretation of spina bifida mortality rates, however, is prone to greater errors. A small error in earlier studies is the inclusion of conjoined twins, cyclopian monsters and rarities in the death code 750.0, "monstrosity", used to estimate anencephalus before the implementation of the 8th revision of the International Code of

5

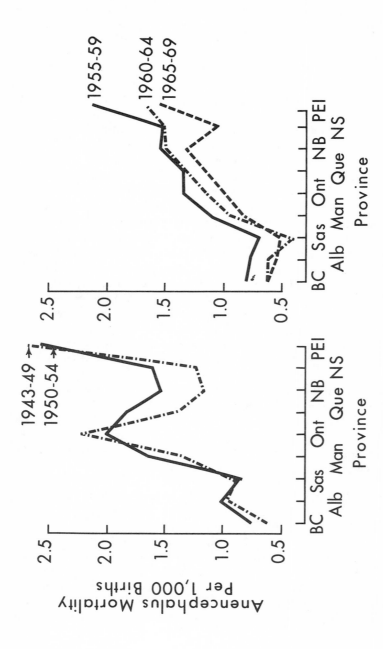

Fig. 1. Mortality rates, as stillbirth and infant deaths per 1,000 total births from anencephalus from 1943 to 1969, in nine provinces of Canada, arranged in west to east order from left to right. *(Courtesy of the American Journal of Epidemiology.)*

6

Diseases in 1969. Over 95% of deaths in this category, however, are, in fact, anencephalus.[8]

Geographical Variation in the Incidence of ASB

Hewitt's data[9] show an east to west decrease in infant death rates from spina bifida in the United States from 1950–59. Kurtze *et al.*[5] observed a concentration of "monstrosity" in northeastern states during 1959–61 but did not include stillbirths. Incidence rates of ASB in Los Angeles[10] and Iowa,[11] furthermore, were lower than in New England, and rates in the southern states of Georgia and Alabama were similar to rates in New England.[12,13] Anencephalus mortality rates since 1955, in Canada, based on infant deaths and stillbirths from 28 weeks gestation, show a decline from eastern to western provinces. Saskatchewan and Alberta, however, have slightly lower rates than the western coastal province of British Columbia. During 1943–54, the rates in Ontario and to a lesser extent in Manitoba and Quebec, were high, producing a different pattern (Fig. 1). Mortality rates from spina bifida since 1950 show a similar pattern. The declivity from east to west is specific to central nervous system abnormalities, at least within the provinces of Alberta, Saskatchewan, Manitoba and New Brunswick, from 1966 to 1969 (Table 2). The incidence of ASB and also of hydrocephalus decreases from east to west, with no difference or an increase in other kinds of malformation.[14,15] Higher mortality from hydrocephalus is also seen in the eastern United States.[5]

Long Term Secular Trends in ASB Mortality

MacMahon and Yen[16] describe a peak of ASB mortality in Boston, Mass. and Providence, R.I. in 1930–36 and a minor one in 1940–46. Mortality rates from 1910 to 1960 can be interpreted as rising to and falling from these peaks. Janerich's data from New York State since 1945[17] shows declining incidence rates which are consistent with a similar epidemic. He also notes a small peak in the 1960–65 period. Spina bifida mortality in England and Wales reached a peak between 1930–44[7] and ASB rates in Birmingham, Scotland and Dublin peaked around 1940,[18,19] suggesting pandemicity.

The Canadian data are similar (Fig. 2): annual mortality rates from anencephalus peaked around 1950, followed by a steady fall since. Spina bifida mortality also declined during this period, with a small increase between 1960 and 1962, as noted also in the United States.[5] That this rise was not an artifact of changing the classification of spina bifida into two categories, with and without hydrocephalus – causing a rise in reports of spina bifida mortality and a fall in those of hydrocephalus deaths – is assured, since the change was not implemented in Canada until 1969. The data of small series by hospitals in

TABLE 2

Incidence of Major Groups of Congenital Abnormalities in Newborns, in Four Canadian Provinces, 1966—1969
Provinces are Arranged in West (Left) to East (Right) Order.[11] Incidence Rates Expressed as Total
Stillbirths Plus Livebirths per 1,000 Total Births

	British Columbia	Alberta	Manitoba	New Brunswick
Total Births	135,730	123,377	71,202	49,031
1. Anencephalus	.58	.58	.90	1.51
2. Spina bifida	.87	1.01	1.33	2.46
3. Hydrocephalus	.63	.86	.69	1.22
TOTAL 1—2	2.08	2.45	2.92	5.19
4. Other central nervous system	.28	.42	.38	.36
5. Cardiovascular system	3.30	2.45	1.63	1.90
6. Genitourinary system	2.50	2.46	2.26	1.45
7. Digestive system	3.65	3.26	2.85	2.14
8. Musculo-skeletal system	4.62	4.34	3.62	3.77
9. Others	5.30	5.40	4.86	3.79
TOTAL 4—9	19.76	18.36	16.74	13.51
All abnormalities	21.84	20.81	19.66	18.70

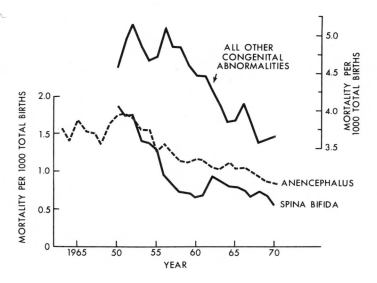

Fig. 2.   Annual mortality rates, as stillbirths plus infant deaths per 1,000 births from anencephalus and spina bifida, Canada.

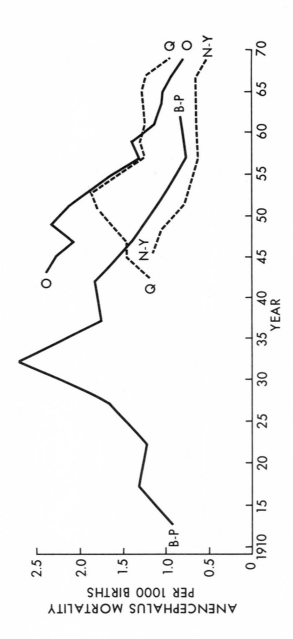

Fig. 3. Comparison of anencephalus mortality rates in Ontario and Quebec with incidence reported from Boston and Providence[16] and New York State.[17]

10

Atlanta,[20] Vermont[21] and Philadelphia,[22] which should be free of this bias, also suggest the rise. The incidence of anencephalus in Virginia[23] was higher, both conditions increased in New York State about this time and a 1960–61 peak occurred in Scotland, Belfast and Dublin.[24] The Canadian data differs in that only infants, not stillbirths, contributed to the rise in mortality from spina bifida and there was no contemporary rise in anencephalus mortality.

The trend of annual mortality rates from anencephalus in Canada differs according to regions. A comparison of mortality rates in New England and in Ontario show similar types of decline (Fig. 3) but a different rate in Quebec. No long term secular trend is apparent in British Columbia, apart from a peak in 1951–52. Rates in the Prairies and the Maritime Provinces decreased less regularly.[4] The trend of annual mortality rates from spina bifida were similar in the five regions of Canada.[8]

Seasonal Variation

Anencephalus in Britain is more frequent and the mortality rate higher in wintertime births than at other seasons,[25] suggesting that a teratogenic agent may have a maximum effect in spring and early summer. The anencephalus mortality rate in Quebec and the Prairies in 1956–1962 also was higher in winter. In contrast to these studies, anencephalus incidence did not vary seasonally in Rhode Island,[26] Boston[27] or Missouri.[28] The seasonal variation was less marked, furthermore, in the other regions and, since 1962, throughout Canada.

Seasonal variation in the incidence of hydrocephalus and ASB in four Canadian provinces from 1966–69 is significant (Table 3), and an excess incidence of spina bifida and hydrocephalus in winter was reported by British general practitioners.[30] The winter excesses of anencephalus or of spina bifida described in several North American studies are not significant[31–34] but larger studies might show significant trends.[29]

Sex Ratio

An excess of girls are born with ASB. The proportion of boys increases with increasing gestational age and is greater in live- than stillborn infants.[26] A greater male abortion rate is thus an unlikely explanation for the excess of affected females.

Although it has been suggested that the sex distribution is nearer equality in areas of low incidence,[35] the proportion of males in Canada does not differ in regions of high or low incidence. There is some evidence in Canada, however, of an increased excess of females at times of high incidence, as suggested by a British study[36] and predicted by Knox's fetus-fetus interaction hypothesis.[37] There is a barely significant increase in the male proportion in Canada since 1943. The time trends for each sex are similar (Fig. 4). In New York State,

11

TABLE 3

Numbers of Cases and Rates per 1,000 Total Births of Central Nervous System Abnormalities by Month of Birth; British Columbia, Alberta, Manitoba and New Brunswick, 1966–1969.41

	March–May		June–August		September–November		December–February		X^2 d.f. = 3	
	No.	Rate	No.	Rate	No.	Rate	No.	Rate		
Anencephalus	84	0.85	64	0.66	75	0.81	66	0.74	2.65	N.S.
Spina bifida	133	1.34	108	1.11	125	1.35	92	1.03	6.13	N.S.
Anencephalus and Spina bifida	217	2.19	172	1.77	200	2.16	158	1.77	7.92	$p < 0.05$
Hydrocephalus	90	0.91	57	0.59	82	0.88	72	0.80	7.86	$p < 0.05$
Total births	99,312		97,366		92,932		89 730			

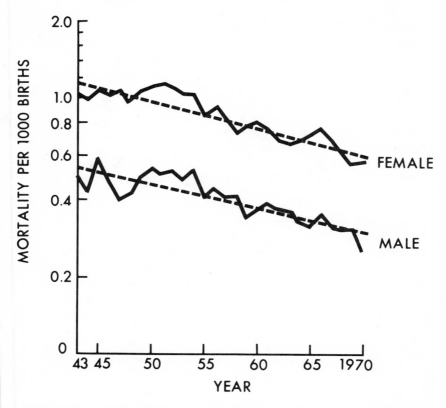

Fig. 4. Annual mortality rates per 1,000 total births from anencephaly by sex, Canada. Semi-logarithmic scale.

however, a rise in male proportion accompanied falling incidence[38] but there was no change in sex distribution during the Boston-Providence epidemic.[39]

Maternal Age and Parity

The incidence of anencephalus and spina bifida in Rhode Island, 1936–1952, showed a stronger association with parity than maternal age.[40] In all age groups, the lowest rate was among second births, with higher rates in primiparae and higher birth orders. An association with age within each parity group was weaker but also u-shaped. During the period of study, however, the higher risk in primiparae decreased and was not seen after 1943.

A u-shaped relationship with parity was also noted in Boston, from 1930 to 1965, without any association with age.[41] The excess risk in primiparae was greatest in Irish mothers, who had high rates, and not seen in Jewish mothers, who had low rates. U-shaped relationships with both age and parity were noted in Quebec.[33]

Analysis of the maternal age effect[42–44] by mother's year of birth, showed that within each maternal birth cohort the incidence of ASB tends to decrease with increasing age.

A u-shaped association with parity, with higher rates in primiparae and in mothers of parity 3 and above, is seen in all age groups in a study of all stillbirths and deaths from anencephalus in fourteen large Canadian cities (Vancouver, Edmonton, Calgary, Regina, Saskatoon, Winnipeg, Hamilton, Kitchener, London, Windsor, Ottawa, Quebec, St. John and Halifax), from 1950 to 1969. The cases were identified from Statistics Canada records and the deaths linked to birth certificates to yield information on age and parity. A comparison group consisting of a random sample of 1,000 livebirths was chosen from the population of all livebirths in these cities in 1952, 1957, 1962 and 1967. The association with age within parity groups is much weaker. Using age alone, without correction for parity, a cohort effect similar to those described by Janerich is clear.[45]

Racial Effects

ASB is more common in the United States in white populations than in blacks.[5,6,26,41,46,47] The incidence in Alabama from 1961–1966 was 1.20 per 1,000 (338 cases) in white and 0.18 (29 cases) in black births.[46] The incidence in Jewish births is low in Boston[41] and Quebec.[33] Miller[48] reported only one case of anencephalus and three of spina bifida in 12,337 Indian births in British Columbia from 1952 to 1958, giving rates of 0.08 and 0.24 per 1,000, compared to 0.67 and 1.08 in the Caucasian population. Although the decline in ASB rates from Boston from 1930 to 1965 was not seen in Jewish births,[41] the number of Jewish cases observed was small.

Possible Reasons for the Geographical and Temporal Variations

1. Genetic factors

Hewitt observed that the distribution of spina bifida mortality in Canada was the opposite of that expected by the major ethnic distribution (French: British).[9] Although a higher level of inbreeding in eastern areas seemed to be a plausible explanation, relative inbreeding data are not available. Other conditions are also higher in the east, *e.g.*, cystic fibrosis and diabetes, yet other malformations, *e.g.*, cleft lip and palate, show a different distribution. Hewitt[9] attempted to estimate the inbreeding levels objectively by using an index of the variance of birth weight of all livebirths; the index, which should increase as levels of inbreeding increase, showed a correlation of +0.56 with the log of state infant death rates from spina bifida, 1950—59. The index for the Canadian provinces during 1965—69, compared to the anencephalus incidence, yielded a correlation of —0.44 (d.f. = p > 0.2). Naggan and MacMahon[41] found no evidence that changing inbreeding levels were involved in the falling incidence rate in Boston.

2. Socioeconomic factors

Nearly all studies have shown an increased incidence of ASB in the less prosperous socioeconomic groups, including those in Quebec[33] and Boston.[41] The decline in incidence in Boston was similar in all occupational groups. Anencephalus rates in fifty large towns in Canada from 1950 to 1969 were correlated significantly with the mean income of the town and geographic differences in incidence could be due in part to income related factors.

3. Water composition

Higher levels of ASB occur in Britain in areas with soft water, an effect which persists after correction for socioeconomic differences.[49] Infant death rates from spina bifida are greater in those states of the United States with soft water supplies.[50] The crude rates of anencephalus in 35 Canadian towns with populations of over 50,000 from 1965—69 are correlated with mean income, rainfall, water hardness and longitude. Only the negative relationship with hardness remains significant after correction for income by indirect standardization procedure. The results are less clear when other variables, *e.g.*, other mineral concentrations, are included or when other time periods are taken.

4. Potato blight

The correlation between Canadian provincial anencephalus mortality rates and potato production, consumption and blight prevalence[51,52] is strongly positive. However, there is no association between annual blight prevalence and

15

anencephalus mortality one or two years later in the same province or between provinces, nor is there an association between the degree of seasonal variation and blight prevalence.[52,53] No temporal association of blight and ASB has been shown in New England,[54] the other high blight area in North America.

Conclusion

The descriptive epidemiology of anencephalus and spina bifida in North America is complex. The two conditions have a marked geographical variation, with incidence rates 1.5 to 3 times higher in eastern than in western areas. The evidence for variation in hydrocephalus incidence is similar but less marked and, in Canada, is shared by no other abnormalities. The incidence of anencephalus and spina bifida shows marked secular variation, which differs regionally. The decline in incidence rates following the New England epidemic in the 1930's, for example, coincided with those in New York State and Ontario but did not parallel those in British Columbia, which remained stable after 1943. Small peaks in anencephalus incidence occurred around 1950 in Canada and in the early 1960's in New York State. The incidence of spina bifida rose in many areas in 1962. The incidence of ASB was higher in winter in Canada and higher also in lower socioeconomic groups. It is lower in Blacks, Jews and American Indians than in Caucasians. The incidence varies with maternal parity and age, the effect of parity being the more marked and may be affected by the mother's year of birth.

REFERENCES

1. K.K. Nakano, *Develop. Med. Child Neurol. 15,* 383, 1973.

2. H. Nishimura, *in* Congenital Malformations, Proceedings of the Third International Conference, Excerpta Medica, 275, 1970.

3. A.D. MacDonald, *Brit. J. Prev. Soc. Med. 25,* 220, 1971.

4. J.M. Elwood, *Amer. J. Epidem. 100,* 288, 1974.

5. J.F. Kurtze, I.D. Goldberg and L.T. Kurland,*in* Epidemiology of Neurologic and Sense Organ Disorders, J.F. Kurtze, I.D. Goldberg and L.T. Kurland (Eds.), Harvard University Press, 169, 1073.

6. A.M. Gittelsohn and S. Milham, *Brit. J. Prev. Soc. Med. 16,* 153, 1962.

7. S.C. Rogers and M. Morris, *Ann. Hum. Genet. 34,* 295, 1971.

8. J.M. Elwood, unpublished data.

9. D. Hewitt, *Brit. J. Prev. Soc. Med. 17,* 13, 1963.

10. G. Smilkstein, *Calif. Med. 96,* 350, 1962.

11. S. Hay, *Amer. J. Epidem. 94,* 572, 1971.

12. National Communicable Disease Center, Metropolitan Atlanta Congenital Defects Program, Report No. 1, 1969.

13. G. Cassady, *Amer. J. Obst. Gyn. 103,* 1154, 1969.

14. P. Banister, *in* Monitoring, Birth Defects and Environment, E.B. Hook, D.T. Janerich and I.H. Porter (Eds.), Academic Press, New York, 1971.

15. J.M. Elwood and J.R. Rogers (a) *Canad. J. Publ. Health* (in press).

16. B. MacMahon and S. Yen, *Lancet 1,* 31, 1971.

17. D.T. Janerich, *Teratology 8,* 253, 1973.

18. I. Leck and S.C. Rogers, *Brit. J. Prev. Soc. Med. 21,* 177, 1967.

19. J.H. Elwood, *Inter. J. Epidemiol. 2,* 171, 1973.

20. M. Boris, R. Blumberg, D.B. Feldman and J.E. Sellers, *J. Amer. Med. Ass. 184,* 768, 1963.

21. J.F. Vucey, R.W. Mann, G.M. Simmons and E. Friedman, *Pediatrics 33,* 981, 1964.

22. T.H. Ingalls and M.A. Klingberg, *Amer. J. Med. Sci. 249,* 316, 1965.

23. M.K. Solowy and F.M. Shepard, *Clinical Pediatrics 10,* 43, 1971.

24. J.H. Elwood and H.A. Warnock, *Irish J. Med. Sci., 7th Series, 2,* 17, 1969.

25. J. H. Elwood, this Symposium, p.

26. B. MacMahon, T.F. Pugh and T.H. Ingalls, *Brit. J. Prev. Soc. Med. 7,* 211, 1963.

27. L. Naggan, *Amer. J. Epidem. 89,* 154, 1969.

28. S.L. Sliberg, F.T. Watson and J.C. Martin, *Canad. J. Publ. Health 59,* 239, 1968.

29. J.M. Elwood, *Brit. J. Prev. Soc. Med. 29,* 22, 1975.

30. B.C.S. Slater, G.I. Watson and J.C. MacDonald, *Brit. J. Prev. Soc. Med. 18,* 1, 1964.

31. D. Hewitt, *Amer. J. Publ. Hlth. 52,* 1676, 1962.

32. M. Alter, *Amer. J. Dis. Child. 106,* 536, 1963.

33. I. Horowitz and A.D. McDonald, *Canad. Med. Ass. J. 100,* 748, 1969.

34. N.W. Choi, F.A. Kaponski, E. Ateah and N.A. Nelson, *in* Drugs and Fetal Development, M.A. Klingberg (Ed.), Plenum Publ. House, 511, 1972.

35. L. Naggan, *Pediatrics 47,* 577, 1971.

36. S.C. Rogers and M. Morris, *Brit. J. Prev. Soc. Med. 27,* 81, 1973.

37. E.G. Knox, *Develop. Med. Child Neurol. 12,* 167, 1970.

38. D.T. Janerich, Annual Meeting, Society for Epidemiologic Research, 1974.

39. S. Yen, personal communication.

40. T.H. Ingalls, T.F. Pugh and B. MacMahon, *Brit. J. Prev. Soc. Med. 8,* 17, 1954.

41. L. Naggan and B. MacMahon, *New Engl. J. MEd. 277,* 1119, 1969.

42. D.T. Janerich, *Amer. J. Epidemiol. 95,* 319, 1971.

43. D.T. Janerich, *Amer. J. Epidemiol. 96,* 389, 1972.

44. D.T. Janerich, *in* Congenital Defects: New Directions in Research, D.T. Janerich, R.G. Skalko and I.H. Porter (Eds.), Academic Press, New York, p. 73, 1973.

45. S. Raman and J.M. Elwood, 7th Annual Meeting, Society for Epidemiologic Research, 1974.

46. G. Cassady, *Amer. J. Obst. Gynecol. 103,* 1154, 1969.

47. C.S. Chung and N.C. Myrianthopoulos, *Amer. J. Hum. Genet. 20,* 44, 1968.

48. J.R. Miller, *in* The Use of Registries and Vital Statistics in the Study of Congenital Malformations, International Medical Congress, New York, 336, 1963.

49. C.R. Lowe, C.J. Roberts and S. Lloyd, *Brit. Med. J. 2,* 357, 1971.

50. J. Fedrick, *Nature 227,* 176, 1970.

51. J.H. Renwick, *Brit. J. Prev. Soc. Med. 26,* 67, 1972.

52. J.M. Elwood, to be published.

53. J.M. Elwood, *Lancet 1,* 769, 1973.

54. B. MacMahon, S. Yen and K.J. Rothman, *Lancet 1,* 598, 1973.

ANENCEPHALY AND SPINA BIFIDA IN THE BRITISH ISLES*

J. Harold Elwood

In this paper I describe some aspects of the epidemiology of anencephaly and spina bifida in the British Isles with particular reference to the occurrence of these defects in Ireland. I have intentionally not considered studies in other countries except where relevant to interpreting the British and Irish data.

Official Statistics

National mortality statistics form the basis of the early investigations of major malformations of the central nervous system conducted by Record and McKeown[1] in Birmingham over twenty years ago. Owing to its obvious appearance and complete fatality, anencephaly is perhaps the only common major congenital malformation which may be satisfactorily studied using death certifications. Fatal cases of spina bifida also may be investigated via this source but as the proportion of such affected infants surviving varies considerably by area within the British Isles, conclusions concerning the epidemiology of this defect from death data only are based on incomplete ascertainment and may be misleading.

Tabulations of stillbirths and infant deaths attributed to anencephaly and spina bifida have been published by the Registrars General for Scotland, England and Wales and Northern Ireland since 1939, 1950 and 1963 respectively and for the Irish Republic by the Director of Central Statistics Office, Dublin, since 1966. Absence of Irish data until comparatively recently is due to the fact that the Registrations of Stillbirths Act (N.I.) was not passed until 1960 and statutory certification of stillbirths in the Irish Republic is not required even yet. There is, however, a voluntary system of stillbirth notification in the Irish Republic and I have made estimates of the incidence of anencephaly after adjusting for the degree of underascertainment[2] (see below). In all the United Kingdom areas and also in the Irish Republic, stillbirths (synonymous with late fetal deaths) are defined as of 28 weeks gestation or

*Supported in part by Grant Number G 972/919/C from the Medical Research Council, United Kingdom.

21

TABLE 1

Official Statistics* Relating to Stillbirths and Infant Deaths Attributed to Anencephaly and Spina Bifida During One Year (1970) in the British Isles

Country	Births (Live and Still)	Anencephaly			Spina Bifida			Both Defects (Live and Still)	
		Still-born	Infant death	Rate	Still-born	Infant death	Rate Rate	No.	Rate
England and Wales	794,831	1201	173	1.7	207	554	1.0	2135	2.7
Scotland	88,569	183	24	2.3	31	83	1.3	321	3.6
Northern Ireland	32,551	88	21	3.3	14	51	2.0	174	5.3
Irish Republic	65,286	106	43	2.3	17	47	1.0	213	3.3
British Isles	981,237	1578	261	1.9	269	735	1.0	2843	2.9

*Sources: Annual Reports of the three U.K. Registrars General and Annual Report on Vital Statistics (Central Statistics Office, Dublin). Anencephaly includes stillbirths (ICD No. P.69) plus infant deaths (ICD No. 740); Spina Bifida stillbirths (ICD No. P70) plus infant deaths (ICD No. 741). Rates are expressed per 1,000 (live and still) births.

22

over.

Taking 1970 as an example (Table 1), official statistics for the British Isles indicate that 1,839 cases of anencephaly (86 percent stillborn) and 1,004 of fatal spina bifida (17 percent stillborn) occurred in a population of 981,237 (live and still) births. Considering anencephaly only, the geographic variation in incidence shows the highest rates in Northern Ireland and the eastern Province of Leinster in the Irish Republic (Fig. 1). High frequencies also occur in those parts of Great Britain bordering the Irish Sea, namely the lowlands of Scotland, Wales and the northwest region of England. The six counties and two county boroughs in Northern Ireland exhibit rates varying from 2.7 per 1,000 (live and still) births in County Londonderry to 4.2 in both Belfast and Londonderry City.[3] While it is possible to calculate an incidence rate for anencephaly in each of the twenty-six counties comprising the Irish Republic, I think these data are inaccurate at present for the following reasons. The proportion of anencephalics registered as liveborn and later as infant deaths in Belfast[4] was 19.2 percent during 1956–66 compared with 21.5 percent in Coffey and Jessop's Dublin survey,[5] 1953–56. These figures are higher than in Great Britain (e.g. Glasgow 10.5 percent and Aberdeen 1.5 percent, 1956–66) and probably reflect different certification practices with respect to distinguishing a stillbirth from a liveborn infant dying shortly after delivery. In the stillbirth notification data for the Irish Republic, 1965–67, there are seventeen areas with a total anencephalic rate of less than 2.0 per 1,000 and 43 percent of these anencephalics reported were liveborn, whereas in the areas with rates of more than 2.0, only 21 percent were reported as liveborn.[6] Undernotification of affected stillbirths, therefore, is highly probable with this voluntary rather than statutory system of notification in operation.

At present it is not possible to construct a map similar to Figure 1 illustrating the frequency of spina bifida in the British Isles because of the lack of information on surviving infants with this defect. Some data are obtainable from the voluntary notification systems for congenital malformations administered by the Department of Health and Social Services and the General Register Office, Northern Ireland, and the Department of Health and Social Security and the General Register Office, England and Wales. Of these two systems in existence since 1964, studies to date suggest considerable undernotification of CNS defects in England and Wales[7] but not in Northern Ireland.[3] No comparable data are collected in Scotland or in the Irish Republic. A detailed analysis of the notifications in England and Wales since 1964 is being prepared.[8]

The latest available official statistics relating to the whole of the British Isles cover the period 1963 to 1970 inclusive. The United Kingdom figures are from annual reports of the three Registrars General; for the Irish Republic

23

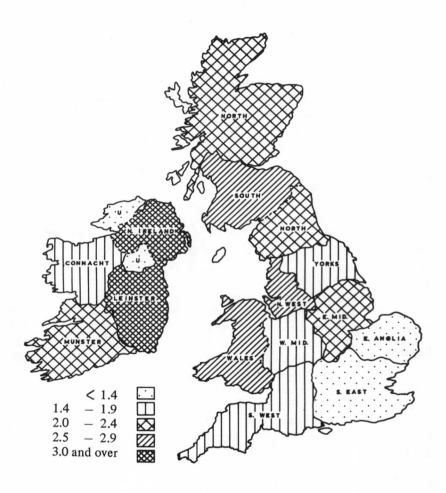

Fig. 1. Geographical variations in the incidence of anencephaly (stillbirths and infant deaths) per 1,000 total births in the British Isles, 1965–67. *(Courtesy of Developmental Medicine and Child Neurology.)*

tabulations of stillbirths and infant deaths from spina bifida date only from 1966 and the anencephalic rates graphed in Figure 2, which were prepared by the Central Statistics Office, Dublin, are those published by Masterson et al.[9]

Mortality Trends

There has been a definite decline in mortality attributable to anencephaly in Scotland and a minimal fall in England and Wales. Owing to the smaller numbers of births annually, rates in Ireland fluctuate more from year to year but there is no obvious trend over the 1963–70 period; mortality from anencephaly in both Northern Ireland and the Irish Republic seems fairly stationary at present (Fig. 2). The death rate from spina bifida, however, has not fallen in Scotland or England and Wales, while there has been a small overall increase in Northern Ireland (Fig. 3).

Incidence

Findings from various community surveys designed to ascertain all affected births within a defined population at risk during a specified time period are summarized in Table 2. Some, but not all listed, used multiple sources of ascertainment. The incidence of anencephaly follows the trend seen in the mortality data (Fig. 2) and shows that the frequency in Belfast[12] is the highest in the world yet reported from a community series. It is three times that found in Greater London by Carter and Evans[23] and 20 percent above the incidence in South Wales.[18] The latest Belfast survey[13] which also included spina bifida indicates the frequency of this malformation to be equally high; some years one defect is more prevalent than the other but over the quinquennium studied, more cases of spina bifida than of anencephaly occurred. Ratios of spina bifida/anencephaly rates suggest the former to be more common in most areas of the British Isles with the exception of Birmingham.[20] Some of the smaller surveys mentioned may not have ascertained all surviving spina bifida children as my experience is that these cases are sometimes missed. Spellman's surveys in Cork City and County[16,17] were based on questionnaires sent to all local doctors, midwives and maternity hospitals; Coffey's study[15] was made by examining records of all hospital and nursing homes registered by the Department of Health in the Irish Republic for the delivery of maternity cases. The earlier studies by Coffey and Jessop[31–32] were based on hospital deliveries only and a community survey of neural tube defects in Dublin has yet to be made.

Secular Trends

Long-term trends in the incidence of anencephaly have been reported from Belfast,[12] Dublin,[33–35] Birmingham,[36] England and Wales[37] and Scotland[38]

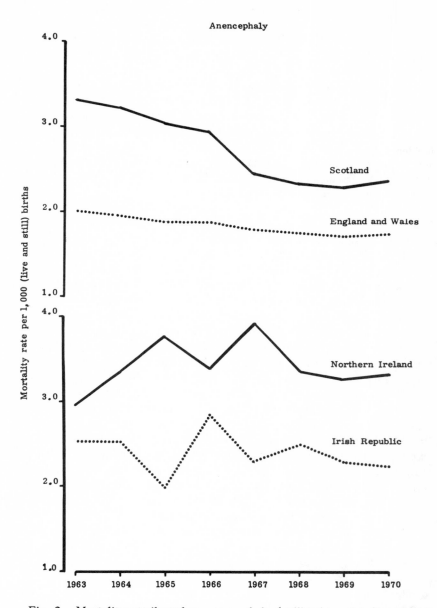

Fig. 2. Mortality attributed to anencephaly (stillbirths and infant deaths based on official statistics in the British Isles, 1963–70.

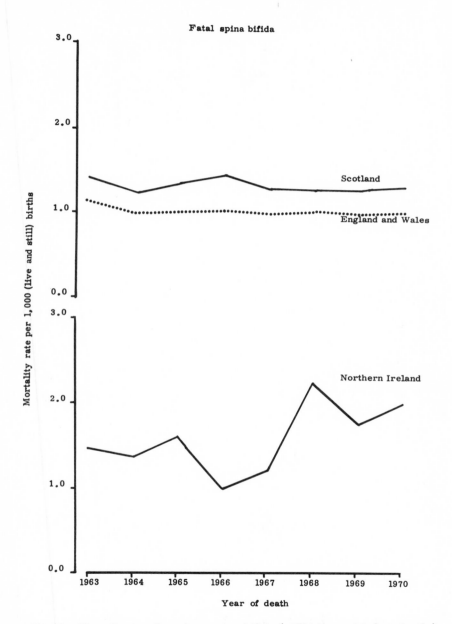

Fig. 3. Mortality attributed to spina bifida (stillbirths and infant deaths) based on official statistics in the British Isles, 1963–70.

TABLE 2

Selected Community Surveys of Anencephaly and Spina Bifida in the British Isles

Area	Period of Observation	Total Births No.	Anencephaly frequency per 1,000 total births		Spina Bifida frequency per 1,000 total births		Ratio of Rates Spina Bifida/ Anencephaly	Reference
			No.	Rate	No.	Rate		
Northern Ireland								
All	1964–66	103,353	371	3.6	382	3.7	1.03	Elwood (1970a)[10]
Belfast	1957	8,519	33	3.5	16	1.7	0.49	Stevenson and Warnock (1959)[11]
Belfast	1950–66	147,825	584	3.9	–	–	–	Elwood (1970b)[12]
Belfast	1964–68	41,351	175	4.2	185	4.5	1.07	Elwood and Nevin)1973)[13]
Irish Republic								
County Galway	1958–60	5,367	21	3.9	–	–	–	Cahalane et al. (1965)[14]
All	1961–62	49,262	–	–	152	3.1	–	Coffey (1970)[15]
Cork City and Co.	1962–66	37,135	76	2.0	91	2.4	1.20	Spellman (1969, 1970)[16,17]
Wales								
South Wales	1956–62	102,786	364	3.5	425	4.1	1.17	Laurence et al.(1968)[18]
Scotland								
All	1939–45	655,812	1,668	2.5	1,512	2.3	0.92	Record and McKeown (1949)[1]
Glasgow	1964–68	100,165	292	2.8	289	2.8	1.00	Wilson (1970)[19]
England								
Birmingham	1950–59	190,236	459	2.4	251	1.1	0.46	Leck et al. (1968)[20]
Camden	1964–67	17,102	21	1.2	24	1.3	1.1	Jepson (1969)[21]
Exeter	1954–60	8,117	24	3.0	6	0.7	0.23	Ward and Irvine (1961)[22]
Greater London	1965–68	409,466	578	1.4	631	1.5	1.07	Carter and Evans (173)[23]
Hertfordshire	1952–55	3,081	8	2.5	7	2.2	0.88	McDonald (1961)[24]
Leicester	1953–62	46,312	107	2.3	122	2.6	1.13	Moss (1964)[25]
Liverpool	1960–64	91,176	286	3.1	306	3.4	1.09	Smithells (1968)[26]
Northampton	1944–57	62,224	64	1.0	116	1.9	1.90	Pleydell (1960)[27]
Reading	1958–63	12,951	28	2.2	34	2.6	0.85	Griffin and Sorrie (1964)[28]
Southampton	1958–62	14,907	29	1.9	48	3.2	1.68	Williamson (1965)[29]

TABLE 3

Incidence per 1,000 Births of Both Defects (Anencephaly and Spina Bifida) in the British Isles and in Offspring of Migrants Resident in North America

British Isles 1950–58		Quebec[45] 1956–65		Boston[46] 1946–65	
Irish[13]	8.7			Irish	2.5
Welsh[18]	7.6	French	3.4	Italian	1.2
Scots[19]	5.6	British	3.2	—	
English[20]	3.5	Jewish	0.6	Jewish	0.8
Mean	6.3	Mean	3.3	Mean	2.2

based on national mortality data, community surveys and studies of hospital births. In the data on all births to women resident in Belfast, 1960—66, it is possible to demonstrate the bias in incidence resulting from estimates calculated on teaching hospital births only (rate 6.3), a widely used source of ascertainment, compared with all births in the community (rate 4.2) — a 50 percent difference. Similar trends, however, are evident in both groups of births. A summary of some of these observations is shown in Figure 4 based on data from the Annual Report of the Registrar General for Scotland, the paper by Leck[36] on Birmingham and the papers by Elwood[10,34] on Belfast and Dublin. The Belfast trend relates to births in the Royal Maternity Hospital and the Jubilee Hospital, the Dublin trend to births in the Rotunda Hospital and the Coombe Lying-In Hospital. The Birmingham rate fell from a peak around 1940—43 to rise again in 1954—55, after which it declined; the interval between peaks is about sixteen years. In Scotland, Belfast and Dublin, the incidence has increased since 1950 and a peak, which is particularly striking in the Irish material, is evident in all three areas in 1960—61.[39]

Further analysis of the Dublin hospital data, 1900—65[33,34] shows two "epidemics" which peaked in 1940—41 and 1960—61. The first resembled the 1930—34 epidemic of anencephaly and spina bifida described by MacMahon and Yen[40] in the northeast United States, although it occurred some five or so years later. Post-war trends, however, are strikingly different, the anencephalic rate having increased steadily in Dublin while declining in Boston,[40] Providence,[40] New York State[21] and Canada[42] (Table 3).

Seasonal Trends

In the British Isles, several authors have reported a significant association between the numbers of affected births and month of delivery. A consistent finding, both in official anencephalic stillbirth registrations and in the surveys from Belfast,[12] Birmingham[38] and Scotland,[38] is the excess of anencephalics born during winter compared with summer. The only exception to this trend, observed to date, is South Wales[43] where more summer births were affected. This relationship with season has changed slowly with time in Scotland, Birmingham and Belfast (Fig. 5). There is much less information about short-term trends in the monthly numbers of spina bifida births but those reported seem similar to anencephaly. In Belfast, a winter excess was more marked with fatal cases compared with non-fatal cases (survivors aged one year or over) of spina bifida.[13]

In most surveys so far conducted in the British Isles and elsewhere, including Hungary,[44] Quebec,[45] the United States[46] and Israel,[47] the incidence of neurological malformations has been found to vary with maternal age, parity,

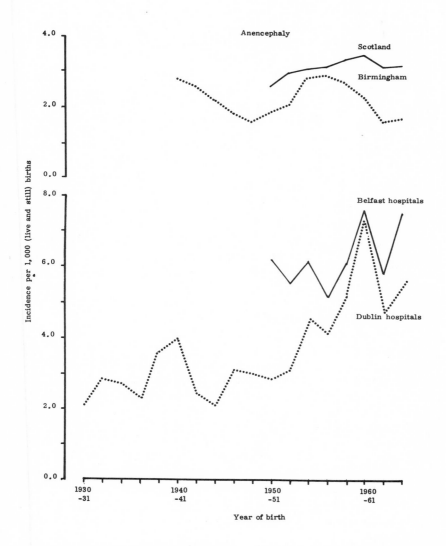

Fig. 4. Secular trends in the incidence of anencephaly (stillbirths and infant deaths) per 1,000 total births in four areas of the British Isles, 1930–65 (see text).

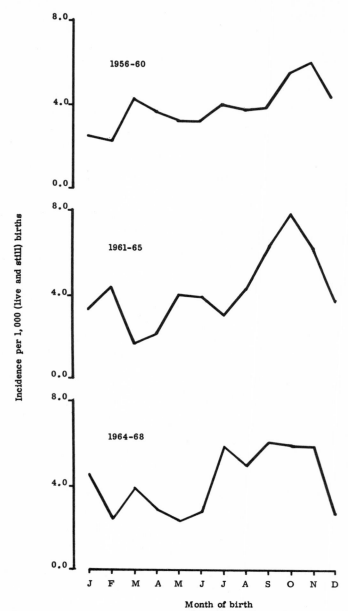

Fig. 5. Monthly incidence of anencephaly (stillbirths and infant deaths) per 1,000 total births in Belfast during three time periods, 1956–60, 1961–65 and 1965–68.

socioeconomic status and the biological factors of sex, twinning and sibship aggregation. Because of the confounding effects between maternal age, parity and socioeconomic status, the independent influence of each factor has not yet been satisfactorily unraveled. However, high rates are associated at a single factor level with primiparity, a history of one or more previous stillbirths or abortions, reproduction after 35 years of age and poor socioeconomic status. The latter, based on the Registrar General's "Classification of Occupations", indicates a low incidence of affected offspring to parents in classes I and II compared with classes III, IV and V in Aberdeen,[48] Glasgow[19] and all Scotland.[1] A similar although less marked gradient is seen in Belfast,[13] Birmingham and South Wales. The high frequency of anencephaly in offspring of unemployed fathers in Dublin[31] was not found in Belfast, where the rate in children of the unemployed was 3.0 in contrast with 4.9 in social class V.

More female than male infants are affected by neural tube defects and as chromosomal studies are normal, this difference is genuine. For anencephaly, 26 percent of cases in Belfast[13] are male and the Dublin figure is 20 percent; 41 percent of spina bifidas in Belfast are male. Leck has stated[49] that the Birmingham epidemic of anencephaly in the 1950's was confined to females, hence it will be important to determine whether this also happened in the 1961 epidemic peak in Ireland and Scotland.[50] Studies of sibship risks show an increased likelihood of recurrence of the same or other defects in subsequent children after one neurological malformation has occurred in a family. Laurence[51] also has demonstrated a greater frequency of spina bifida occulta in sibs of children having spina bifida aperta compared with controls. The risk for other living children in the British Isles is about 1 in 20 and this rises to 1 in 10 in families where two affected births have already occurred. No estimates of risk are available yet for births to women resident in Ireland but preliminary data from a pedigree study of Belfast infants in progress suggest recurrence rates higher than those just quoted, which are calculated from the surveys made in Glasgow,[52] South Wales,[53] Greater London[23] and Southampton.[29] The occurrence of neural tube defects in both infants of a twin pair, whether monozygotic or dizygotic, is rare. Leck[49] has recently calculated the concordance rate as 1.45 percent, based on 212 pairs assembled from the literature. The incidence of spina bifida in twins seems to be less than in singletons but anencephalic rates are similar.

Conclusion

The high incidence of both anencephaly and spina bifida in communities resident in the British Isles contrast with the much lower frequencies in populations of similar genetic stock now living in North America; frequencies in the migrant groups have declined by over 50 percent during periods of one or two generations or less. Offspring of Boston-Irish have a significantly lower risk of being affected than births to Irish mothers resident in Ireland[35] and Leck has shown the incidence in Birmingham children of Irish parents to be closer to the rate for infants of British origin in Birmingham than in the Irish born.[54] Thus, comparisons of frequencies in communities of alike stock but living under different geographic conditions indicate an alteration of malformation risk by environment. Furthermore, the relatively brief time periods over which these changes have occurred seem to exclude certain genetic causes such as selective outbreeding or other alterations of marriage patterns.

Many attempts have been made to identify these environmental determinants and among the factors so far studied are: trace elements (*e.g.* zinc deficiency),[15] softness of water,[56] nitrites and nitrates in cured meats,[57] tea intake;[58] drugs taken during pregnancy (*e.g.* phenytoin),[59] analgesics[60] and antidepressants;[61] and infections (*e.g.* influenza),[62] Renwick's hypothesis[63,64] based on ingestion of blight-infested potatoes has been examined using Irish[65] and Scottish[66] data and found to be unacceptable. Also short-term avoidance of potatoes does not prevent neural tube defects.

A perspective potato avoidance trial has recently been carried out in Belfast[67,68] based on 88 high risk mothers, each of whom previously had given birth to one or more offspring with a neural tube defect. These mothers were divided into two groups and their subsequent pregnancies followed up at regular intervals until delivery. In group one, 27 mothers who excluded potatoes from their diet prior to conception and throughout pregnancy, there were 4 abortions (none had a CNS defect) and 23 births; 2 out of these 23 were born with a neurological malformation. In group two, 61 mothers who ate a normal diet, including potatoes, prior to and throughout pregnancy, there were 5 abortions (one had a CNS defect) and 56 births; 2 out of these 56 had a neural tube defect. The original estimate that 95 percent of the anencephalic and spina bifida births in the United Kingdom were prevantable by potato avoidance has now been modified by Renwick[69] to a much lower proportion. Janerich's hypothesis[70,71] that certain cohorts of mothers identifiable by their year of birth are responsible for the secular variations in incidence observed during this century could be further tested with respect to the 1961 epidemic in Scotland and Ireland. A study of the age at which females became landed immigrants in North America linked to subsequent marriage and birth records along the lines of the 1972 research by Dean and Kurtzke on disseminated sclerosis in South Africa might permit isolation of the age group most susceptible to environment influence.[72]

Genetic factors also are important and various models have been proposed including a multifactorial hypothesis in which genes at a number of loci with additive effects are operating.[73] Knox,[74] however, has postulated that these defects occur in pregnancies which were initially multiple. One twin is eliminated and the other damaged due to differences in their genetic constitution, specifically in a diallelic gene system situated on the X-chromosome. Destruction of one fetus is because of absence of one gene possessed by the surviving fetus. Some support for this view is the observation[75] of anencephaly in pregnancies induced by clomid, a drug which causes multiple ovulations; also, the twinning rate in the Irish Republic[76] is high. If Knox's hypothesis were proven, it would have important implications for prevention. Primary prevention would be virtually impossible except in terms of genetic engineering or else selective mating because an environmental factor may not be required to trigger a fetus-fetus interaction.

At present, research is in progress in the United Kingdom into secondary prevention of anencephaly and "open" spina bifida cases by identifying prior to 20 weeks gestation, elevated levels of alpha-fetoprotein in the amniotic fluid and in maternal blood. In Belfast[77,78] at the time of writing, quantitative estimates of this substance have been made on 400 samples of amniotic fluid and 1200 samples of maternal blood. Some 21 pregnancies associated with anencephaly or spina bifida have been studied in detail prospectively. A small number of terminations of pregnancies associated with neurological malformations have been carried out but, to date, very high levels of amniotic alpha-fetoprotein have been the main indication in only two instances — each therapeutic abortion had anencephaly on examination post-operatively. Assessment of results to date suggest that elevated levels of alpha-fetoprotein in amniotic fluid may be associated with fetal malformations, both of the central nervous system and of other body systems. Elevated levels of alpha-fetoprotein in maternal blood, on the other hand, may not be specific for fetal malformations but may be influenced by other obstetric conditions including rhesus disease, multiple pregnancy, intrauterine death, threatened abortion and antepartum hemorrhage, pre-eclampsia, hypertension and diabetes mellitus. Research aimed at clarifying these questions has been initiated.

A secondary prevention program of identifying potentially abnormal fetuses by elevated maternal blood levels of alpha-fetoprotein together with further investigations by amniocentesis, ultrasound scanning and, finally, selective termination of pregnancy is possible. Potentially, these measures can reduce the number of infants having neural tube defects at term and result in only children with "closed" spina bifida lesions being born. Four communities in the United Kingdom have so far been surveyed to estimate the proportion of spina bifida children, expressed as a percentage of all (live and still) cases ascertained, surviving to one year of age; the reported percentages are 43, 36, 24 and 18 for Belfast,[79] Liverpool,[80] Birmingham,[81] and South Wales[82] respectively. Such findings indicate the necessity of considering a secondary prevention program for spina bifida in Belfast and other high risk areas in the British Isles as a matter of urgency.

REFERENCES

1. R.G. Record and T. McKeown, *Br. J. Soc. Med. 3,* 183, 1949.

2. J.H. Elwood, *Dev. Med. Child. Neurol. 12,* 582, 1970.

3. J.H. Elwood, *Dev. Med. Child. Neurol. 14,* 731, 1972.

4. J.H. Elwood and G. MacKenzie, *Br. J. Prev. Soc. Med. 25,* 17, 1971.

5. V.P. Coffey and W.J.E. Jessop, *Irish J. Med. Sci., Sixth Series, 393,* 391, 1958.

6. J.H. Elwood, unpublished data.

7. J.A.C. Weatherall, *Med. Offr. 121,* 65, 1969.

8. S.C. Rogers, personal communication.

9. J.G. Masterson, C. Frost, G.J. Bourke, N.M. Joyce, B. Herity and K. Wilson-Davis, *Br. J. Prev. Soc. Med. 24,* 78, 1970.

10. J.H. Elwood, *Br. J. Prev. Soc. Med. 24,* 78, 1970.

11. A.C. Stevenson and H.A. Warnock, *Ann. Hum. Genet., Lond. 23,* 382, 1959.

12. J.H. Elwood, *Med. Offr. 123,* 33, 1970.

13. J.H. Elwood and N.C. Nevin, *Brit. J. Prev. Soc. Med. 27,* 73, 1973.

14. S.F. Cahalane, J.D. Kennedy, B. McNicholl and E. O'Dwyer, *J. Irish Med. Ass. 57,* 135, 1965.

15. V.P. Coffey, *J. Irish Med. Ass. 63,* 343, 1970.

16. M.P. Spellman, *J. Irish Med. Ass. 62,* 316, 1969.

17. M.P. Spellman, *J. Irish Med. Ass. 63,* 339, 1970.

18. K.M. Laurence, C.O. Carter and P.A. David, *Br. J. Prev. Soc. Med. 22,* 146, 1968.

19. T.S. Wilson, *Hlth. Bull., Edin. 28,* 32, 1970.

20. I. Leck, R.G. Record, T. McKeown and J.H. Edwards, *Teratology 1,* 263, 1968.

21. A.M. Jepson, *Med. Offr. 121,* 15, 1969.

22. I.V. Ward and E.D. Irvine, *Med. Offr. 106,* 381, 1961.

23. C.O. Carter and K. Evans, *J. Med. Genet. 10,* 209, 1973.

24. A.D. McDonald, *Br. J. Prev. Soc. Med. 15,* 154, 1961.

25. B.J.L. Moss, *Med. Offr. 112,* 79, 1964.

26. R.W. Smithells, *Br. J. Prev. Soc. Med. 22,* 36, 1968.

27. M.J. Pleydell, *Br. Med. J. 1,* 309, 1960.

28. G.V. Griffin and G.S. Sorrie, *Med. Offr. 112,* 197, 1964.

29. E.M. Williamson, *J. Med. Genet. 2,* 161, 1965.

30. V.P. Coffey and W.J.E. Jessop, *Irish J. Med. Sci., Sixth Series, 349,* 30, 1955.

31. V.P. Coffey and W.J.E. Jessop, *Br. J. Prev. Soc. Med. 11,* 174, 1957.

32. V.P. Coffey and W.J.E. Jessop, *Lancet 1,* 748, 1963.

33. I. Leck and S.C. Rogers, *Br. J. Prev. Soc. Med. 21,* 177, 1967.

34. J.H. Elwood, *Irish J. Med. Sci., Seventh Series, 142,* 346, 1973.

35. J.H. Elwood, *Int. J. Epidemiol. 2,* 171, 1973.

36. I. Leck, *Lancet 2,* 791, 1966.

37. S.C. Rogers and M. Morris, *Ann. Hum. Genet., Lond. 34,* 295, 1971.

38. T. McKeown and R.G. Record, *Lancet 1,* 192, 1951.

39. J.H. Elwood and H.A. Warnock, *Irish J. Med. Sci., Seventh Series, 2,* 17, 1969.

40. B. MacMahon and S. Yen, *Lancet 1,* 31, 1971.

41. D.T. Janerich, *Teratology 8,* 253, 1973.

42. J.M. Elwood, *Canad. Med. Assoc. J.* (in press).

43. K.M. Laurence, P.A. David and C.O. Carter, *Br. J. Prev. Soc. Med. 22,* 212, 1968.

44. A. Czeizel and C. Revesz, *Br. J. Prev. Soc. Med. 24,* 205, 1970.

45. I. Horowitz and A.D. McDonald, *Canad. Med. Assoc. J. 100,* 748, 1969.

46. L. Naggan and B. MacMahon, *New Eng. J. Med. 277,* 1119, 1967.

47. L. Naggan, *Pediatrics (Springfield) 47,* 577, 1971.

48. W.J.R. Anderson, D. Baird and A.M. Thomson, *Lancet 1,* 1304, 1958.

49. I. Leck, *Br. Med. Bull. 30,* 158, 1974.

50. S.C. Rogers and M. Morris, *Br. J. Prev. Soc. Med. 27,* 81, 1973.

51. K.M. Laurence, *Arch. Dis. Child. 45,* 274, 1970.

52. I.D.G. Richards, T.H.McIntosh and S. Sweenie, *Dev. Med. Child. Neurol. 14,* 626, 1972.

53. C.O. Carter, P.A. David and K.M. Laurence, *J. Med. Genet. 5,* 81, 1968.

54. I. Leck, *Teratology 5,* 303, 1972.

55. L.E. Sever and I. Emanuel, *Teratology 7,* 117, 1973.

56. C.R. Lowe, *Br. Med. J. 3,* 515, 1972.

57. E.G. Knox, *Br. J. Prev. Soc. Med. 26,* 219, 1972.

58. J. Fedrick, *Proc. Roy. Soc. Med. 67,* 356, 1974.

59. M.M. Nelson and J.O. Forfar, *Br. Med. J. 1,* 523, 1971.

60. I.D.G. Richards, *Br. J. Prev. Soc. Med. 23,* 218, 1969.

61. C.A. Clarke, O.M. McKendrick and P.M. Sheppard, *Br. Med. J. 3,* 251, 1973.

62. I. Leck, *Br. J. Prev. Soc. Med. 17,* 70, 1963.

63. J.H. Renwick, *Br. J. Prev. Soc. Med. 26,* 67, 1972.

64. J.H. Renwick, *New Scientist 56,* 277, 1972.

65. J.H. Elwood and G. MacKenzie, *Nature 243,* 476, 1973.

66. L. Kinlen and A. Hewitt, *Br. J. Prev. Soc. Med. 27,* 208, 1973.

67. J.H. Elwood and N.C. Nevin, *Pediatrics Digest (Illinois)* (in press).

68. N.C. Nevin, unpublished data.

69. J.H. Renwick, A.M. Possami and M.R. Munday, *Proc. Roy. Soc. Med. 67,* 360, 1974.

70. D.T. Janerich, *Am. J. Epidemiol. 95,* 319, 1972.

71. D.T. Janerich, *in* Congenital Defects, D.T. Janerich, R.G. Skalko and I.H. Porter (Eds.), Academic Press, Inc., New York, p. 73, 1974.

72. G. Dean and J.F. Kurtzke, *Br. Med. J. 3,* 725, 1971.

73. World Health Organization, *Tech. Rep. Ser.,* World Health Organ. No. 438, 1970.

74. E.G. Knox, *Br. J. Prev. Soc. Med. 28,* 73, 1974.

75. M.J. Whitelaw, C.F. Kalman and L.R. Grams, *Am. J. Obstet. Gynec. 107,* 865, 1970.

76. G. Dean and T. Keane, *Br. J. Prev. Soc. Med. 26,* 186, 1972.

77. N.C. Nevin, W. Thompson and S. Nesbitt, *Br. J. Obstet. Gynaec.* (in press).

78. B. Bond, unpublished data.

79. J.H. Elwood and N.C. Nevin, *Ulster Med. J. 42,* 213, 1973.

80. P.P. Rickham and T. Mawdsley, *Dev. Med. Child. Neurol., Suppl. 11,* 20, 1966.

81. E.G. Knox, *Dev. Med. Child. Neurol., Suppl. 13,* 14, 1967.

82. K.M. Laurence and B.J. Tew, *Arch. Dis. Child. 46,* 127, 1971.

I. METHODOLOGY OF ASCERTAINMENT IN INTERNATIONAL COMPARISONS
II. ANENCEPHALY AND SPINA BIFIDA IN ISRAEL

Lechaim Naggan

I. INTERNATIONAL COMPARISONS – VARIATIONS DUE TO THE METHODOLOGY OF ASCERTAINMENT OF CASES

I have been asked to discuss two subjects: anencephaly and spina bifida in Israel and on international comparisons. I shall start with the latter and since several good reviews of the world literature have been published,[1-4] rather than add yet another one, I chose to elaborate on a specific methodologic issue of the data collection in several national studies, which greatly complicate international comparisons; namely, differences in the methods of ascertainment of cases.

The neural tube defects are probably the most "convenient" group of congenital anomalies to be studied. There are two main reasons for this:

1. Anencephaly and spina bifida cystica are readily diagnosed at birth and are practically always recorded in obstetric records. Thus, the many problems of definition and diagnosis commonly associated with many congenital malformations are greatly reduced.

2. The variation of these anomalies with regard to many demographic variables is quite remarkable and therefore most intriguing in the search for etiology. The great geographic and ethnic variation of these anomalies makes them ideal for international studies and studies in migrant populations.

It is my intention to attempt to show that it is possible that a sizable proportion of the international variation may be due to the varying degrees of completeness of ascertainment of cases. I must stress that most authors recognize and many stress the shortcomings of the used method but the rates are published, recorded and then later used as estimates of the prevalence rates in these countries. A classic example is the excellent international study of[24] centers by Stevenson et al.[5] The authors very carefully stressed the shortcomings of a study limited to hospital births, especially in countries where hospital deliveries represented only a biased proportion of the total number of births in the population. Yet, this study and its rates are quoted and compared in practically every relevant paper published and the authors' own warnings on the limitations of their data are quickly forgotten.

Much emphasis is placed in the epidemiologic literature on whether a study is prospective or retrospective. In my experience, this does not affect the quality and completeness of ascertainment in the case of anencephaly and spina bifida. Of much greater importance is the number of sources of ascertainment and whether the case finding is "active" or "passive". My definition of "active" case finding is a search for cases made by a limited number of qualified and highly motivated personnel who look for cases in all possible sources.

A "passive" case finding is one which relies on information either routinely collected, such as vital statistics, or information collected upon request from many or all sources by people who usually have no incentive or knowledge of data collection. This is often done with the aid of instruments such as questionnaires and forms sent to physicians or hospitals.

I shall give several examples of both active and passive methods to try to make my point clear. These examples were chosen purposely from some of the best studies in the field, so that there will be no doubt as to the value of each study in itself but only as to its contribution to international comparison.

High prevalence rates were reported in Bombay — 2.97 per 1,000 for both anomalies in the W.H.O. study.[5] These were later analyzed by Master-Notani and Kolah[6] who found that while the total prevalence for the two anomalies among women who registered for antenatal treatment in the Wadia Maternity Hospital was only 1.15 per 1,000, it was 5.88 per 1,000 for women who were admitted through the emergency ward. A later study that included all births in Bombay during December 1968[7] showed a significantly lower rate of 1.55 per 1,000 for both anomalies (compared to 2.97 per 1,000) — half the frequency obtained by the W.H.O. study. The same artifact of high rates was probably operating in Alexandria, Egypt, because both the Shatby Hospital in Alexandria and the four hospitals surveyed in Bombay are highly specialized referral centers where the prevalence of these anomalies is expected to be much greater than in the general population, especially so in countries where the total proportion of hospital deliveries is relatively low.

Even in developed countries where hospital deliveries approach 100%, it can be seen that relying on hospital records alone yielded only 52.6% of all cases in Budapest[8] and 83.6% in Israel[9] although an active search through all hospital records was made in both studies.

When one relies on information "passively" collected through questionnaires sent to hospitals, clinics and obstetricians, such as in the study in France by Frézal et al.,[10] the rates are quite surely going to be greatly underestimated because of both lack of response and lack of motivation among the physicians involved, in addition to incomplete records. The large variation found within the country in that study may very well reflect variation in completeness of ascertainment and reporting rather than true regional variation. Again, I must stress that the authors discussed these possible biases in their paper and yet these rates have remained our only estimate of the rate of anencephaly in France.

Another example of the difference between "passive" and "active" ascertainment may be seen in the Israel data. A prospective pilot study[11] conducted in 1959–1960 relied on reporting from hospitals, without any active search for cases. It produced only 73% of the cases of anencephaly and spina bifida that were later ascertained for the same two years by the retrospective study which I am about to present.[9] The Jerusalem Perinatal Study[12,13], in which all pregnant women in Jerusalem are followed from early pregnancy to birth and the children further into childhood, developed precisely the same roster of cases as this retrospective study in which active search for cases was made using practically all possible sources.

The point I wish to make is that if international comparisons are made, they should only be made on as completely ascertained data as possible or they may be quite misleading. The second point is that such ascertainment should be done by actively looking for cases by a small number of highly motivated personnel and that all possible sources should be investigated thoroughly to increase the probability of complete ascertainment. There are, of course, some practical constraints to this and I would like to quote a paragraph from a paper by Smithells on this issue.[14]

"The final and most important decision concerns the ascertainment of the defects. Who is to detect them? Who is to inform the registering organization? Here there is a paradox which can only be resolved by compromise. The smaller the number of observers, the higher will be the standard of ascertainment, the highest standard being achieved by a single enthusiast. But the larger the population surveyed, the more information will be obtained. The one extreme will produce a negligible quantity of completely reliable data; the other will provide vast quantities of suspect information."

With this quotation, I would like to leave the question of ascertainment and turn to the second part of my discussion and present some data on anencephaly and spina bifida in Israel.

II. ANENCEPHALY AND SPINA BIFIDA IN ISRAEL

Previous studies[15,16] have indicated that Jews in the U.S. have low prevalence rates of anencephaly and spina bifida and that there might be some ethnic variation among the Jews in Israel.[11,17] The present study included

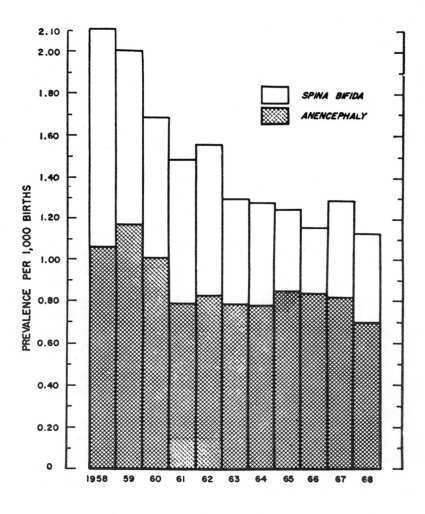

Fig. 1. Prevalence of anencephaly and spina bifida in Israel by year of birth, 1958–1968. (Reprinted from *Pediatrics*, Vol. 47, No. 3. *Courtesy of the American Academy of Pediatrics.*)

532,000 Jewish births that occurred between 1958–1968 (Fig. 1). An active search for cases from multiple sources increased the completeness of ascertainment. The main sources were death and stillbirth certificates from the Central Bureau of Statistics and all diagnostic indices, birth books and P.M. reports of all hospitals in the country which have either a maternity or a neurosurgery ward, or both.

The total population of Jewish births was used as a comparison group. This allowed us to compute reliable rates for population subgroups but also confined the analysis to routinely collected items only. Detailed information was not usually available on stillbirths but these represent only 1.4 percent of the total births and their exclusion from the denominator should not lead to appreciable bias.

FINDINGS

The first table shows the distribution of prevalence rates per 1,000 total births by diagnosis, sex and sex ratio. Sex ratio is defined here as the proportion of males out of the total number of propositi.

776 cases were ascertained, giving a prevalence rate for the two anomalies combined of 1.46 per 1,000 births. (The term prevalence at birth is preferred to incidence because of the known prenatal wastage of these anomalies.)

In most studies, the sex ratio for anencephaly varies between 20 and 35 percent male. This high sex ratio of 44.1 percent male is unusual and was also observed among the Jewish anencephalics in Boston.[18]

There were no significant variation of sex ratio among the various birth orders or ethnic group. The previously described pattern of increasing sex ratio with increasing duration of gestation was observed in this study as well.

The second table shows the prevalence rates per 1,000 live births by birth order. The relatively high risk for first-born, observed in most studies, was not found in Israel.

A very marked association with birth order can be seen. Rates are markedly and uniformly high for both anomalies after the fifth child and uniformly lower within the lower birth orders.

The number of grand multipara in Israel is quite sizable and over 83,000 women had 6 or more live born children during the study period.

The mean maternal age for the cases was 28.4 years, with a standard deviation of 6.1, and for the total population of mothers, the mean age was 27.6 years, with a standard deviation of 6.0. While this difference is highly significant ($p < 0.001$), it is seen from Table 3 that, on the whole, the effect of maternal age disappears with adjustment for birth order and is probably accounted for on that basis. On the other hand, the birth order effect remains unchanged by adjustment for maternal age. However, women having their

TABLE 1

Distribution and Prevalence Rates per 1,000 Total Births According to Diagnosis and Sex

Diagnosis	Number of Cases				Sex ratio (%male)	Prevalence per 1,000 births
	Male	Female	Sex not determined	Total		
Anencephaly	189	233	6	428	44.8)	0.80
Anencephaly with Spina Bifida	12	22	0	34	35.3) 44.	0.06
Spina Bifida	129	177	8	314	42.2	0.60
Total Cases	330	432	14	776	43.3	1.46
Total Number of Births	273,896	258,089	—	531,985	51.5	—

TABLE 2

Numbers and Prevalence Rates per 1,000 Live Births for Anencephaly, Spina Bifida and Both Anomalies, by Birth Order

Birth Order	Anencephaly		Spina Bifida		Total		
	Cases	Rate	Cases	Rate	No. of Births	Cases	Rate
1	102	0.72	73	0.53	145,338	175	1.25
2	109	0.82	61	0.48	134,290	170	1.31
3	66	0.80	45	0.57	83,470	111	1.37
4	43	0.96	29	0.67	45,466	72	1.63
5	24	0.79	18	0.62	30,906	42	1.40
6	36	1.46	22	0.93	24,978	58	2.40
7–8	44	1.32	28	0.87	33,941	72	2.19
9+	29	1.21	20	0.87	24,371	49	2.07
Total	453	0.88	296	0.60	522,760	749	1.48

Birth order was unknown for 27 (3.5%) of the cases (9 cases of anencephaly and 18 cases of spina bifida and for 2,144 (0.4%) of the total number of births.

X^2 (7.D.F.) = 40.25, P < 0.001.

46

TABLE 3

Prevalence Rates per 1,000 Live Births for Both Anomalies by Maternal Age
And Birth Order

| Maternal Age (1) | Birth Order | | | | Total* |
	1	2–3	4–5	6+	
Up to 24	1.14 (117;106,999)	1.37 (105;79,524)	1.10 (13;12,235)	1.90 (3;1,641)	1.40
25–29	1.35 (36;27,646)	1.26 (97;80,211)	1.80 (53;30,562)	2.19 (38;18,019)	1.51
30–34	2.19 (16;7,584)	1.43 (57;41,438)	1.63 (34;21,646)	2.40 (72;31,113)	1.66
35+	1.71 (5;3,043)	1.26 (20;16,441)	1.23 (14;11,844)	2.02 (63;32,396)	1.36
Total	1.40	1.34	1.47	1.91	1.48

Numbers in parentheses represent first, the number of cases and second, the number of all births in each cell.

*The totals for birth order are adjusted for differences between the birth order groups in distribution by maternal age. The totals for maternal age groups are adjusted for differences in birth order distribution.

(1) For maternal age summary X^2 (I.D.F.) = 0.39, P > 0.50.

(2) For birth order summary X^2 (I.D.F.) = 16.03, P < 0.001.

47

TABLE 4

Numbers and Prevalence Rates per 1,000 Live Births for Anencephaly, Spina Bifida and Both Anomalies by Maternal Ethnic Group

Ethnic Origin	No. of births	Anencephaly		Spina Bifida		Both Anomalies	
		No. of cases	Rate	No. of cases	Rate	No. of cases	Rate
Israel	111,182	76	0.69	50	0.47	126	1.15
North Africa (1)	146,674	124	0.86	83	0.59	207	1.45
Yemen	37,183	39	1.07	26	0.73	65	1.79
Iraq – Iran	83,502	104	1.27	67	0.83	171	2.10
Ashkenaz (2)	93,092	71	0.77	44	0.49	115	1.27
Sepharad (3)	52,962	40	0.77	32	0.63	72	1.39
Total	524,595	454	0.88	302	0.60	756	1.48

For 20 (2.6%) of the (12 cases of spina bifida and 8 cases of anencephaly) maternal ethnic origin was unknown.

Total X^2 (5 D.F.) = 34.14, P   0.001

(1) Mothers born in Morocco, Algeria, Tunisia and Libya.

(2) Mothers born in East and West Europe as well as in America and Oceania.

(3) Mothers born in Southern Europe and the Middle East (other than Iraq) and all "others".

first liveborn child late in life seem to be at increased risk of bearing a child with one of these anomalies.

In Table 4, the prevalence rates by maternal ethnic origin are shown. The grouping is based on the historical migration of the Jews in the Diaspora, as well as on known genetic differences.[19]

More detailed analysis by maternal country or origin did not reveal any variations that cannot be seen from this table.

Highest rates are observed among immigrants from Iraq, Iran and Yemen. The lowest risk groups are the Israeli and the European born.

The Israeli born mothers are, of course, themselves heterogenous. Table 5 shows the rates for children of Israeli born mothers by maternal grandfather's continent of birth. Of major interest is the observation that ethnic differences have disappeared among this group. The low rate observed among Israeli born mothers of Asian-African origin is especially striking because this group is derived mainly from grandfathers born in Iraq, Persia and Yemen, a group, originally, with the highest prevalence rates.

Table 6 shows a more detailed classification of continent of birth, unfortunately available for only 4 years of the study period and adjusted for parity. The rates among Asian born remain high after adjustment for parity, while this same adjustment effaces the variation observed among the other groups. The birth order effect, however, remains unchanged.

There is no adequate method of socioeconomic classification in Israel. One classification used the period of immigration into Israel as an index, but this proved to give completely misleading results because of the distinct ethnic composition of each wave of immigration. An attempt to classify rates by paternal occupational class is seen in Table 7. The variation is due only to differing rates for spina bifida. Professional and administrative personnel do have the lowest rates for both anomalies but the reasons why traders and farmers share the highest prevalence rates with unskilled workers are not clear. The ranking of the groups is that used by the Central Bureau of Statistics and may not accurately reflect a social class gradient.

Figure 1 shows the change in prevalence rates of anencephaly and spina bifida during the study period. The obvious decline in prevalence is due mainly to spina bifida. Table 8 shows a summary of the analysis resulting after division of the study period into a high prevalence period (1958–1962) and a low prevalence period (1963–1968). Because of the difference between anencephaly and spina bifida with regard to this decline, rates and X^2 values are given separately for each. For spina bifida, all rates have diminished and most of them markedly so. For anencephaly, significant decline is observed within the first birth order, after the seventh child and for Jews from Iraq and Iran. Interestingly, quite a sizable decline is manifest among North African

TABLE 5

Numbers and Prevalence Rates per 1,000 Live Births for Children of Israeli Born Mothers
By Maternal Grandfather's Continent of Birth

Maternal grandfather's continent of birth	Number of Cases			Total of of births	Rates		
	Anencephaly	Spina Bifida	Total		Anencephaly	Spina Bifida	Total
Asia – Africa	11	7.	18	22,640	0.63	0.40	1.02
Europe, U. S. A. and Oceania	37	20	57	59,555	0.80	0.44	1.23
Israel	11	12	23	28,987	0.49	0.53	1.02
Total	59	39	98	111,182	0.68	0.45	1.13

For 28 (22%) of the cases (17 cases of anencephaly and 11 cases of spina bifida) maternal grandfather's continent of origin was unknown.

Total X^2 (2 D.F.) = 0.83, P > 0.50

50

TABLE 6

Prevalence Rates per 1,000 Live Births for Both Anomalies by Maternal Continent of
Birth and Birth Order for the Years 1958, 1960, 1961 and 1962

Maternal continent	Birth Order (1)				
of birth (2)	1 − 2	3 − 5	6 − 7	8+	Total*
Israel	1.41 (34;24,196)	1.16 (8;6,909)	1.46 (1;687)	− (0;399)	1.49
Asia	1.72 (37;21,519)	1.75 (33;18,846)	2.42 (18;7,444)	4.10 (24;5,859)	1.97
Africa	1.09 (20;18,412)	1.53 (27;17,590)	2.04 (16;7,846)	2.80 (19;6,782)	1.48
Europe, U.S.A. and Oceania	1.38 (37;26,786)	0.82 (9;11,003)	− (0;724)	2.60 (1;384)	1.35
Total*	1.49	1.38	1.88	2.95	1.62

Numbers in parentheses represent first, the number of cases and second, the number of all births in each cell.

*The totals by birth order are adjusted for differences between the distributions of maternal continent of birth. The totals by maternal continent of birth are adjusted for differences in birth order distribution.

(1) For birth order summary X^2 = 13.91 (1 D.F.), P < 0.001.

(2) For maternal continent of birth summary X^2 between Europe plus Israel and Asia = 6.21(1 D.F.), P < 0.025
   Between Europe plus Israel and Africa X^2 = 0.31 (1 D.F.), P > 0.50.

TABLE 7

Prevalence Rates per 1,000 Live Births by Occupational Class, Both Anomalies, 1963–1968

Occupational Class	Total number of births	Number of Cases			Prevalence Rates		
		Anencephaly	Spina Bifida	Both	Anencephaly	Spina Bifida	Both
Professional and administrative	65,619	43	18	61	0.66	0.27	0.93
Traders and farmers	41,748	33	29	62	0.79	0.69	1.49
Workers in transportation and construction	47,430	38	16	54	0.80	0.34	1.14
Craftsmen and services	71,838	48	21	69	0.67	0.29	0.96
Unskilled workers	49,498	41	28	69	0.82	0.57	1.39
Total	276,133	203	112	315	0.74	0.41	1.14

65 cases and 25,823 of the total population of births were classified as army, students and unknowns. These were completely excluded from the computation of rates.

For spina bifida total $X^2 = 17.32$ (4 D.F.), $P < 0.001$.

For anencephaly total $X^2 = 2.05$ (4 D.F.), $P > 0.70$.

TABLE 8

Comparison of Rates in Two Periods

Variable	Anencephaly Prevalence rates per 1,000 live births 1958–62	1963–68	X^2 values (with 1 degree of freedom)	Spina Bifida Prevalence rates per 1,000 live births 1958–62	1963–68	X^2 values (with 1 degree of freedom)
Total prevalence	0.97	0.79	4.67	0.80	0.44	29.01
Ethnic origin						
Israel	0.81	0.61	1.45	0.53	0.40	0.92
N. Africa	0.97	0.76	1.79	0.87	0.38	14.75
Yemen	1.01	1.09	0.05	1.01	0.41	4.70
Iraq–Iran	1.45	1.07	2.41	1.00	0.63	3.52
Ashkenaz	0.81	0.72	0.21	0.54	0.41	0.75
Sepharad	0.75	0.76	1.05	0.71	0.52	0.80
Birth order						
1	0.89	0.58	4.57	0.68	0.39	5.79
2	0.89	0.75	0.79	0.64	0.32	7.54
3	0.62	0.91	2.05	0.71	0.42	3.09
4	1.16	0.78	1.75	0.66	0.62	0.02
5	0.69	0.86	0.28	0.62	0.55	0.06
6	1.17	1.69	1.16	1.17	0.61	2.19
7–8	1.61	1.03	2.12	1.28	0.44	7.35
9+	1.59	0.91	2.28	0.99	0.70	0.62

For $X^2 > 3.85$, $P < 0.05$; $X^2 > 6.64$, $P < 0.01$; $X^2 > 10.83$, $P < 0.001$.

53

Jews in the first birth order for both anomalies and in the second and third for spina bifida alone — low prevalence subgroups originally.

Analysis of the seasonal variation showed only slight, non-significant trends that disappeared completely when the season of conception was substituted for season of birth.

Familial Incidence

Twenty-six women gave birth to more than one affected child. Altogether these 26 mothers gave birth to 55 affected children, five of whom were born before the study period and, therefore, were not included among the cases. Among the 21 mothers who had more than one child included in the study, 18 had 2 affected children and 3 had 3 affected children. The estimated prevalence among siblings of affected children is 13.4 per 1,000 total births, nine times that of the general population.

Among the 19 sets of twins included in the study, only one, an unlike-sex pair, was found concordant for neural tube defect, both having spina bifida. The sex distribution of the 19 sets of twins was as follows: 2 pair of identical twins, 2 pair of like-sex (dizygous), 9 pair of like-sex (zygosity unknown) and 6 pair of unlike-sex (dizygous) twins.

DISCUSSION

The high sex ratio of 44.1% male observed among anencephalics in this study is unusual. Such high ratios were also observed in Mexico City, Singapore and Manila.[5] These high sex ratios seem to prevail mainly in populations with low prevalence rates of neural tube defects. And a recent study by Rogers and Morris[20] seems to indicate that the sex ratio within the same population goes up as the prevalence of anencephaly declines. The rates among the non-Jewish population of Israel (predominantly Arab) were found to be about twice as high as for the Jews and the sex ratio was 32%.[18] There is a possibility that only one of several causes of anencephaly affects females primarily and that this cause is important among high prevalence populations but of lesser importance where prevalence is low.[21]

The Jews from Iraq and Iran, representing 70% of the high risk group, are known to differ genetically from other ethnic groups with regard to frequency of such characteristics as glucose-6-phosphate dehydrogenase (G6PD) deficiency.[19] They are also known to have remained genetically isolated and to have the highest rate of consanguinity in the country, about 15–20 percent of marriages being between first cousins. A high consanguinity rate is also found among the Jews from Yemen (10% first cousin marriages). Among Jews from Europe and the United States, first cousin marriages account for about

1% of the total.[22]   A relationship between rate of consanguinity and the prevalence rates of neural tube defects seems attractive but would imply much greater differences than observed, even before adjustment for birth order.

The rapid disappearance of the ethnic variation and adoption of rates characteristic of the host country, as manifested among Israeli born mothers, is in accord with other recent observations.   Such groups are the Irish in Boston,[16] the Irish, Hindu and Pakistani in Birmingham, the French in Quebec[24] and migrants in South Wales.[25] Intermarriage among the various Israeli born ethnic groups is not yet common and could not account for any major portion of the observed changes.   The cohort approach suggested by Janerich[26,27] may provide some clues to this phenomena and should be tried, provided maternal age is also adjusted for parity effect.

Birth order stands out in this analysis as a most important variable and is completely independent of maternal age and ethnic variations. It accounts for the differences observed between Jews from Europe, Africa and Israel. Despite the inadequacy of the present analysis of socio-economic variation, there is little doubt that birth order and ethnicity in Israel are very closely associated with socioeconomic status.

The downward trend observed during the study period is additional evidence for an environmental cause. Declines in the prevalence of the neural tube defects were observed in New York State between 1946 and 1972[28,29] and in Boston, Massachusetts, between 1930 and 1950.[30]   Such declines require examination of possible changes in the pertinent variables, besides errors in methodology. They may, in fact, represent part of huge epidemic declines such as the one manifested in Boston and Rhode Island.[31]   In Israel, there has been very little change in the birth order trends during the study period and the most striking decline is, in fact, observed within several of the birth order groups. The ethnic composition of the population of mothers has changed somewhat during the study period.   Mothers from Iraq, Iran and Yemen constituted 25.2 percent during the period 1958–1962, as compared with 21.6 percent for the period 1963–1968. Thus, the proportion of high risk mothers in the population has decreased slightly and this may account for a small proportion of the observed decrease.   Interestingly enough,   the strongest decline was observed among North African Jews.

The difference between spina bifida and anencephaly with regard to the secular trend is puzzling, as in most studies the rates of the two anomalies have seemed to vary together. Analysis of the socioeconomic variation indicates a stronger relation between this variable and spina bifida. There was major improvement in the socioeconomic status of the average Israeli citizen during the study period and this may explain the decline in the prevalence of spina bifida. Anencephaly, however, is more strongly associated with birth order and ethnic variation and these change more slowly. This dissociation with regard to the secular trend supports the hypothesis that several etiologic agents may be involved and that the several patterns in the distribution of these anomalies may have different explanations.

These results do not implicate a specific etiology but several of the commonly suspected environmental causes are largely excluded. The lack of major seasonal variation or clustering in space or time make infections unlikely as a possible cause. The secular decline tends to exclude drugs, alcohol and tobacco, as well as exposure to x-rays, since use of all these has increased in recent years. The observation of different rates among various ethnic groups makes environmental pollution unlikely as a possible cause. A deficiency of some nutrient or a contaminant of certain foods can not be excluded on the basis of our present knowledge. Many controversial papers have been reported recently about the possible association with blighted potatoes[32,33] and other nutrients.[34–36] Dietary habits vary in time and place and may change among migrant populations or remain unchanged among certain ethnic groups. In Israel, a nutritional deficiency which is aggravated by depletion through multiple pregnancies but which is diminishing, may explain the association with parity, ethnic group and the rapid decline.

Finally, it is not necessary that any single hypothesis explain all the observations. It may well be that several different etiologic agents are involved and that the several patterns in the distribution of these anomalies have different explanations.

I believe that future investigations should concentrate on more sensitive measures than "social class" or "ethnic group". Biochemical determinations and blood levels of electrolytes and vitamins or other factors associated with nutrition should be compared between cases and controls and between mothers of cases and controls as well as between high and low risk groups.

REFERENCES

1. M. Lamy and J. Frezal, *in* Abstracts, 1st International Conference on Congenital Malformations, London, 1960, M. Fishbein (Ed.), J.B. Lippincott Co., Philadelphia.

2. A.M. Lilienfeld, *Excerpta Medica International Congress Series 204*, 251, 1970.

3. .L. Naggan, *Isr. J. Med. Sci. 8*, 549, 1972.

4. W.P. Kennedy, *Birth Defects, Orig. Art. Series 3, No. 2*, 1967.

5. A.C. Stevenson *et al.*, *Bull. W.H.O.*, *Suppl. 34*, 9, 1966.

6. P. Master-Notani, P.J. Kolah and L.D. Sanghvi, *Acta Genet. (Basel) 18*, 97, 1968.

7. A.R. Rustom and C.T. Vasant, *J. Ind. Med. Assoc. 60*, 18, 1973.

8. A. Czeizel and C. Revesz, *Br. J. Pres. Soc. Med. 24*, 205, 1970.

9. L. Naggan, *Pediatrics 47*, 577, 1971.

10. J. Frezal *et al.*, *Amer. J. Hum. Genet. 64*, 336, 1964.

11. H.S. Halevi, *Br. J. Prev. Soc. Med. 21*, 66, 1967.

12. S. Legg *et al.*, *Isr. J. Med. Sci. 5*, 1107, 1969.

13. S. Harlap *et al.*, *Isr. J. Med. Sci. 7*, 1520, 1971.

14. R. W. Smithells, *Isr. J. Med. Sci. 7*, 1515, 1971.

15. B. MacMahon, T.F. Pugh and T.S. Ingalls, *Br. J. Prev. Soc. Med. 7*, 211, 1953.

16. L. Naggan and B. MacMahon, *New Eng. J. Med. 277*, 1119, 1967.

17. S. Merin and M. Davies, *in* The Genetics of Migrant and Isolate Populations, E. Goldschmidt (Ed.), Tel-Aviv, p. 313, 1962.

18. L. Naggan, unpublished data.

19. S. Shiba, *M.A.D.A. (Hebrew) 13*, 94, 1968.

20. S.C. Rogers and M. Morris, *Br. J. Prev. Soc. Med. 27*, 81, 1973.

21. L. Naggan, Dr. P.H. Thesis, Harvard School of P.H., Boston, Mass., 1970.

22. E. Goldschmidt and A. Ronen, *Bull. Res. Counc. Israel 58*, 317, 1969.

23. I. Leck, *Br. J. Prev. Soc. Med. 23*, 166, 1969.

24. I. Horowitz and A.D. McDonald, *Can. Med. Ass. J. 100*, 748, 1969.

25. I.D.G. Richards, C.J. Roberts and S. Lloyd, *Br. J. Prev. Soc. Med. 26*,

26. D.T. Janerich, *Am. J. Epidemiol. 95, 319*, 1972.

27. D.T. Janerich, *Am. J. Epidemiol. 96, 389*, 1972.

28. A.M. Gittelsohn and S. Milham, *Br. J. Prev. Soc. Med. 16,* 153, 1962.

29. D.T. Janerich, *Teratology 8, 253,* 1973.

30. L. Naggan, *Amer. J. Epidemiol. 89,* 154, 1968.

31. B. MacMahon and S. Yen, *Lancet 1,* 131, 1971.

32. J.H. Renwick, *Br. J. Prev. Soc. Med. 26,* 67, 1972.

33. B. MacMahon, S. Yen and K.J. Rothman, *Lancet 1,* 598, 1973.

34. E.G. Knox, *Br. J. Prev. Soc. Med. 26,* 219, 1972.

35. Leading Article, *Br. Med. J. 4,* 684, 1972.

36. J.H. Elwood and N.C. Nevin, *Br. J. Prev. Soc. Med. 27,* 73, 1973.

DISCUSSION

K. MICHAEL LAURENCE: First of all, spina bifida is more serious in girls. By the age of nine or ten, more boys have survived, although more girls are affected at birth. The surviving girls, furthermore, are more handicapped.

I doubt that the difference in survival rate is intrinsic, since there are unrecognized variables among the different series, such as the effect of surgical intervention and standards of care. We have data from a water survey in Wales, for example, that shows that aluminum is the only heavy metal or pollutant looked at that has etiologic significance.

Finally, we have evidence from Japan and from our own studies in South Wales suggesting that we are probably dealing not with an increased number of malformations conceived or developed but with its prevalence *in utero*. In Japan, the incidence of these malformations is low and abortion material shows an incidence of neural tube malformation far in excess of that found at birth. In South Wales, where we have a high incidence of malformations, we, too, have a relationship between miscarriage and incidence at birth (after 28 weeks). In areas in South Wales where the incidence is high, we have a slightly lower abortion rate than where the incidence is high. This, I think, is an observation to which we should direct our efforts, because we are really looking at what is not being rejected by the usually efficient maternal organ.

J. HAROLD ELWOOD: I quite agree with the interpretation of the ASB survival data. Undoubtedly, more recent clinical series will give higher survivals. The importance of our report is that it gives some information on the numbers of children with spina bifida that are surviving in the community, because this is relevant to any form of prevention. Again, the aims of epidemiology are to discover the primary cause of these defects and if the primary etiology is known to be genetic, apart from eugenics and selective breeding, etc., there would be no practical method of preventing these babies from being born. Therefore, secondary prevention — termination of pregnancy — would be the only option and that, as Dr. Edwards in Birmingham has said, is not prevention, it's eviction. I think this is important.

I don't think we can make any judgment about mineral deficiencies at present. Recent epidemiological studies show, however, that there are environmental contaminants which are not only associations but causally related and, if this is so, it will have important implications for public health programs. This is something we are concerned with in the United Kingdom and Ireland.

J. MARK ELWOOD: Thank you for emphasizing the fact that all the descriptive epidemiological differences could reflect different early fetal losses. In fact, all of us are making semantic errors by using the term "incidence". The rates under discussion should strictly be called prevalence at birth.

I have no North American data on survival rates by sex. This is normally not seen in neural tube defects and a number of other congenital defects, such as Down's syndrome and aortic coarctation, which show still different survival rates by sex.

ARTHUR D. BLOOM: Will you please review the question of whether spina bifida and anencephaly are caused by genetic factors alone?

J. HAROLD ELWOOD: The method of determining this problem is to set up a mathematical genetic model and apply the appropriate data to it. That has not been done with sufficient accuracy. The family studies — with the exception of some recent ones — are deficient, as they have been incompletely ascertained. Dr. Knox in Birmingham thinks that his fetus-fetus interaction model, which is basically a genetic model related to twinning, fits the data and explains various epidemiological findings. I think the approach by multiple recessive genes has not been adequately studied. We have a large pedigree study underway in Ireland and Dr. Carter is working on this problem in London.

TRACY B. PERRY (McGill University, Montreal, Canada): Dr. Elwood, have you any data on the incidence or prevalence at birth of these neural tube defects in the eastern provinces since 1970?

J. MARK ELWOOD: Dr. Lennon and Shambrook have recorded a localized increase in their own area.

LAWRENCE SHAPIRO (Letchworth Village, Thiells, New York): Dr. J.H. Elwood, if the incidence in October and November is three-fold, isn't the recurrence risk for that period of time for conceptions dating back to January and February three-fold and, if so, should we not take this into consideration when counseling parents at risk for recurrence?

J. HAROLD ELWOOD: Yes. Our medical geneticists do this. Seasonal variation has changed in Belfast over the past 15 or 20 years and the changes are similar to those Dr. Lennon has shown in Birmingham; i.e., the winter peak declined slightly and the summer trough decreased, forming a plateau and more even distribution. The seasonal variation in Belfast is still significant and shows an excess of cases in winter.

SECTION II

PRENATAL DIAGNOSIS OF ANENCEPHALY AND SPINA BIFIDA*

K. Michael Laurence

To prevent a condition it is necessary to know the cause or causes which, in neural tube malformations, are undoubtedly multifactorial in nature. A genetic predisposition, almost certainly polygenic, interacts with environmental trigger mechanisms probably as early as the 3rd or 4th week of gestation to produce an affected fetus.[1] The evidence for this comes from family studies, epidemiology and experimental teratology. As nothing can be done as yet to reduce the genetic predisposition, every effort has been concentrated on identifying the environmental trigger mechanisms. The indications are that there may be many of these trigger mechanisms, each playing a relatively small part, probably largely dietary or infective in nature and that drugs probably play little or no role. In spite of intensive research and much speculation, none have been identified with any certainty. In view of this, prevention of neural tube malformations altogether is not yet within our grasp and we have to resort to early prenatal detection of abnormal fetuses and selective abortion as a second best if the birth incidence of these malformations is to be reduced at term.

The possible methods of detection available before the 20th week of pregnancy consist of radiology, fetoscopy, ultrasonography and alpha fetoprotein estimation (AFP) after amniocentesis.

Radiology

X-rays carry a risk to the developing fetus of causing leukemia in childhood and a potential risk of mutation in the gonads of the mother. Also, although it will identify anencephaly quite readily, at least after 25 weeks, spina bifida is very difficult to see on a radiograph of the pregnant abdomen even near term, let alone before 20 weeks. For these reasons radiology is not used in the early prenatal diagnosis of this group of disorders.

---

*Supported in part by a grant from the National Fund for Crippling Diseases and by money donated by the Tredegar Branch of the South Wales Association for Spina Bifida and Hydrocephalus.

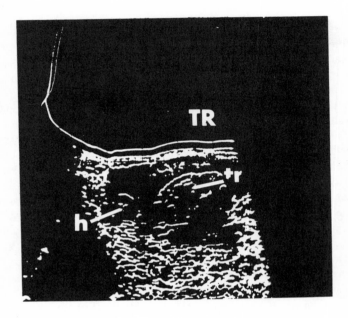

Fig. 1. Ultrasonograph in a case of anencephaly at 16 weeks (transverse section). The small head (h) and the trunk (tr) are indicated.

Fetoscopy

This type of investigation was pioneered by Scrimgeour[2] and Valenti,[3] using a variety of fibre-optic and other instruments inserted into the amniotic cavity usually at laparotomy. It is largely experimental in nature and has been carried out on only very few occasions when continuation of the pregnancy was planned. Fetoscopy seems to be both chancy and hazardous. It is chancy because there is some danger of not seeing the parts of the fetus required for diagnosis, either because the amniotic fluid is opalescent or because the fetus does not present the relevant parts for inspection. It is hazardous because there seems to be a considerable chance of abortion and of some other complications.[4] It has been found that when carrying out fetoscopies during the 5th month, the fetus at this stage is presenting by the breech and is lying with its back to the uterine wall facing the placenta and that no amount of manipulation enables a good view to be obtained of the back.[5] Fetoscopy, therefore, cannot be expected to be a useful investigation for spina bifida and has now been abandoned, especially after Scrimgeour has had a number of disappointments.[6]

Ultrasonography

This is a quick and non-invasive investigation, which though requiring expensive apparatus and considerable skill in interpretation of the results, is safe for the mother and the pregnancy and almost certainly also for the fetus, though there has been some concern about possible ultrasound damage to the fetal chromosomes,[7] which now appears to have been dispelled.[8]

With ultrasonography it is possible to identify anencephaly as early as 12 weeks. At 16 weeks the diagnosis can be made with certainty[9] (Fig. 1). It may be possible to identify encephalocele (Fig. 2a, 2b) with the equipment available at present. Spina bifida has escaped detection by this technique so far (Fig. 3).

However, with improvements in the technique and apparatus being developed (such as the "grey scale method"), abnormalities of the spine may possibly be visualized in the future. Hydrocephalus, not associated with spina bifida which is relatively rare though theoretically amenable to this approach, has yet to be diagnosed by this method.[9]

Amniocentesis and Alpha Fetoprotein Estimations

In the two years since Brock and Surcliffe first reported the association between anencephaly and raised AFP levels in the amniotic fluid in 1972,[10] this relationship has become firmly established even though it is still a matter of speculation as to whether the AFP, which is produced by the fetal liver up to about 22 weeks, enters the amniotic fluid by leakage of cerebrospinal fluid

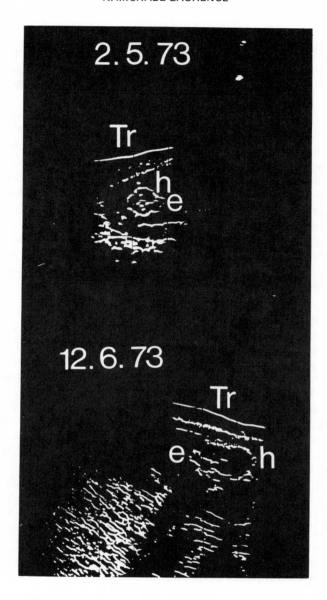

Fig. 2a. Transverse ultrasonographs at 27 and 33 weeks of the case of encephalocele reported briefly by Laurence *et al.* In the scans, the encephalocele (e) was outlined but it was not recognized for what it was. The main clinical problem was growth retardation.

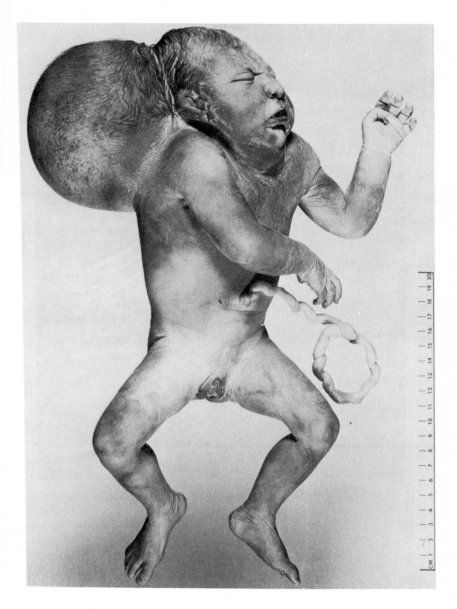

Fig. 2b. Aborted 34 week fetus with the large closed encephalocele. There was a 2 cm defect in the skull and a large amount of the cerebellum and the occipital poles as well as meninges and cerebrospinal fluid filled the sac.

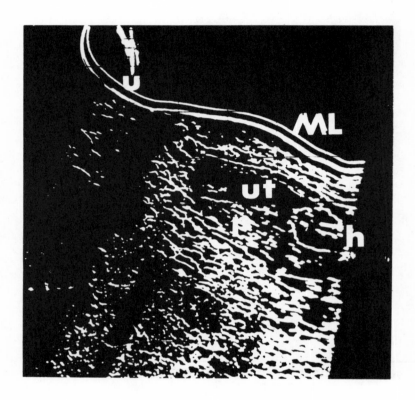

Fig. 3. Midline ultrasonograph at 16 weeks of a fetus with spina bifida. A normal picture is shown with a normal sized head (h). The uterine (ut) and the umbilical (u) shadows are indicated.

or by transudation of fetal serum from the exposed neural tissue. In a number of centers in Britain, amniocentesis at between 15 and 20 weeks of pregnancy, followed by AFP estimations, is now part of the routine antenatal diagnostic armamentarium for antenatal detection of major neural tube malformations in high risk situations.[11] Using any of the immunodiffusion techniques, there is considerable difference between the upper level of amniotic AFP in normal pregnancies and that of pregnancies with a neural tube malformation (Fig. 4). In Cardiff, the AFP estimation is carried out by the Electro-immunodiffusion "Rocket" technique, where a number of standard fluids containing known amounts of AFP are compared with fluids under investigation (Fig. 5). The test costs no more than 50 cents and is relatively easy to carry out. So far, no false positives have been reported in the United Kingdom, except when there has been an intrauterine death, despite the caution expressed by some[12,13] that false negatives are expected in association with certain of the neural tube abnormalities, predominantly the closed.

It is expected that at the 16 to 18 week stage of pregnancy nearly all cases of anencephaly (Fig. 6) will be associated with considerably raised AFP levels.[10,14—19] The only exceptions are the rare cases of exencephaly acrania and of iniencephaly, as reported by Nevin,[20] where there is no exposed neural tissue.

Encephaloceles (Fig. 7), most of which are "closed" lesions and which account for only about 3 percent of cases of neural tube malformations compatible with survival,[21] are also liable to be missed, as in the case reported by Laurence and his co-workers[22] (Fig. 2b). The rare skin-covered myeloceles (Fig. 8), which form no more than 3 percent of all serious cases of spina bifida, are unlikely to be detected. The same will probably be true for the small puckered "open" but much less serious lesion (Fig. 9), which again makes up about 3 percent of cases of spina bifida cystica.[23] To date, however, there appear to be no reports of examples of the last two having been missed. The true meningoceles (Fig. 10), which account for about 5 percent of cases of spina bifida cystica and which are usually covered by a thick membrane, will, in all likelihood, also remain undetected — as in the case reported by Ferguson-Smith.[24] On the other hand, the common open myeloceles — 95 to 90 percent of all cases of spina bifida cystica — (Fig. 11, 12) seem to be consistently associated with high AFT levels.[14,15,25]

At about 16 weeks, amniocentesis ought to be a quick, simple and safe procedure, requiring no general or local anesthetic and no special apparatus other than a needle with a trochar (Fig. 13). However, it would be preceded by an ultrasound scan for placental localization, identification of twins, confirmation of fetal maturity and the detection of anencephaly. Placental localization is essential[9] so that the placenta can be avoided, thus reducing

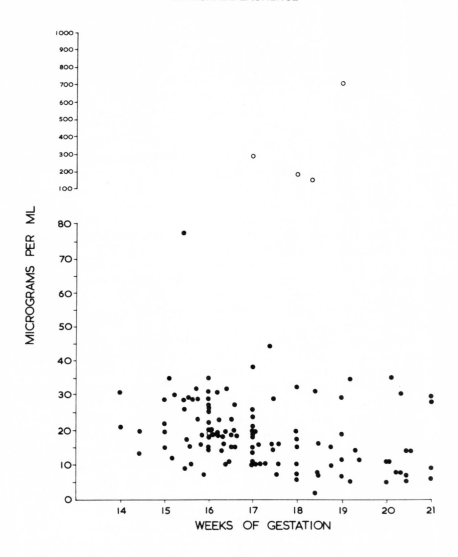

Fig. 4. Scattergram of amniotic fluid AFP results in 122 pregnancies. Estimations have been carried out by the "Rocket" method of Allen *et al.*[15] using the Behringewerke standard. Open circles are of cases resulting in a neural tube malformation. The high result (μgm/ml) at 19 weeks was in a case of threatened abortion. *(Reprinted from "Special Education in the New Community Services", courtesy of the National Council for Special Education, 17 Pembridge Square, London, England.)*

70

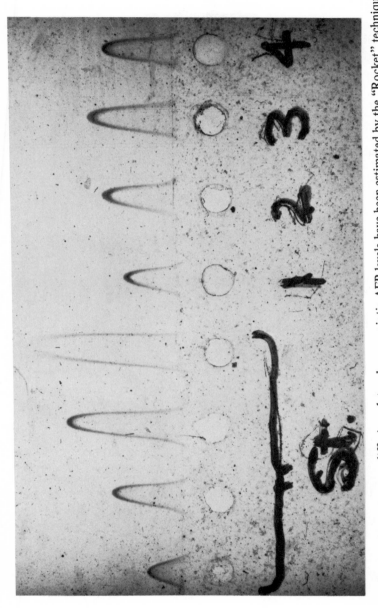

Fig. 5. An electro-immunodiffusion plate where amniotic AFP levels have been estimated by the "Rocket" technique of Allen *et al.*15 Five unknowns (1, 2, 3, 4) have been tested against four dilutions of Behringewerke standard of about 12, 24, 50 and 100 μgm/ml.

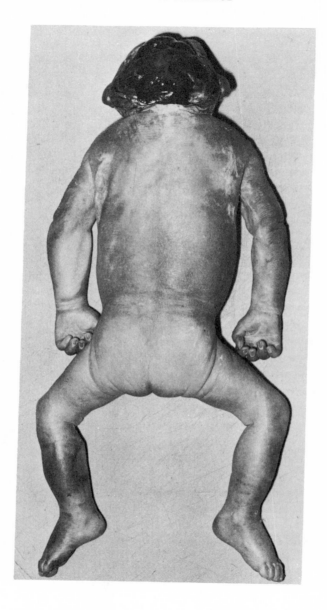

Fig. 6. An anencephalic fetus at term. A large open lesion incompatible with survival.

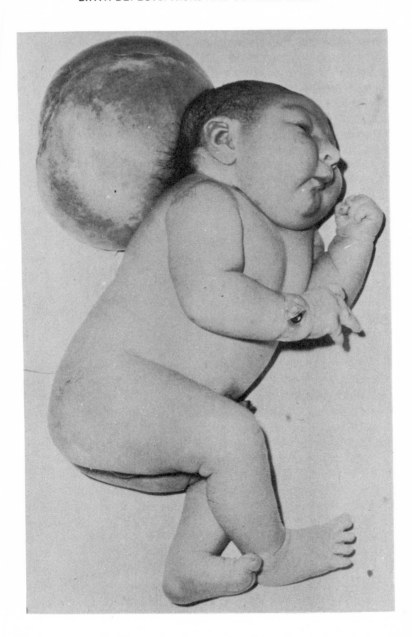

Fig. 7. An infant with a large closed encephalocele. This is a very serious lesion often associated with severe mental retardation.

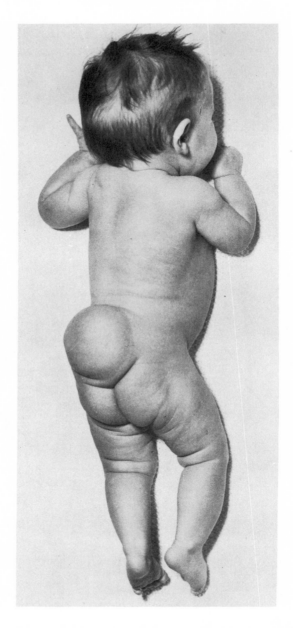

Fig. 8.   An infant with a myelocele with complete whole skin cover. These patients are frequently severely paralyzed and incontinent.

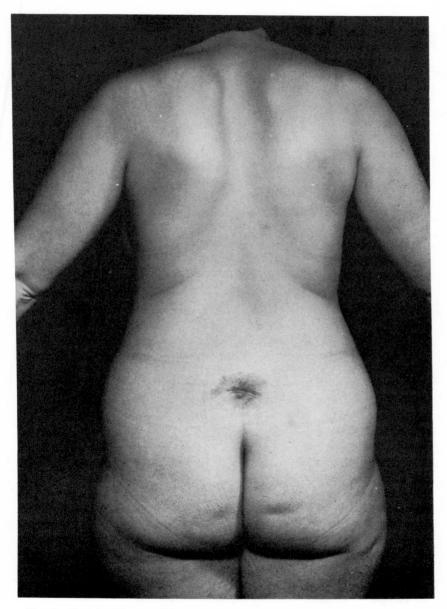

Fig. 9. A girl with a small but originally open myelocele which has become secondarily epithelialized over. These patients are often only minimally affected.

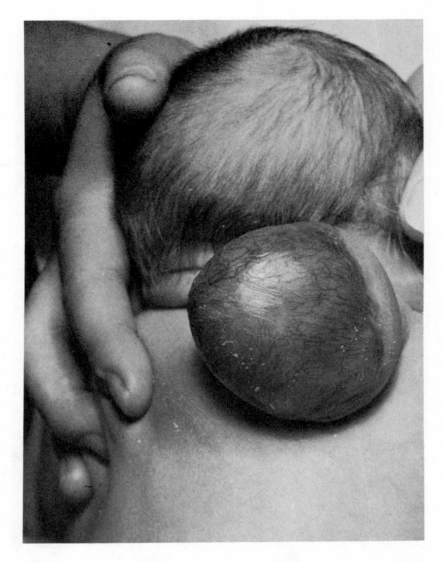

Fig. 10a. A true meningocele in an infant. This is usually a closed lesion even though the membrane is relatively thin and most of these patients having this relatively rare form of spina bifida are physically and mentally normal once the sac is removed. *(Reprinted from "Special Education in the New Community Services", courtesy of the National Council for Special Education, 17 Pembridge Square, London, England.)*

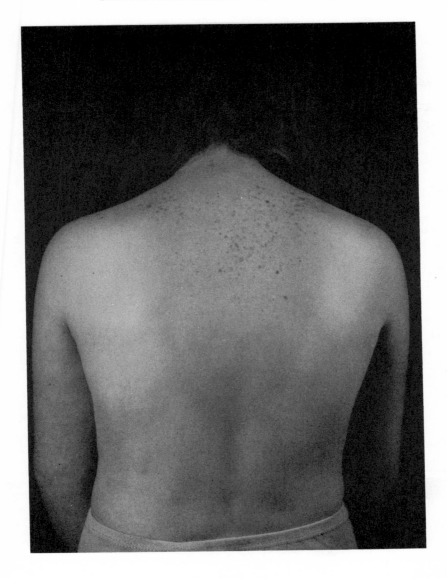

Fig. 10b. The same individual now age 15 years, after the sac had been removed. *(Reprinted from "Special Education in the New Community Services", courtesy of the National Council for Special Education, 17 Pembridge Square, London, England.)*

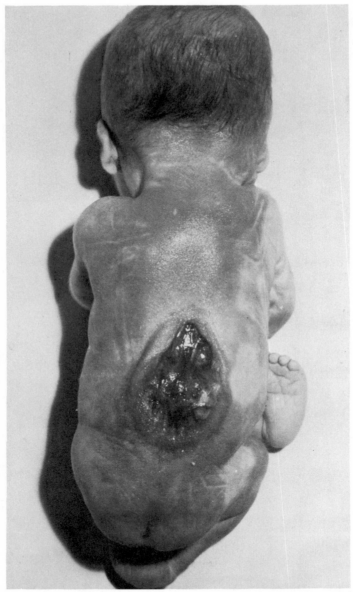

Fig. 11. A newborn infant with a large open myelocele. Most of these are severely paralyzed and incontinent and usually also have hydrocephalus. *(Reprinted from "Special Education in the New Community", courtesy of the National Council for Special Education, 17 Pembridge Square, London, England.)*

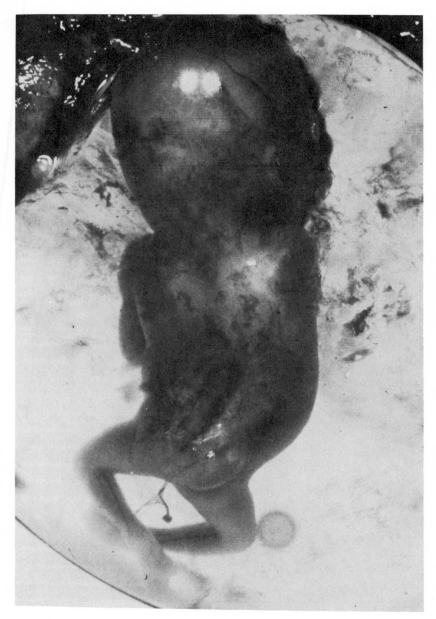

Fig. 12. A 14–15 week fetus with a large open myelocele. The fetus is still within the amniotic sac.

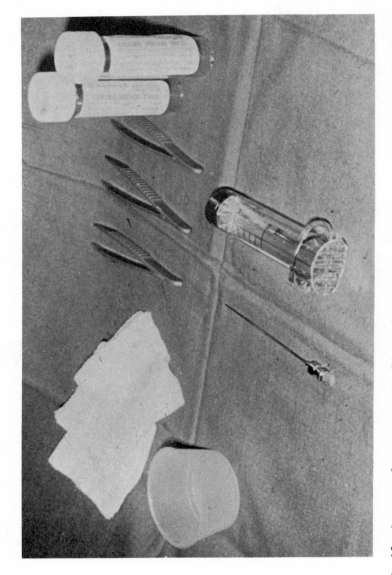

Fig. 13. Apparatus for amniocentesis after an ultrasound scan has been carried out. The essential items are skin cleaning materials, needle and trochar, syringe and specimen bottles.

the risk of hemorrhage and of rhesus iso-immunization. The problems presented by a twin pregnancy are obvious — when only one of the amniotic cavities may be entered and the fluid examined. Estimation of fetal maturity is essential so that the timing of the amniocentesis is correct, when the uterus has emerged from the pelvis and when there is sufficient amniotic fluid present for some 10—20 ccs to be taken without danger. If performed too early and in the presence of only a small amount of amniotic fluid, it could result not only in faulure but also in possible fetal damage[26] and, if too late, there may be problems in the timing of a possible termination. Finally, there is always a risk of precipitating a miscarriage but, in competent hands, this would appear to be a risk of less than 1 percent.[27]

The amniotic fluid removed should be yellowish and free from blood. When blood is present, this may have occurred as a result of the amniocentesis and may cause difficulties in interpretation of the results, especially if it is present in quantity and is of fetal origin. Occasionally, the blood may be there as a result of a recent fetal death. Usually under these circumstances, however, the blood is "altered", especially if the fetus has been dead for any length of time. The fluid should be kept sterile as it is now the policy in most centers not only to carry out the AFP estimations but also to do amnion cell culture and cytogenetics on the centrifuged cell deposit on all amniocenteses from pregnancies of 20 weeks duration or less. This followed an unfortunate case where a high risk pregnancy in a young woman that had been pronounced free from neural tube malformation was found to end in a child with Down's syndrome.

Amniocentesis for the prenatal diagnosis of neural tube malformations should normally be undertaken only if both the obstetrician and the parents will act on the results and accept termination of pregnancy if it is indicated. It would be a wise precaution to have a thorough discussion with both parents prior to attempting the investigation, to make quite sure that they appreciate what is involved[11] and to allay worries which the parents will often have. They should realize that it might involve a termination of the pregnancy. They should have it made clear to them that there is a small risk of precipitating a miscarriage and that the investigations to be carried out will only detect "open" neural tube malformations and chromosome abnormalities and leave undetected the large number of other malformations which may occur from time to time. It may be wise to obtain a signed consent form.

In Cardiff, to date, 100 pregnancies at high risk for a neural tube malformation have had an amniocentesis carried out: 4 have been terminated for a neural tube malformation; 2 have been terminated for chromosomal abnormality (2 for anencephaly and 2 for "open" spina bifida); 1 was terminated at 34 weeks and was found to have a "closed" encephalocele associated with

81

growth retardation;[22] and 1 had an unplanned abortion which very likely resulted from the amniocentesis. The other 102 ended in infants free from neural tube malformations or obvious chromosome abnormality. A further 12 women whose pregnancies were not particularly at risk for either neural tube malformations or chromosome abnormalities had an amniocentesis carried out because of maternal anxiety about malformation which, in our opinion, is a perfectly valid indication in certain circumstances. One of these turned out to have a fetus with Down's syndrome, terminated at 18 weeks; the others ended in normal infants (Table 1).

With the above approach, nearly all cases of anencephaly and about nine out of ten serious cases of neural tube malformation compatible with survival should be detectable at about the 16th week of pregnancy, which is early enough for a termination to be carried out.[11] It should be possible therefore to eliminate almost all recurrences. Instead of giving the recurrence risk of about 1 in 20 after one affected child, as in the past, one is able to give a risk of less than 1 in 150 for a major neural tube malformation which would not be detected.[14] Such relatively small odds should not deter a couple from starting another pregnancy if they really want more children.

Possible Screening for Neural Tube Malformations

Monitoring all pregnancies in women who have had a previous child with a neural tube malformation or who have some family history, would only reduce the community incidence of neural tube malformations compatible with life at term by about 10 percent. To reduce the incidence further would mean screening all pregnancies. However, subjecting all pregnancies to an amniocentesis, even if logistically feasible, would not be justifiable in view of the possible risks. Probably, departments of obstetrics would find it difficult to cope with the vastly increased work load and inevitably many amniocenteses would be carried out by relatively inexperienced staff, probably without a previous ultrasound scan and with the resultant risk of all sorts of mishaps and almost certainly a greatly increased number of miscarriages. Cytogenetics laboratories would certainly be in great difficulties with the extra cell cultures though the AFP estimations would not present any insuperable problems.

Indications that AFP estimation in maternal serum might be of help as a diagnostic test — first reported by Leek and his co-workers[28] in the autumn of 1973, and later by others,[14,17,29–32] were welcome in that they seemed to hold out hope of a possible screening procedure in all pregnancies. Simultaneous estimations of amniotic and maternal serum AFP suggest that there is come correspondence between the two. Often a high amniotic fluid level is associated with a raised maternal serum level but when the amniotic

TABLE 1

Amniocentesis for Neural Tube Malformation

Indication	Outcome						Total
	Abortion	Spina Bifida	Anencephaly	Encephalocele	Down's	Normal	
High Risk	1	2*	2*	1**	2*	102	110
Anxiety	—	—	—	—	1*	11	12

*Terminated before 21 weeks.

**Terminated at 34 weeks

83

AFP is falling (at about 22 weeks) the maternal serum level is still high and seems to remain so for 8–10 weeks longer. The concentration of AFP in the serum is 500 times lower than it is in the amniotic fluid (*i.e.,* in ng instead of μg amounts), therefore, accurate determination requires radio-immunoassay methods sensitive to less than 100 ng/ml. Further, the need for accuracy is increased by the apparently smaller difference between the upper limit of levels associated with normal fetuses and the levels associated with those with neural tube malformations (Fig. 14).

Workers from a number of centers met in the spring of 1974 and again toward the end of the year, to collate the published and unpublished results derived from a large number of pregnancies, both normal and at high risk for neural tube malformations. Taking only values between the 15th and 20th week of gestation, it was found that 12 of 15 anencephalic and 10 of 17 open spina bifida fetuses were associated with maternal serum AFP levels above the highest value for normal pregnancies.[33] These results were thought to be sufficiently encouraging to warrant the launching of a multi-center research program in order (a) to refine and standardize AFP assay techniques, (b) to obtain more AFP results from women who are at risk for neural tube malformation and women who are not, (c) to study the effects of maternal illness and pregnancy abnormalities and to discover what factors might determine a false positive or negative and, (d) by means of serial serum estimations, to establish the best time for differentiating abnormal pregnancies. So far, the indications are that the serum AFP levels in affected pregnancies do not begin to rise until after 16 weeks, while in threatened abortions the level rises and then falls (Fig. 15).

It now seems possible that the test may be sufficiently sensitive not to miss too many affected pregnancies and sufficiently specific not to call to question too many normal ones; for a pilot screening project of all pregnancies in a circumscribed area to be undertaken and for a careful "cost benefit" analysis, taking into account anxieties relieved and generated, as well as "hard cash", to be undertaken. Presumably, a portion of the usual blood sample taken for various antenatal tests at about the beginning of the 4th month could be sent for AFP radio-immunoassay. Should the AFP result be high, it may be well to repeat the test. If the high level is confirmed, the obstetrician would be informed of the result and he would then have to decide whether to carry out an ultrasound scan and amniocentesis for amniotic fluid AFP estimation and a termination if the diagnosis is confirmed. Such a screening procedure would probably call for a revision of confinement "booking" arrangements but would, in itself, not be costly – the clinical side being part of the normal routine antenatal testing. The laboratory costs (provided there was full automation) both in equipment and data processing,

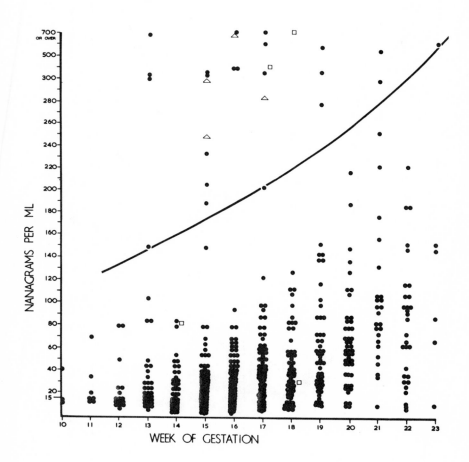

Fig. 14. Scattergram of serum AFP estimations carried out by a modification of the method of Rouslahti and Seppälä.[36] The line denotes the 95% normal confidence limit derived from a Finnish population.[14,37] The triangles denote pregnancies which have either aborted or have threatened to abort; the squares are those which have ended in a neural tube malformation. The remainder have resulted in a normal child or have not yet come to term.

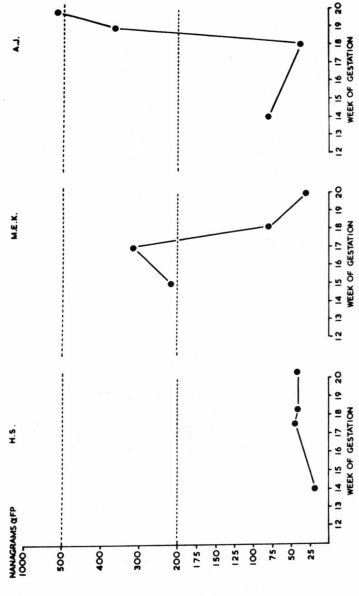

Fig. 15. Serial maternal serum AFP measurements in a normal pregnancy (left), a threatened abortion (center) and a spina bifida pregnancy (right).

are minimal. On present evidence, the indications are that although most cases of anencephaly would be detected, it is unlikely that more than 50% of spina bifida would. However, in view of the seriousness of spina bifida, even detection of somewhat less than 50% would probably be worthwhile.[11] On the other hand, a considerable number of women with borderline levels of AFP would undoubtedly be subjected to an unnecessary amniocentesis with all its attendant anxieties,[34] risks and costs, for the sake of a relatively small number of cases detected, especially in relatively low incidence communities, but this difficulty is common to most screening procedures.

Finally, in selective screening in high risk situations where there has been a previous case in the family, usually parents will be only too aware of the risks and they enter the screening procedures only if they agree to termination of an abnormal fetus. A woman having a blood test which is part of a routine antenatal diagnostic regime will not have given prior permission for a possible termination. Indeed, she will probably be completely unaware of the risk of an abnormality and would presumably not have given the possibility of a termination any thought. Under these circumstances, the approach to a woman with a possible abnormal fetus would have to be cautious as it might turn out to be a "false alarm" and there might be religious or moral objections to a termination.

Summary

X-rays and fetoscopy do not seem too useful as methods for the early prenatal diagnosis of neural tube malformations. Ultrasonography, apart from being a necessary preliminary for amniocentesis, will identify anencephaly and possibly encephalocele.

Estimation of alpha fetoprotein (AFP) in amniotic fluid obtained by amniocentesis in the fifth month of pregnancy seems to be the most useful and reliable method. Almost all cases of anencephaly and widely-open myelocele can be detected by high levels of AFP.

Because estimations of AFP in amniotic fluid are usually only undertaken in women at risk for neural tube malformations, prenatal detection will reduce the incidence of spina bifida by less than 10 percent. However, if estimation of AFP in maternal serum fulfills its initial promise, screening of all pregnancies may become possible and may lead to a substantial reduction in the incidence of spina bifida.

ACKNOWLEDGMENTS

The assistance of Dr. M. Addison, Department of Clinical Biochemistry, University Hospital of Wales, and Dr. J. Keyser, Department of Clinical Biochemistry, Cardiff Royal Infirmary, in estimating amniotic and serum AFP values respectively, and Mr. T.J. Cooke in drawing the charts, is gratefully acknowledged. Drs. Hugh Gavelle and Margaret Jones[35] of the Department of Radiology, University Hospital of Wales, kindly gave permission for the inclusion of ultrasonographs.

REFERENCES

1. C.O. Carter, *Dev. Med. Child Neurol. 16, Suppl. 32,* 3, 1974.

2. J.B. Scrimgeour, *in* Prenatal Diagnosis, A.E.M. Emery (Ed.), p. 26, Edinburgh, 1973.

3. C. Valenti, *Int. Congress Series. No. 297,* 26, 1973.

4. K.M. Laurence, J.F. Pearson, R. Prosser, C. Richards and I. Rocker, *Lancet 2,* 1120, 1974.

5. K.M. Laurence, R. Prosser, I. Rocker, J.F. Pearson and C. Richards, *J. Med. Genet.* (in press).

6. *J.B. Scrimgeour, in* Birth Defects, A.O. Motulsky and W. Lenz (Eds.), 234, Amsterdam, 1974.

7. I.J.C. MacIntosh and D.A. Davey, *Br. Med. J. 4,* 92, 1970.

8. W.T. Coakley, J.S. Slade, J.M. Braeman and J.L. Moore, *Br. J. Radiol. 45,* 328, 1972.

9. S. Campbell, *in* Birth Defects, A.O. Motulsky and W. Lenz (Eds.), 240, Amsterdam, 1974.

10. D.J.H. Brock and R.G. Sutcliffe, *Lancet 2,* 197, 1972.

11. K.M. Laurence, *Lancet 2,* 939, 1974.

12. A.M. Ward and C.R. Stewart, *Lancet,* 345, 1974.

13. L. Wisniewski, Z. Skrzydlewski and J. Orcluch, *Br. Med. J. 3,* 742, 1974.

14. R. Harris, R.F. Jennison, A.J. Barson, K.M. Laurence, E. Ruoslahti and M. Seppälä, *Lancet 1,* 522, 1973.

15. L.D. Allen, M.A. Ferguson-Smith, I Donald, E. Sweet and A.A.M. Gibson, *Lancet 1,* 522, 1973.

16. M.J. Seller, S. Campbell, T.M. Coltart and J.D. Singer, *Lancet 2,* 73,

17. D.J.H. Brock, A.E. Bolton and J.M. Monahan, *Lancet 2,* 923, 1973.

18. J. Lorber, C.R. Stewart and A. Milford Ward, *Lancet 1,* 1187, 1973.

19. B. Field, G. Mitchell, W. Carrett and C. Kerr, *Lancet 2,* 798, 1973.

20. N.E. Nevin, W. Thompson and S.J. Nesbitt, *Obstet. Gynaec. Br. Commonw. 81,* 757, 1974.

21. K.M. Laurence, B.J. Tew, *Arch. Dis. Child. 46,* 127, 1971.

22. K.M. Laurence, A.C. Turnbull, R. Harris, R.F. Jennison, E. Ruoslahti and M. Seppala, *Lancet 2,* 860, 1973.

23. K.M. Laurence, *Lancet 1,* 301, 1974.

24. M.A. Ferguson-Smith, Personal Communication.

25. N.E. Nevin, S. Nesbitt and W. Thompson, *Lancet 1,* 1383, 1973.

26. A. Milunsky, Prenatal Diagnosis of Hereditary Diseases, Springfield, Illinois, 1973.

27. A.B. Gerbie, H.L. Nadler and M.V. Gerbie, *Am.J. Obstet. Gynecol. 109,* 765, 1971.

28. A.E. Leck, C.R. Ruoss, M.K. Kitan and T. Chard, *Lancet 1,* 385, 1973.

29. D.J.H. Brock, A.E. Bolton and J.B. Scrimgeour, *Lancet 1,* 767, 1974.

30. M.J. Seller, J.D. Singer, T.M. Coltart and S. Campbell, *Lancet 1,* 428, 1974.

31. N.J. Wald, D.J.H. Brock and J. Bonnar, *Lancet 1,* 765, 1974.

32. F.S. Cowchock and L.G. Jackson, *Lancet 2,* 48, 1974.

33. *Lancet 1,* 907, 1974.

34. A.E. Leck and T. Chard, *Lancet 1,* 876, 1974.

35. H. Gravelle and M. Jones, *Br. J. Radiol.* (in press).

36. E. Ruoslahti and M. Seppälä, *Int. J. Cancer 8,* 374, 1971.

37. M. Seppälä and E. Ruoslahti, *J. Perinat. Med. 1,* 107, 1973.

COHORT RELATED RISK FACTORS AND CONGENITAL MALFORMATIONS: A COMPUTER GRAPHIC METHODOLOGY

Charles E. Lawrence
Eric E. Blair

It has recently been suggested that congenital malformations may be the result of environmental factors which affect the mother early in life and predispose her to neural tube defects.[1,2] The purpose of this paper is to present a computer graphic methodology for the simultaneous cross-sectional and longitudinal analysis of congenital malformations and potential predisposing maternal factors.

The description of a large epidemic of anencephaly and spina bifida by MacMahon and Yen[3] strongly suggests that these malformations have an environmental etiology. Several environmental explanations have been hypothesized as the possible cause of the epidemic. These explanations may be grouped in two categories. The first category centers on an insult during gestation. For example, MacMahon and Yen[4] have hypothesized that the epidemic may have been caused by the consumption of abnormal constituents of illicit alcohol during the Prohibition era. Also, Renwick[5] has suggested that potato blight may have been a causal factor.

The second category deals with preconditioning events. Emanuel and Sever[2] refer to this type of mechanism as an intergenerational effect. They suggest that non-specific interference in the normal growth and development process may cause an alteration in the development of the reproductive and/or endocrine system which contributes to the later production of ASB. Janerich[6] suggested that the 1918–1919 influenza pandemic may have been a preconditioning event. Subsequently, he has advanced this line of argument and suggested an endocrine dysfunction as an epidemiologic hypothesis.[7]

The value of longitudinal studies in epidemiology has long been recognized but their use in the study of congenitally defective offspring has been infrequent. This shortcoming has been caused by both data limitations and the procedural difficulties associated with these studies. However, Janerich[8] reported an analysis of spina bifida incidence which examines both a longitudinal and cross-sectional data perspective. While the two analyses should yield similar results when the underlying phenomena are static, a dynamic etiologic phenomenon would produce analytic differences. These complimentary analyses illustrated clear differences in the maternal age-specific pattern of the rate of spina bifida when viewed from the longitudinal and the cross-sectional perspectives.

The study compares the results of these two analytic techniques. The analysis we will present considers them simultaneously. A simultaneous analysis which considers the age-temporal population dynamics should enhance our understanding of the etiologic mechanisms. It could contribute to the resolution of the controversy between etiologic explanations centered around teratogens versus preconditioning events.

Fortunately, recent developments in the area of computer graphics include the development of three-dimensional plotting algorithms with hidden line subroutines. We have three such algorithms available and will present plots from one of these. This technique gives the projection of a three-dimensional object onto a plane perpendicular to the user's viewpoint vector (Fig. 1). A hidden line subroutine removes the lines which correspond to that proportion of the three-dimensional object that we would be unable to see in reality.

With this technology we can view incidence rates simultaneously as a function of time and age (Fig. 1). By selecting a specific point in time and looking across the surface at various ages, we obtain a cross-sectional view. By slicing a vertical plane from the three-dimensional object along this line, we obtain the conventional cross-sectional graph. Longitudinal rates are projected on the surface along cohort lines. Since the current time (t) is the year of birth of a cohort (c) plus its age (a), we obtain a longitudinal view by looking along a line in which the age and time increase at the same rate or a 45° line. Such cohort lines are used by demographers[9] in lexis diagrams.

Consider the following example. Let us assume that we have observed a minor epidemic wave rising above level background incidence rates. If the epidemic wave is caused by an insult to pregnant mothers during the epidemic period we would expect to see a rising wave in the surface across several ages at the time of the epidemic (Fig. 2). An alternate explanation suggests that these epidemic results are from a preconditioning insult to cohorts of women. In the latter case we would observe a rising wave of defects along cohort lines (Fig. 3).

We are now analyzing ASB rates for New York State from 1945 to 1970 using this method. As expected, our raw data plot by single years contains numerous random fluctuations. Aggregation and/or smoothing of the data will be necessary before any type of recognizable surface emerges from the three-dimensional plot.

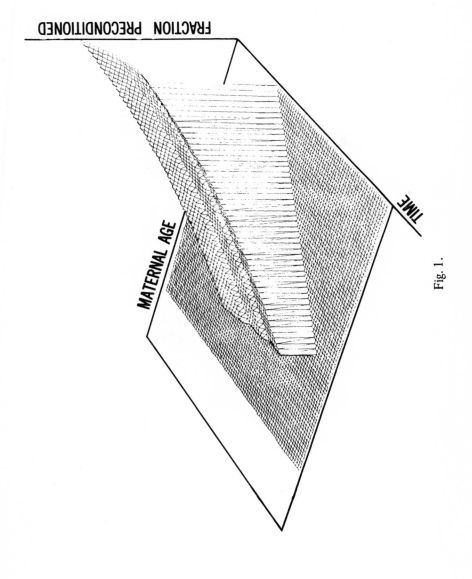

Fig. 1.

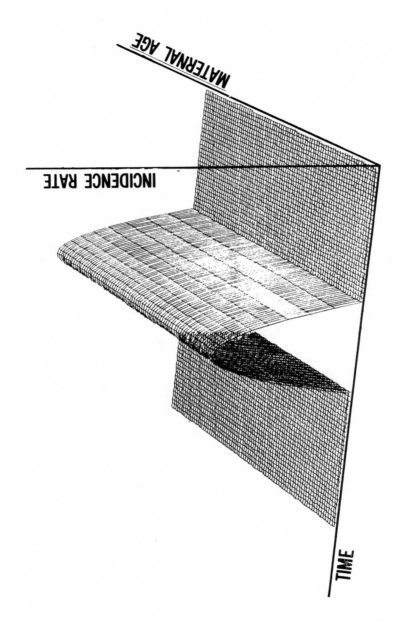

Fig. 2.

94

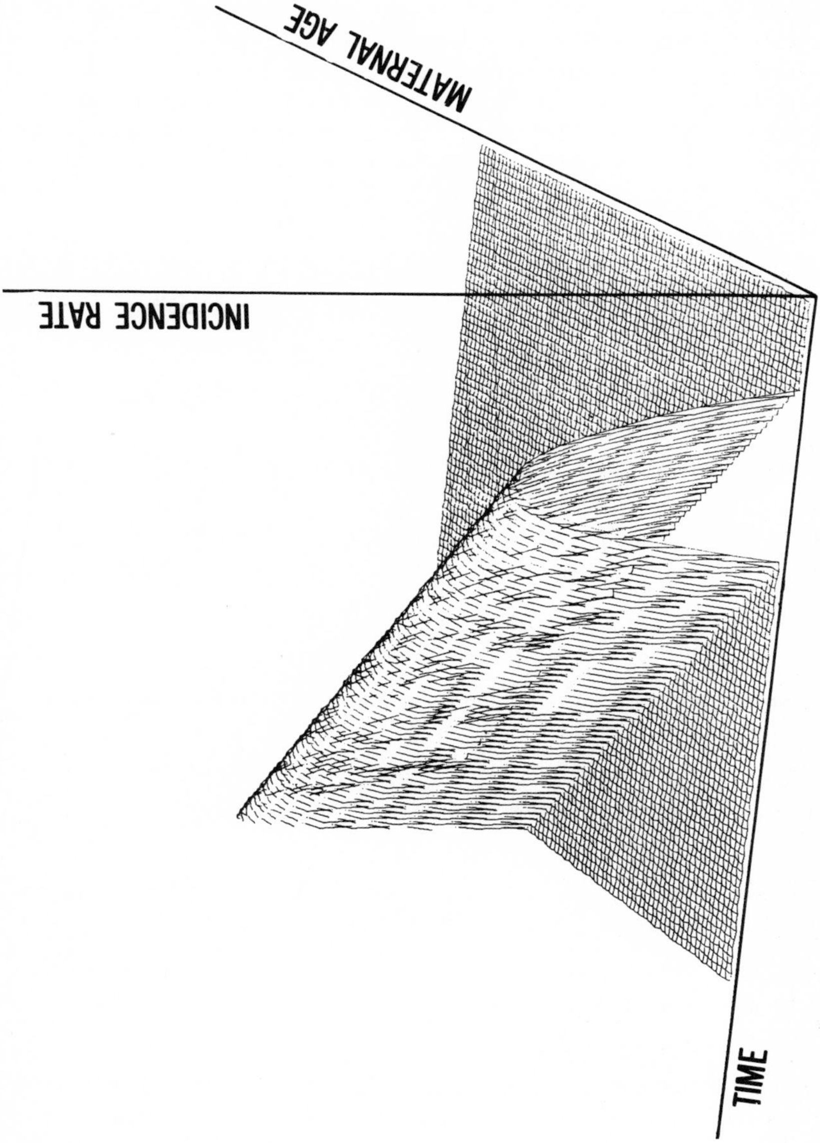

Fig. 3.

To establish the connection between the preconditioning event(s) and the incidence of the congenital malformations, it is necessary to trace back from the birth incident or forward from the preconditioning event. In essence we would be moving backwards or forward through time. Since the preconditioning affects cohorts of women, the age changes are equivalent to the time changes, or the motion is on 45⁰ lines of the time-age plane. The establishment of this relationship will be greatly enhanced through the formulation of a specific mathematical model. First, some notational definitions are in order.

Let:

$O(a, t)$ = the observed ratio of defective births to women of age (a) in the time period (t) to the total births to women of age (a) in time period (t).
(defect fraction)

$Z(a, t)$ = number of women of age (a) in time period (t) to be in a preconditioned state.

$N(a, t)$ = total number of women of age (a) in time period (t) in the population.

We start by assuming that the defect fraction is proportional to the fraction of preconditioned women in the population. Mathematically this is described as follows:

$$(1) \qquad O(a, t) = K_1 \; \frac{Z(a, t)}{N(a, t)} \qquad \begin{array}{l} a = 1 \ldots A \\ t = 1 \ldots T \end{array}$$

As noted above, the current time for a cohort is the cohort's age plus their year of birth or:

$$(2) \qquad t = c + a.$$

The number preconditioned as a function of time and age is:

$$Z(a, t) = g(a, t).$$

However, since the preconditioning events affect cohort groups, the parameters of this relationship depend on the cohorts of:

$$(3) \qquad Z(a, t) = g_c (a, t).$$

Substituting (2) into (3) we obtain

$$Z(a, a + c) = g_c (a, a + c).$$

The primary issue in this exercise relates to the nature of this preconditioning function and how its parameters may be determined. There are two techniques which can be used to define the relationship. First, an hypothesized mechanism for the preconditioning may suggest a form that is consistent

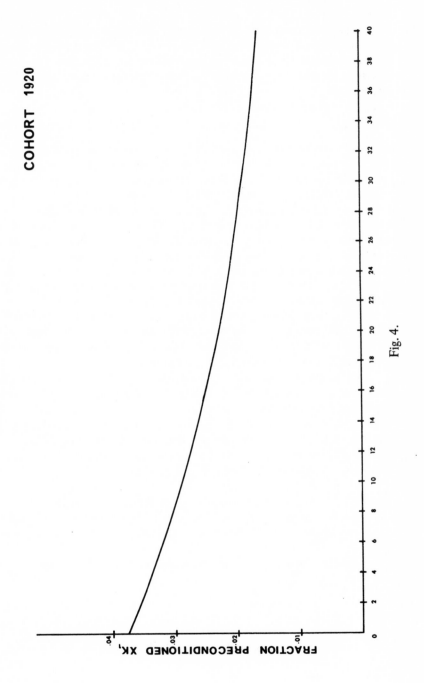

COHORT 1920

FRACTION PRECONDITIONED XK,

Fig. 4.

97

with a specific potentially causal event. The other potential source is the incidence surface itself. In the case of ASB, Janerich[8] has presented longitudinal data for cohorts in five-year intervals. The form of these data seems to suggest an exponential decline as a function of age for cohorts through age 39.

Let us explore this lead. In this case,

$$Z(a, a + c) = B(c)e^{-\varkappa(c)a}.$$

Such curves have a form as shown in Fig. 4. A three-dimension view of the number preconditioned can be obtained by plotting $Z(a,t)$. This is equivalent to viewing several of these cohort declining curves placed on the age-time plane, on $45°$ lines. The resulting surface is pictured in Fig. 1.

As with the incidence surface discussed above, slices from this figure yield cross-sectional and longitudinal data. The cohort data presented above constitutes a view from a longitudinal perspective. For a cross-sectional perspective, we slice through the surface at a fixed time (Fig. 5). If the hypothesized cause of the insult is an event that occurred over a relatively short period of time, the resulting cross section gives the age-specific distribution of the impact of the insult (Fig. 6).

If the preconditioning function $g_c(a, a + c)$ is estimated from the underlying biological mechanism, we may extend our analysis to provide estimates of the age-specific distribution of the impact within a hypothesized time distribution of the insult, under a broader set of conditions.

Taking several cuts through our three-dimensional surface at fixed ages, we obtain curves of the number of preconditioned women for a fixed age as a function of time (Fig. 6).

The secular trend of the hypothesized insult yields another curve as a function of time. The question remains, how can we make a set of time-specific preconditioning cuts at fixed ages most compatible with the time distribution of this hypothesized environmental insult.

Let:

$E(t) = $ number of women affected by insult at time (t)

$y(a) = $ fraction of the total women of age (a) who were affected by the insult that became preconditioned (age-specific impact of the insult).

Assuming the age-specific impact is independent of time, yields:

$$Z(a, t) = y(a) E(t)$$

$$y(a) = \frac{Z(a, t)}{E(t)}.$$

To obtain the best estimate of $y(a)$ we would seek to find the $y(a)$ that

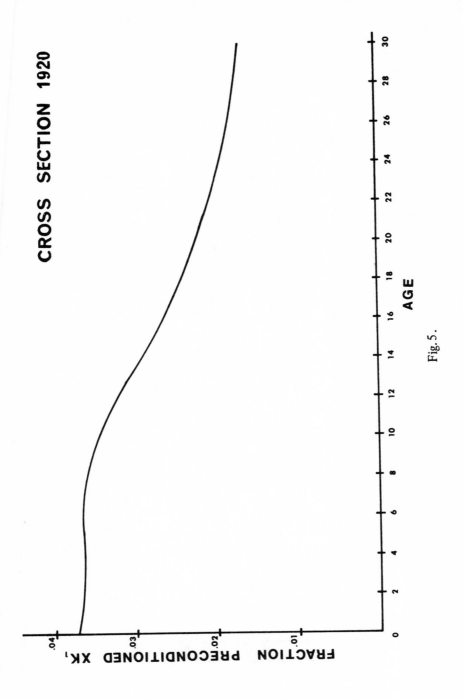

CROSS SECTION 1920

FRACTION PRECONDITIONED XK,

AGE

Fig. 5.

99

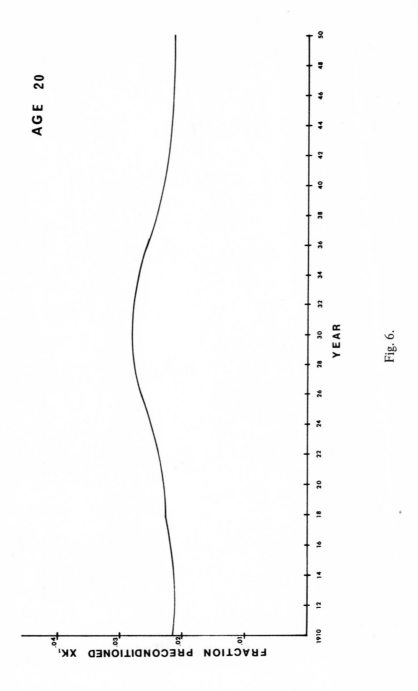

Fig. 6.

minimized the sum of the squared errors as follows:

$$\min_{y} v = \min_{y} \left[\sum_{t} \sum_{a} \left[Z(a,t) - y(a)\, E(t) \right]^{2} \right]$$

The result is the age distribution of the impact of the environmental insult that is most compatible with the hypothesized time distribution of the insult.

In conclusion, a methodology for the simultaneous cross-sectional and longitudinal analysis of incidence rate data has been presented. Building on this base, an approach has been suggested for estimating the age temporal distribution of potential preconditioning etiological events.

REFERENCES

1.   D.T. Janerich, *Lancet 1*, 1165, 1971.

2.   I. Emanuel and L.F. Sever, *Teratology 8*, 325, 1973.

3.   B. MacMahon and S. Yen, *Lancet 1*, 31, 1971.

4.   *Ibid.*

5.   J.H. Renwick, *Lancet 2*, 967, 1972.

6.   D.T. Janerich, *Lancet 1*, 1165, 1971.

7.   D.T. Janerich, *Amer. J. Epid. 99*, 1, 1974.

8.   D.T. Janerich, *Amer. J. Epid. 96*, 389, 1973.

9.   N. Keyfitz, *Mathematics of Populations*, 1970.

MATERNAL-FETAL ENDOCRINE FUNCTION IN ANENCEPHALY AND SPINA BIFIDA — EPIDEMIOLOGICAL CONSIDERATIONS

Dwight T. Janerich

This annual symposium is intended to provide a mechanism whereby new ideas can be presented or discussed, in the hope of providing information which will lead to the development of improved programs for the prevention of birth defects. In past years, many speculative and innovative ideas have been presented at these meetings. In keeping with this theme, my objective will be to outline a very broad and a very speculative etiological mechanism which is based upon the epidemiology of anencephaly and spina bifida. Specifically, I will explore the epidemiological support for the idea that maternal-fetal endocrine dysfunction is responsible for inadequate closure of the neural tube and produces the classical malformations of anencephaly and spina bifida in the human.

In the development of this outline I will focus on four important epidemiological characteristics related to anencephaly and spina bifida: (1) the unexplained association between dizygotic twinning and these malformations, (2) the female excess among cases, (3) the maternal age dependent risk and (4) epidemic waves in the incidence rates of these malformations.

Our first concern will be with twinning. Dizygotic twinning represents an event produced by multiple concurrent, or nearly concurrent, ovulations. It occurs spontaneously in apparently normal, healthy females and is generally not considered to be a sign of underlying reproductive pathology in the mother. Dizygotic twinning, or multiple ovulation, can also be produced by controlled supplemental treatment of subfertile women with the pituitary gonadotrophins or with compounds which stimulate the production of endogenous gonadotrophins.

Anencephaly and spina bifida (ASB), on the other hand, are obvious signs of reproductive pathology and in general are thought to be different developmental manifestations of the same etiological mechanism. Several studies which have examined the relationship between ASB and twinning have produced results which pose interesting questions about the population genetics of ASB, as well as the familial inheritance of ASB. On the population level, ASB and dizygotic twinning are positively correlated. Some degree of correlation can be seen in the fact that both the ASB rate and the dizygotic twinning rate have been concurrently declining in several western countries but we have no precise explanation for the decline in either case. The apparent population correlation between ASB and dizygotic twinning is one of the major unexplained epidemiological observations of the multi-nation study by A.C. Stevenson *et al.,* in the early 1960's.[1] This observation is particularly curious because the association is not apparent at the family level; that is, families which have a high risk for ASB do not appear to have an unusually high risk for dizygotic twinning. In view of the positive population correlation, the subtle implication here is that the conditions which cause ASB can protect against dizygotic twinning. Since ASB does not appear to be unusually common among dizygotic twins, we can conclude that, in high risk populations, the conditions which cause dizygotic twinning are somewhat protective for ASB. This latter point is dramatically underscored by an observation made by Yen and MacMahon in 1968.[2] They assembled 108 sets of twins from consecutive series. In all instances, only one member was affected. They noted that this lack of concordance is quite arresting when one considers that the sibling recurrence risk for these malformations is approximately 5 percent while the risk is apparently less when the sib is a dizygotic twin. Their data suggests that the conditions which produce twins may very well protect against ASB. To exclude the possibility that the lack of concordance among twins is the result of selective intrauterine mortality among concordant twin sets, Yen and MacMahon compared the expected and observed frequency of twin sets in their entire data base. The two values were similar enough to exclude the possibility that differential mortality was the sole explanation for the lack of concordance in the twin pairs which were included in their study series.

The low concordance rate in twin pairs is peculiar for yet another reason. It is not compatible with any conventional genetic etiological scheme, including the idea of polygenic inheritance. Nance has summarized the twin data and concluded that the pattern can only be explained on the basis of cytoplasmic inheritance.[3] However, this idea assumes that the basic etiological mechanism is the mutation of cytoplasmic genes, a mechanism whose existence has not yet been established. In an earlier publication we developed the rationale for attributing the inheritance mechanism for ASB to the intergenerational endowment of membrane-bound hormone receptors for the gonadotrophin hormones.[4] The etiological concept is based on the assumption that the gonadotrophins are responsible for spontaneous, as well as induced, multiple ovulations. Theoretically, the receptor mechanism can explain why the conditions which produce dizygotic twinning can protect against ASB.

Stated simply, the concept suggests that ASB can be caused by a deficiency in gonadotrophin production in relation to the level of fetal sensitivity to gonadotrophin.　The excess production of gonadotrophin which leads to dizygotic twinning can compensate for inherited deficiencies in hormone sensitivity, thus explaining why the concordance rate among dizygotic twins is less than that found among ordinary sites.

The etiological role of gonadotrophins is based entirely on indirect evidence and is derived entirely from epidemiological observations. It assumes that the number of functioning receptor sites on the cell membrane of reproductive cells is a function of a normal distribution. It is important to emphasize that nearly all characteristics in the biological world follow this type of distribution and that the mathematical reasoning associated with the development of the polygenic inheritance-threshold model for ASB is equally valid for a receptor function-threshold model.　It is also important to point out that both the polygenic model and the receptor model are unproven at the laboratory level. This conceptual outline leaves many questions unanswered.　One of the most important is, "How can the gonadotrophins actually be involved in fetal development?".

Data on sex ratios of ASB cases may suggest some partial answers and we have presented the data in a separate report.[5] We will briefly comment on the data because they are an important part of our broad outline. We have observed a pattern of change in the sex-specific rates of anencephaly and spina bifida, which appears to be directly related to the wave-like waning of the major epidemic of ASB that occurred during the earlier part of this century.[6,7] The interrelationship between the epidemic waves and the sex ratio patterns is quite complex and will not be redescribed here.　The interested reader should refer to the original report.[5] The results of that study indicate that the sex specific rates for anencephaly and for spina bifida are quite different but appear to be interrelated to the epidemic waves in the incidence of both malformations.

We believe that the observed relationship provides some indirect evidence suggesting that one of the gonadotrophins, specifically human chorionic gonadotrophin or HCG, is involved in the process which leads to improper closure of the neural tube. The basis for this speculation lies in the observed sex-specific HCG levels which have been determined during several stages of pregnancy. Maternal plasma levels of HCG have been shown to be higher when the fetus is female compared to the HCG levels in pregnancies which produce male offspring. This difference was generally detectable only during the latter part of pregnancy. It has recently been shown that during earlier stages of pregnancy the level of HCG in amniotic fluid is also higher when the fetus is female. The following explanation assumes that the observed excess of HCG in pregnancies which resulted in females is an indication that the female fetus has a greater need for HCG even during the early states of development.

During all human pregnancies, HCG can be detected in the maternal plasma and urine about ten days after ovulation. The level increases rapidly to its maximum at about 45–50 days after ovulation, dropping to lower levels for the remaining months of the pregnancy. Closure of the anterior neuropore occurs at about 25 days and closure of the posterior neuropore occurs somewhat later, at about 45 days.

Anatomically and embryologically, the anterior neuropore corresponds to the site of development of the lesions which causes anencephaly, while the posterior neuropore corresponds to the site of development of the lesion which causes spina bifida. Therefore, neural tube closure occurs during the major period of increasing HCG output.

If the female embryo has a greater need for HCG in order to produce closure of the neural tube, any given degree of reduction in hormone receptor function would have a greater likelihood of causing a malformation when that receptor defect occurred in a female embryo. Thus, a receptor defect which is not in itself sex-specific, could produce a developmental abnormality which is sex-specific. Since the levels of HCG increase from near zero to day ten of pregnancy, to maximum amounts by the end of the second month, the deficiency should be greatest during the early part of that interval. Therefore, one would expect the percentage of females to be greater among anencephalics because HCG levels are lower at the 25th day of pregnancy when the anterior neuropore is closing than at the 45th day when the posterior neuropore is closing.

Therefore, the mechanism of expression of the maternal hormone deficiency, which we theorize to be responsible for ASB, may produce its effect on the fetus through HCG. This mechanism assumes that the levels of production of each of the gonadotrophins (FSH, LH, HCG) are correlated within the mother.

Using a crude cohort approach, we have attempted to show that it is reasonable to interpret the epidemiological patterns shown in studies of the variability risk of ASB related to maternal age as suggesting that environmental events during the mother's early life play an important role in determining her risk of having a child with ASB. I will not detail the reasoning or data to support this view. The available data are suggestive of this possibility but the methodological approach needs much work before a definitive data analysis can be attempted. The basis for the idea that events during the early life of the mother can influence her risk of having a malformed infant involved a hypothesized relationship between the severe illness which accompanied the 1918 influenza pandemic and the major peak of the ASB epidemic.[8] The biological basis for that hypothesis has never been established.

Using epidemic influenza as an example of an environmental factor which could cause this type of predisposition in a mother, I will attempt to show how the actual mechanism could work and how the epidemiological data supports this view.

The proposal is based on the close anatomical proximity of the anterior pituitary gland to the upper respiratory mucosa lining the sphenoidal sinus, plus the fact that influenza is a respiratory virus which occasionally exhibits neurotropic properties. Figure 1 shows the close proximity of the sphenoidal sinus and the pituitary fossa is illustrated in the slide. Lockhart, Hamilton and Fyfe[9] in their description of the anatomy of this area show that anteriorly and inferiorly, the pituitary gland is separated from the mucus membrane of the sphenoidal air sinuses merely by a thin layer of bone. The thin separation of the air sinus and the anterior lobe of the pituitary provides two potential ways by which influenza could affect the function of the anterior pituitary gland. First, the neurotropic properties of the virus could allow direct invasion of the gland from the respiratory mucosa through the thin bony layer which separates the sinus and the pituitary fossa. Second, toxic effects associated with the reproduction of the virus in the mucosal cells of the lining of the sphenoidal sinus could produce conditions which assert physical pressure on the anterior pituitary and thereby alter the normal functioning of the gland. Lockhart et al.[9] draw specific attention to the potential effect of inflammation in the sphenoidal sinus on the structures immediately surrounding it. They observed that structures surrounding the sphenoidal sinus may be readily affected by conditions in the sinus or by fluids introduced into the sinus through inflammation. Therefore, it is reasonable to suggest that influenza has the potential, as well as the opportunity, to influence the function of the anterior pituitary gland.

The way that influenza affects a host cell may explain how it could interfere with hormone receptor function in the cells of critical host tissue. Holland and Kiehn[10] have shown that during infection by influenza virus, viral proteins become firmly attached to the host cells, plasma membranes and other cell membranes. Virus shell proteins can completely replace host membrane proteins in some portion of the plasma membrane. If the portion of the cell membrane which is replaced contains a significant number of gonadotrophin receptors, the host's endocrine balance for those hormones will be impaired, not only for those specific cells but perhaps also in the progeny of those cells. The suggestion that influenza is involved in the etiology of ASB is supported by a degree of secular correlation between periodic influenza epidemics and observed peaks in ASB incidence. Figure 2 is the composite of ASB incidence in the U.S. during this century.[6,7] As

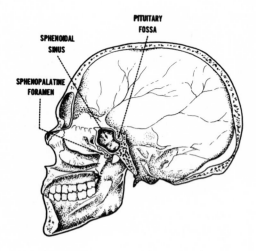

Fig. 1. Illustration of the close anatomical relationship between the sphenoidal sinus and the anterior lobe of the pituitary gland.

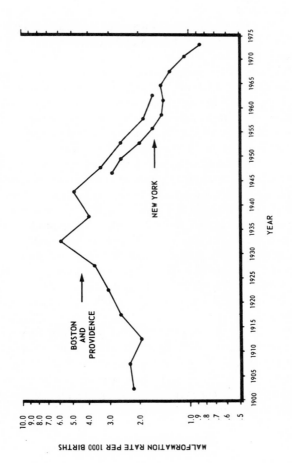

Fig. 2. Prevalence of anencephaly and spina bifida at birth. Northeastern U.S., 1900 through April 1974. (References 1 and 11.)

many as four "epidemic" peaks are apparent: a small one just after the turn of the century, the major one about 1930, another in the 1940's and probably a fourth in the 1960's. Influenza also has its milestone epidemics during this period. Hoyle[11] historically groups these into five distinct categories which appear to enjoy almost universal agreement. These are: the pandemic of 1889–1890, the pandemic of 1918–1919, the era of prevalence of the A type viruses of 1932–1946, the period of prevalence of A prime or A_1 viruses of 1946–1955 and the 1957 pandemic of Asian or A_2 influenza.

In four instances out of five, an epidemic peak in ASB incidence followed approximately ten years after the beginning of a new period of influenza activity. The single exception follows the period of the A_1 viruses in 1946–1956, which was perhaps the least prominent of the new virus strain introduction during the entire period. The most significant period of influenza activity was the 1918–1919 pandemic and it precedes the most significant peak in ASB incidence by approximately ten years.

This proposal is a very broad and speculative outline. It attempts to show how specific environmental events could operate early in the mother's life to later affect her risk of having a child with ASB. Influenza need not be the only agent capable of producing this type of effect. The mechanism is attractive because an environmental agent would be able to produce an effect which would mimic a genetic mechanism. This mechanism could provide the current debate on genetic versus environmental factors in the etiology of ASB with an opportunity to move away from the present stalemate. There are many gaps in this outline, many assumptions to be proven and many questions left unanswered. My admitted objective is to spark interest rather than to provide a definitive answer.

We have labeled this concept *Environmental Preconditioning.* If the mechanism is proven to exist for ASB, even in the general sense, it will probably also have relevance to other malformations and similar disease processes. In essence, it is a replacement or specific extension of the polygenic inheritance and multifactorial concepts which are presently used to explain the etiology of these malformations.

REFERENCES

1. A.C. Stevenson, H.A. Johnston, M.I.P. Stewart *et al., Bulletin of W.H.O., Suppl. Vol. 34,* 127, 1966.

2. S. Yen and B. MacMahon, *Lancet 2,* 23, 1968.

3. W.E. Nance, *Nature 224,* 373, 1969.

4. D.T. Janerich, *Amer. J. Epidemiol. 99,* 1, 1974.

5. D.T. Janerich, *Amer. J. Epidemiol. 101, No. 1.,* 70, 1975.

6. B. MacMahon and S. Yen, *Lancet 1,* 31, 1971.

7. D.T. Janerich, *Teratology 8,* 253, 1973.

8. D.T. Janerich, *Lancet 1,* 569, 1974.

9. R.D. Lockhart, G.F. Hamilton, F.W. Fyfe, Anatomy of the Human Body, Lippincott, Philadelphia, pp. 697, 1959.

10. J.J. Holland and E.D. Kiehn, *Science 167,* 202, 1970.

11. L. Hoyle, *in* Virology Monographs, S. Gard, C. Hallauer and K.F. Meyer (Eds.) Springer-Verlag, New York, pp. 375, 1968.

DISCUSSION

GODFREY P. OAKLEY: Dr. Laurence, are there data on the debatable question of having more than one person performing ultrasound scan and amniocentesis in a community?

K. MICHAEL LAURENCE: A large medical research council investigation going on now in Great Britain indicates that amniocentesis not done by an experienced person and not preceded by an ultrasound scan runs a much higher risk of ending in miscarriage.

Performing amniocentesis without ultrasound scan is running a considerable risk. Blood in the amniotic fluid − apart from everything else − may well cause misinterpretations.

H. LAWRENCE VALLET (Birth Defects Institute, Albany, New York): The preconditioning concept may have a parallel in adult onset or acquired obesity. The lymphocytes of these patients have an increased number of receptor sites for insulin; they also develop diabetes mellitus. When they diet, the number of receptor sites and lymphocytes decreases markedly and the diabetes mellitus is ameliorated.

I'm not sure we can assume HCG in the feedback mechanism has a marked effect in shutting off maternal LH early in pregnancy when, at the same time, fetal LH appears and seems to be a factor in its own sexual development, at from 8 to 14 weeks. How HCG could affect maternal LH and not fetal LH, when it is on both sides of the placenta, I don't know.

Dr. Janerich, in early radioimmunoassays it was difficult to differentiate human prolactin, HCS and HGH immunologically. Is it not possible that we've been looking at the biological effect on growth of HCG rather than a sexual effect?

HERBERT JACOBSON (Albany Medical College, Albany, New York): Are you suggesting that the effect of HCG would be a reflection of inadequate amounts?

DR. VALLET: No, but perhaps an altered hormone. For example, the beta subunit of HCG and the sequencing of the subunit which may make it similar biologically to, let us say HCS, may be missing or perhaps so changed by a previous viral infection that the specific biological action of that subunit of HCG is different.

DR. JANERICH: We postulated a growth hormone effect when we noted a relationship between stature and the risk of ASB recurrence. Ossen and Byrd's data suggest an association between the responsible hormone and growth hormone.

JONATHAN LANMAN: Dr. Janerich, in your postulate of a ten year interval between an influenza epidemic — notably the 1918 epidemic — and an epidemic of anencephaly, what happened during that interval? Why weren't there abnormal babies sooner? Was the current group of pubertal girls so affected that, years later, they had abnormal pregnancies? If so, the age distribution of the women with anencephalic babies should indicate this.

DR. JANERICH: I think that puberty is probably the most critical time for a severe preconditioning environmental insult. Since there appears to be no age threshold and the distribution tails off somewhat later, a broad range of women were at risk. Although the relative risk would vary by age, it reaches an apex with puberty. By superimposing the bimodal age-specific risk curve on the unimodal age-specific fertility curve, one sees the epidemic curves in the composite. Thus, the reason for the ten year delay is not because a single cohort reached its top reproduction. The interval, furthermore, may not be identical because we have superimposed a series of epidemic waves, including the huge epidemic of the 1930's.

STEVEN H. LAMM (National Institutes of Health, Bethesda, Maryland): The implications that the period of puberty would be the period of great sensitivity suggest that the greatest incidence is most marked in early parity. Dr. Naggan's data indicated that incidences were far greater in the period of high parity. Is this not so in your area?

DR. JANERICH: Not only in our area, but the international data suggest that the impact of risks on first births is highest where the overall incidence is highest.

DR. BLOOM: Dr. Janerich, is there direct evidence that influenza virus invades the pituitary?

DR. JANERICH: No, except that it reproduces in the mucosal cells lining the upper respiratory system.

DR. JACOBSON: The problem may be even more complicated than it looks. In addition to the five age periods which Dr. Janerich mentioned as potentially susceptible to this insult, other factors within the cohort may be

114

preconditioned. We hope to associate the preconditioning with certain cohorts and then follow their subsequent course.

ROBERT J. DESNICK: Dr. Janerich and Dr. Jacobson's hypothesis reminds me of Ashwell and Morell's attempt to identify some of the specific concepts of susceptibility to teratogenic procedures with animal studies of the mode of inheritance. They indicate multigenic control, indisputably, although the linkage relationships, gene products and the thresholds are unknown. If you could demonstrate the truth or substantiate the theory, would it eliminate the multifactorial hypothesis?

DR. JANERICH: No. The new hypothesis extends the multifactorial concept of etiology.

D.J. McCALLION (McMaster Medical Center, Hamilton, Ontario): Without adjusting for parity, the value is doubtful in the cohort approach. In this regard, I see no cohort effect in the Boston data.

THEODORE KRUSHNICK (New Jersey Medical School, Berkley Heights, New Jersey): Will Dr. Janerich comment on the possibility of HLA specificity in producing malformations?

DR. JANERICH: We have no information on the hypothesis.

DR. DESNICK: We know that the enzymes affecting glycoproteins and glycolipids are changed in virus-transformed cells — these presumably are components of receptors on the cell membrane. If the mother undergoes a preconditioning event or virus infection transmissible to the fetus, and if neural tube closure is governed by receptor interactions, including altered receptors, then an endocrinologic basis is not necessary to explain the failure of neural tube closures. One might test the proposal by measuring reverse transcriptase activity or other viral-induced proteins in appropriate fetal tissue.

SECTION III

PROBLEMS OF OUTCOME OF PREGNANCY: SOME CLUES FROM THE EPIDEMIOLOGIC SIMILARITIES AND DIFFERENCES*

Irvin Emanuel

Many diseases are related to socioeconomic factors. Tables 1 and 2 list conditions which contribute to excessive mortality of lower and higher occupational groups in England and Wales respectively.[1] The higher risk for several problems of pregnancy outcome — early and late fetal mortality, neonatal and postneonatal mortality, prematurity and anencephaly and spina bifida (ASB) — in the lower economic classes is also noteworthy.[2-11] The factors responsible for the greater abundance of disease among the poor are still only poorly understood; the reasons summoned usually relate to extrinsic factors — specific toxic substances, deficiencies or infectious agents. This choice is to be expected, perhaps, since prevention is easier if specific extrinsic factors can be found, rather than searching for possible intrinsic factors. Indeed, some of the best etiologic models pertain to specific extrinsic agents. On the other hand, there is considerable evidence that specific agents are far from the whole answer and that host factors may often be of considerable importance.

Most problems of pregnancy outcome are probably multifactorial. The search for causal factors for the non-genetic component usually relates to the mother's external environment. Since the mother is the immediate environment of the developing embryo and fetus, it is important to unravel the maternal host factors and to place in perspective the roles of internal and external environment.

The dramatic examples of rubella and thalidomide as human teratogens have perhaps led to an overemphasis on other infectious agents and drugs as possible etiologic factors in congenital malformations. A few other infectious and chemical agents have been implicated in birth defects. Further reinforcement comes from several decades of experimental teratology which has shown the possibility of producing almost any malformation in some strain of animal with some chemical. Although several studies have revealed that pregnant

---

*Supported in part by Public Health Service Grant 2-PO1 HD02274-09 from the National Institute of Child Health and Human Development.

TABLE 1

Causes of Death Inversely Related to Social Class for Men and Married
Women, 15-64 Years, 1959-1963, England and Wales

Tuberculosis	Seizure Disorders
Syphilis	Otitis Media & Mastoiditis
All Cancers	Rheumatic Fever
Tongue Cancer**	Rheumatic Heart Disease
Mouth Cancer**	Coronary Disease, Angina**
Pharyngeal Cancer (except oral	Chronic Endocarditis (non-rheum.)
mesopharynx)	Acute & Subacute Endocarditis**
Esophageal Cancer	Other Myocardial Degeneration
Stomach Cancer	General Arteriosclerosis
Colonic Cancer**	Aortic Aneurysm, non-luetic**
Rectal Cancer	Disease of Veins
Liver Cancer (2º & unspec.)*	Hypertension
Nasal Cancer	Influenza & Pneumonia
Laryngeal Cancer	Other Chron. Interstitial Pneumonia*
Lung Cancer	Bronchitis
Cervical Cancer**	Pneumoconiosis, occupational *
Uterine Cancer (except Cx & Corpus)**	Bronchiectasis
O & U Female Genital Cancer**	Peptic Ulcer
Benign Ovarian Tumors**	Diarrheal Diseases
O & U Male Genital Cancer*	Appendicitis
Kidney Cancer	Abdominal Hernia
Bladder Cancer	Intestinal Obstruction
Skin Cancer n.e.c.**	Cholecystitis**
Bone Cancer	Nephritis & Nephrosis
Benign NS Tumors	Rheumatoid Arthritis
Neoplasm of NS, Unspec.*	Osteoarthritis**
Thyroid Cancer**	Motor Accidents*
Thyrotoxicosis	Home Accidents*
Diabetes Mellitus**	Other Accidents*
Anemias (P.A. & other hyperchromic)	Suicide*
Psychoses*	Complications of Pregnancy and
Stroke	Childbirth**
Parkinsonism	

*Men only.
**Women only.
No asterisk denotes both men and women.
Source: Reference No. 1.

TABLE 2

Causes of Death Directly Related to Social Class for Men and Married
Women, 15—64 years, 1959-1963, England and Wales

Infectious Hepatitis**

Testicular Cancer*

Malignant Melanoma*

Brain Cancer**

Hodgkins Disease**

Other Lymphomas**

Aortic Aneurysm, non-luetic*

Cholecystitis*

*Men only

**Women only.

No asterisk denotes both men and women.

Source: Reference No. 1.

women commonly take a variety of medicines, few additional drugs have been implicated as human teratogens,[12–21] and there is little evidence that congenital malformations have increased concomitantly with the recent widespread proliferation of chemicals and drugs. Additionally, congenital malformations existed long before this explosive proliferation and exist today in communities minimally influenced by it. I do not wish to minimize the potential importance of chemical teratogenesis in humans, and I hope that monitoring will prevent another disaster like thalidomide and will help to clarify the role drugs and chemicals play in abnormal pregnancy outcome, but it seems fairly clear that the human embryo and fetus are relatively less susceptible to teratogenic response than some other animals. One may speculate about the reasons: the greater degree of inbreeding in many strains of laboratory animals than in man, for example; the different metabolism of drugs in man compared to other mammals; and the possible protective effect of the larger size and longer gestational period of the human fetus. A one-day exposure to a drug, for instance, affects about 1/12 of the embryonic period of a mouse but only about 1/50 of the comparable period in the human. On the other hand, malformations of the human fetus might possibly result from massive doses of certain drugs given during a major part of the embryonic period, which fortunately are rarely administered to pregnant women in that fashion.

There is a commonly held view that no matter what the malformation, extrinsic chemicals are the likely etiology. But each human malformation has its own unique epidemiologic pattern. It is unlikely that the different patterns can be explained primarily by different distributions of different environmental teratogens. Other types of etiologic factors are sometimes suggested by the epidemiologic findings. Down's syndrome, for example, demonstrates one overpowering epidemiologic finding whenever and in whatever population it has been studied: the relationship to maternal age. While there is some evidence that radiation may be a factor,[22–24] clearly it cannot totally explain the maternal age relationship. Nor does it appear likely that an infectious agent is a major factor, since immunity levels increase rather than decrease with age. The invariable maternal age relationship seems to indicate that the major etiologic factor is probably intrinsic to the mother rather than extrinsic, possibly involving physiological aging.[25]

The story of cleft lip with or without cleft palate is somewhat different. Epidemiologic relationships have been variable and not very impressive, with the exception of ethnic group differences. Much of the variability is probably related to the etiologic variability of the malformation itself. Cleft lip is a feature in several dozen syndromes of different etiologies,[26] yet few epidemiologic studies have dealt with the heterogeneity. We made a careful effort in our King County population study[27] to obtain accurate clinical diagnoses and analyzed cases of isolated clefts separately from those with other associated malformations. No significant maternal age, birth order, seasonal, secular change or time-space clustering effects were found in the isolated cleft series. If confirmed, these negative findings suggest that genetic rather than environmental factors are probably of prime importance in this malformation. The high concordance rate in identical twins further supports this view, as do data compatible with polygenic inheritance,[28-31] although the major importance of polygenic factors does not rule out a minor role of non-genetic factors.

In contrast to the rather simple epidemiologies of Down's syndrome and cleft lip, a complex and fascinating epidemiologic pattern has emerged for anencephaly and spina bifida (ASB). Apparently, the complexity cannot be simply explained on the basis of a single factor or teratogen. We have proposed that the complex epidemiologic pattern in ASB indicates a complex "web of causation" involving three categories of etiologic factors: genetic, "immediate" and "intergenerational".[32] The importance of genetic factors relates to the sibling recurrence risk, the risk in other relatives and probably also ethnic group differences.[28-34] The importance of "immediate" factors — those which relate to the pregnancy in question — is supported by the frequent finding of a maternal age effect[6,7,33] and of seasonality,[35] and the usual finding of a parity effect, usually a primogeniture effect.[6,7] Intergenerational factors relate to the period of growth and development of the mothers. The notion that events during the early lives of mothers were related to the production of neural tube defects has been with us for a long time, but has been largely ignored in the quest for extrinsic immediate factors. In 1958, the first investigators to document a social class effect in neural tube defects suggested such a possibility, based on their additional finding of an inverse relationship between maternal stature and rates of anencephaly.[36] Members of the same Aberdeen group have subsequently reiterated the probable importance of childhood maternal growth disturbance as a causal factor in ASB.[37-39] Other workers also suggested that childhood events might later play a role in ASB.[2,33,40-43] Recently, we have proposed that the epidemiologic pattern of socioeconomic gradient, inverse relationship of ASB rates to maternal stature, the timing of the epidemic waves, the cohort effect, geographic variation and changes with migration is consistent with a growth disturbance during childhood which later places women at high risk for producing babies with ASB and which is a major — perhaps *the* major — environmental influence.[32] A growth disturbance which results in the stunting of stature may also be expected to be related to a concomitant growth disturbance of internal organs, including the reproductive and/or endocrine systems, thereby suggesting possibilities for specific mechanisms for the production of the malformation. Other recent work offers further support for an intergenerational concept. Carter and Evans[44] found that in families with an ASB proband the proportion of affected children was unrelated to the social class of the father but was

123

significantly related to the social class of the maternal grandfather. Baird,[39] analyzing data from Aberdeen and Scotland, found that for different maternal age, parity and social class groupings, the epidemic peaks of anencephaly were produced largely by births to women who themselves were born during periods of severe economic depression.

Other problems of reproductive outcome, such as low birth weight and perinatal mortality, have epidemiologic patterns very similar to those of the neural tube defects. Indeed, it has also been proposed by the Aberdeen group,[3–5,10,45] based on a considerable body of evidence, that these other problems of pregnancy outcome relate significantly to childhood deprivation and resultant growth disturbance of the mothers. The intergenerational concept may also provide insight into the causes of the leveling off of the decline in the infant and fetal mortality rates during the 1950's and 1960's, which so far has defied adequate explanation. Women growing up during the Great Depression were at the height of reproductive activity during that period.

While the evidence strongly indicates the major importance of intergenerational factors in the etiology of some of these problems, there seems little question that immediate factors are also important. For instance, in the United Kingdom the rate of stillbirths and early neonatal deaths due to unknown causes immediately plummeted after the inception of a government food priority program in 1940.[46] Famine during the Hunger Winter in the Netherlands[47,48] and more dramatically during the Siege of Leningrad[48,49] was related to decreased birth weight and, in addition, to markedly increased fetal mortality in Leningrad but not in the Netherlands. Several studies show a significant gradient in birth weight related to maternal weight gain.[50–52] But it is not clear whether the weight gain is influenced only by the quality and quantity of food intake or whether intrinsic maternal characteristics are also operating. There is conflicting evidence concerning the value of food supplementation in increasing birth weight.[48]

A number of studies, like that of Dr. Chase, are concerned with the influence of prenatal care on the outcome of pregnancy. It is appealing, of course, to contemplate the solution of major health problems by instituting categorical or even comprehensive medical care programs, although historically there is little justification for such optimism.[53–56] Quite clearly mortality rates of both infectious and non-infectious diseases have fallen dramatically during eras in which neither specific preventive nor therapeutic measures were available and mortality rates from various causes have risen during periods of increasingly proficient and available medical care.

With respect to problems of interest to this conference, there has been little detectable change in the decline of the infant mortality rate after the institution of the National Health Service in the United Kingdom. For industrial countries, the population per physician ratio, the population per obstetrician ratio and the population per pediatrician ratio unexpectedly significantly relate in a negative way to the infant mortality rate.[57] The population per nurse and population per nurse and midwife ratios are, interestingly, positively related to the infant mortality rate.[57] It is not clear what these statistical relationships mean but they offer little support for the importance of medical care as distributed by physicians in reducing infant mortality.

The data from individual countries (Table 3) suggest some interpretations as to which factors might be important in reducing infant mortality. There is perfect correspondence in the United Kingdom between improvement in the population per physician ratio and decline in infant mortality, while in the United States and Canada there is only fair correspondence. On the other hand, although Japan had almost no change in the physician ratio between 1958–1968, there was a 56% reduction in the infant mortality rate. Taiwan, Chile and New Zealand experienced deterioration of the population/physician ratio but, nevertheless, saw a substantial reduction in infant mortality. Thus, several countries with little or no change, or with a deterioration of the physician ratio, had marked improvement in infant mortality. It is unlikely that increased physician efficiency or improved medical technology and health care delivery were responsible for this sharply reduced infant mortality over rather short periods of time. Some of these countries, on the other hand, saw dramatic socioeconomic improvement during this period which, in some way, was doubtless important in the decline in infant mortality. Improvement in nutrition, housing, education and sanitation are the usual factors proposed as related to improved health, but the reasons for the relationship between improving socioeconomic conditions and improved health of the population are not at all well understood.

In the United States, there is a good relationship between the live birth per obstetrician ratio and infant (Fig. 1) and neonatal mortality rates (Fig. 2). On the other hand, there is no relationship between the live birth per obstetrician ratio and the rate of low birth weight (Fig. 3). In spite of a 31% improvement in the obstetrician ratio, low birth weight has been constant since 1963, with a suggestion of a new downward trend beginning in 1970. In fact, the low birth weight rate of white babies has been constant since 1950, while the rate in non-white babies has increased about 30%.[62]

In one of the earliest studies of the possible relationship between prenatal care and outcome of pregnancy, Eastman[63] found an inverse relationship between the number of prenatal visits and rate of low birth weight. He doubted, however, that prenatal care was the crucial factor but suggested that more general living habits were important. Other studies which do not

125

TABLE 3

Relationship Between Infant Mortality and the Population Per Physician Ratio

| Country | Percent Change in Comparative Years | | |
	Infant Mortality	Population Per Physician Ratio	Years
England & Wales	−19	−19	1968-1958
Canada	−30	−20	1968-1958
U.S.A.	−30	−16	1973-1963
Japan	−56	− 3	1968-1958
New Zealand	−20	+ 2	1968-1958
Chile	−23	+ 7	1968-1959
Taiwan	−38	+50	1968-1959

Source of data: References 58−61.

TABLE 4

Relationship Between Prenatal Care and Anencephaly and
Spina Bifida in Taiwan

| Trimester Prenatal Care Began | Normal Babies | | Anencephaly and Spina Bifida | |
	No.	%	No.	%
1st	262	30.5	7	17.5
2nd	319	37.2	14	35.0
3rd	195	22.7	10	25.0
No Care	82	9.6	9	22.5

x^2 for progression = 7.1, d.f = 1, $P < 0.01$.

Source: Reference No. 16.

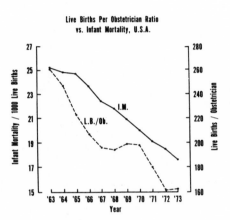

Fig. 1.   Live births per obstetrician ratio and infant mortality, U.S.A., 1963-1973. Source of data: References 59—61.

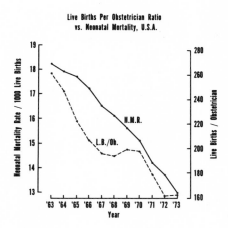

Fig. 2.   Live births per obstetrician ratio and neonatal mortality, U.S.A., 1963-1973. Source of data: References 59–61.

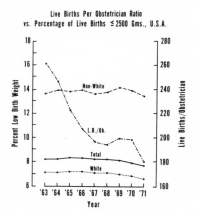

Fig. 3.   Live births per obstetrician ratio and low birth weight rate, U.S.A., 1963-1971. Source of data: References 59-61.

account for other important demographic characteristics also show a similar and striking relationship between prenatal care and pregnancy outcome.[64] Studies which attempt to control various relevant factors, on the other hand, seem to yield somewhat different results. For instance, Schwartz and Vinyard[65] and Terris and Glasser,[66] using life table techniques which accounted for relevant demographic variables, found significant relationships between time of beginning prenatal care and prematurity in some categories of babies but concluded that even if there is a causal relationship, the absence of prenatal care can only account for a minor portion of the problem. Other studies have not shown a significant relationship between the number of prenatal visits and low birth weight[67,68] and perinatal mortality.[69] On the other hand, a two-way simultaneous relationship of both socioeconomic variables and prenatal care with pregnancy outcome has been reported.[70,71]

Two studies[8,9] used an index of adequacy of care which required delivery on the private service as a criterion for adequacy. Whether the private service in itself denotes adequate care has not been demonstrated.[71,72] However, there is evidence that women delivering on the private service are different from those delivering on the ward service in important ways unrelated to prenatal care. For instance, Naggan and MacMahon[73] found that rates of ASB in ward patients were almost twice those of private patients. Furthermore, in Taiwan,[16] the occurrence of these malformations was related to time of onset of prenatal care (Table 4). Compared to controls, only about half the percentage of case mothers began prenatal care in the first trimester, while more than twice the percentage of case mothers received no prenatal care. Since these malformations are established before most women seek antenatal care, it does not seem likely that the relationship to prenatal care is a causal one. Rather it appears that, whatever else it may be, the prenatal care pattern is a social and/or behavioral indicator.

In fact, the prime independent variables in studies of prenatal care have been the number of visits and time of pregnancy the visits commenced. These variables certainly relate to the behavior of the mothers but there is no good evidence that they relate to the activities of the physicians which are crucial in evaluating the efficacy of prenatal care. The process of prenatal care has not been adequately analyzed with respect to the treatment aspects.[72] Therefore, the possible relationship between prenatal care and pregnancy outcome is still a moot point but one worthy of clarification. There does seem to be such a thing as effective prenatal care related, for instance, to the ever increasing survival of babies of diabetic mothers.[74] At the same time there are suggestions that certain common practices in prenatal care may be detrimental. For example, it has been suggested that less severe dietary restriction during pregnancy may reduce the low birth weight rate and infant mortality rate, since maternal weight gain is directly related to birth weight.[50,52,75] If some studies fail to show a relationship between prenatal care and outcome, it may be that the benefits to a small number of women with special problems may be counterbalanced by common practices to the many which are not beneficial.

While there are many compelling reasons for comprehensive prenatal care and drug and chemical monitoring, such measures even at best probably will deal with only a small portion of the overall problem. On the other hand, each problem of pregnancy outcome has its own unique epidemiologic pattern, which, in turn, suggests unique patterns of causal factors. At the same time, some problems share common epidemiologic features or differ only slightly in specific features, which suggests that they may also share some common etiologic factors. It would seem unlikely, for instance, that the similar epidemiologic patterns would relate primarily to a chemical teratogen in ASB but to other causes in low birth weight and fetal mortality. Similarly, there is no particular reason to believe that the mechanism producing identical twin discordance in one malformation is fundamentally different from that in others.

Furthermore, since there is substantial epidemiologic evidence which suggests that maternal host factors relating to the mother's own childhood are important in some problems of pregnancy outcome, particularly some of the problems which are related to poverty, the search for environmental factors should not be restricted to extrinsic toxic or infectious agents relating directly to the pregnancy in question.

Finally, the common problems of pregnancy outcome are found in all contemporary human groups so far studied, living under an almost infinite variety of social, cultural and physical conditions. Therefore, it seems reasonable that they relate primarily to fundamental biosocial processes universally present in all human groups.

ACKNOWLEDGMENTS

Thanks are due to Drs. Richard Ward, E. Russell Alexander, Gerald LaVeck and Ms. Janet Daling for their critical review.

REFERENCES

1. *Registrar General's Decennial Supp. 1961,* Occupational Mortality Tables, London, Her Majesty's Stationery Office, 1971.

2. I. Emanuel, *Postgrad. Med. 51,* 144, 1972.

3. D. Baird, *New Eng. J. Med. 246,* 561, 1952.

4. D. Baird and R. Illsley, *Proc. Roy. Soc. Med. 46,* 53, 1953.

5. D. Baird and A.M. Thomson, *in* Perinatal Problems. The Second Report of the 1958 British Perinatal Mortality Survey, N.R. Butler and E.D. Alberman (Eds.), Livingstone, Edinburgh, p. 211, 1969.

6. J. Fedrick, *Ann. Hum. Genet. 34,* 31, 1970.

7. Editorial Team and W.H. Schutt, *in* Perinatal Problems. The Second Report of the 1958 British Perinatal Mortality Survey, N.R. Butler and E.D. Alberman (Eds.), Livingstone, Edinburgh, p. 283, 1969.

8. D.M. Kessner, J. Singer, C.E. Kalk and E.F. Schlesinger, Infant Death: An Analysis by Maternal Risk and Health Care, Institute of Medicine, National Academy of Sciences, Washington, D.C., 1973.

9. H.C. Chase (Ed.), *Am. J. Pub. Health 63 (Suppl.),* 1-56, 1973.

10. J.C. Kincaid, *Brit. Med. J. 1,* 1057, 1965.

11. C. Daly, J.A. Heady, J.N. Morris, *Lancet 1,* 445, 1955.

12. T.H. Shepard, Catalog of Teratogenic Agents, Johns Hopkins University Press, Baltimore and London, 1973.

13. J.G. Wilson, *Teratology 7,* 3, 1973.

14. M.M. Nelson and J.O. Forfar, *Brit. Med. J. 1,* 523, 1971.

15. I. Emanuel, *in* Methods for Detection of Environmental Agents Which Produce Congenital Defects: Proceedings of the Guadaloupe Conference Sponsored by l'Institute de la Vie, T.H. Shepard, J.R. Miller and M. Marois (Eds.), Amsterdam, North Holland Scientific Publishers (in press).

16. I. Emanuel, *in* Medicine in Chinese Culture: Comparative Studies, A. Kleinman, P. Kunstadter, E.R. Alexander and J.L. Gale (Eds.), Fogarty International Center, National Institutes of Health (in press).

17. A. Klemetti, L. Saxen, *Am. J. Pub. Health 57,* 2071, 1967.

18. J. Warkany, *Pediatrics 53, Pt. II, Suppl.,* 820, 1974.

19. J.J. Nora, A.H. Nora, R.J. Sommerville, R.M. Hill and D.G. McNamara, *J. A. M.A. 202,* 1065, 1967.

20. I.D.G. Richards, *Brit. J. Prev. Soc. Med. 23,* 218, 1969.

21. I.D.G. Richards, *in* Drugs and Fetal Development, M.A. Klingberg, A. Abramovici and J. Chemke (Eds.), Plenum Publishing Corporation, New York, 441, 1972.

22. N. Wald, J.H. Turner and W. Borges, *Ann. New York Acad. Sci. 171,* 454, 1970.

23. E. Alberman, P.E. Polani, J.A. Fraser Roberts, C.C. Spicer, M. Elliott, E. Armstrong, R.K. Dhadial, *Ann. Hum. Genet. (London) 36,* 185, 1972.

24. E. Alberman, P.E. Polani, J.A. Fraser Roberts, C.C. Spicer, M. Elliott, E. Armstrong, *Ann. Hum. Genet. (London) 36,* 195,1972.

25. I. Emanuel, L.E. Sever, S. Milham, Jr. and H.C. Thuline, *Lancet 2,* 361, 1972.

26. R.J. Gorlin, J.J. Pindborg and M.M. Cohen, Jr., Syndromes of the Head and Neck, McGraw-Hill, Second Edition, New York, 1975.

27. I. Emanuel, B.H. Culver, J.D. Erickson, B. Guthrie and D. Schuldberg, *Teratology 7,* 271, 1973.

28. C.O. Carter, *in* Second International Conference on Congenital Malformations, International Medical Congress, Ltd., New York, p. 306, 1964.

29. C.O. Carter, *Prog. Med. Genet. 4,* 59, 1965.

30. C.O. Carter, *in* Congenital Malformations, F.C. Fraser, V.A. McKusick and R. Robinson (Eds.), Excerpta Medica, Amsterdam-New York, p.227,1970.

31. D.W. Smith and J.M. Aase, *J. Pediatr. 76,* 653, 1970.

32. I. Emanuel and L.E. Sever, *Teratology 8,* 325, 1973.

33. C.O. Carter, *J. Biosoc. Sci. 1,* 71, 1969.

34. W.E. Nance, *Nature, 224,* 373, 1969.

35. I. Leck and R.G. Record, *Brit. J. Prev. Soc. Med. 20,* 67, 1966.

36. W.J.R. Anderson, D. Baird and A.M. Thomson, *Lancet 1,* 1304, 1958.

37. D. Baird, *J. Pediatr. 65,* 909, 1964.

38. D. Baird, *in* Horizons in Perinatal Research, N. Kretchmer and E.G. Hasselmeyer (Eds.), Wiley, New York, p. 10, 1974.

39. D. Baird, *J. Biosoc. Sci. 6,* 113, 1974.

40. M.S.T. Hobbs, *Brit. J. Prev. Soc. Med. 23,* 174, 1969.

41. D.T. Janerich, *Am. J. Epid. 96,* 319, 1972.

42. D.T. Janerich, *Am. J. Epid. 99,* 1, 1974.

43. D.T. Janerich, *in* Congenital Defects, D.T. Janerich, R.G. Skalko and I.H. Porter (Eds.), Academic Press, New York, p. 73, 1974.

44. C.O. Carter and K. Evans, *J. Med. Genet. 10,* 209, 1973.

45. R. Illsley, *in* Childbearing: Its Social and Psychological Aspects, S.A. Richardson and A.F. Guttmacher (Eds.), Williams & Wilkins Company, Baltimore, p. 75, 1967.

46. E.H.L. Duncan, D. Baird and A.M. Thomson, *J. Obst. Gyn. Brit. Emp. 59,* 183, 1952.

47. C.A. Smith, *J. Pediatr. 30,* 229, 1947.

48. L. Bergner and M. Susser, *Pediatrics 46,* 946, 1970.

49. A.N. Antonov, *J. Pediatr. 30,* 250, 1947.

50. N.J. Eastman and E. Jackson, *Obst. & Gyn. 23,* 1003, 1968.

51. J.E. Singer, M. Westphal and K. Niswander, *Obst. & Gyn. 31,* 417, 1968.

52. K.R. Niswander, J. Singer, M. Westphal and W. Weiss, *Obst. & Gyn. 33,* 482, 1969.

53. W. Winkelstein and F.E. French, *Calif. Med. 113,* 7, 1970.

54. E. Kass, *J. Infect. Dis. 123,* 110, 1971.

55. C.L. Marshall, R.E. Brown and C.D. Goodrich, *Clin. Pediatr. 10,* 363, 1971.

56. R.A. Stallones, *W.H.O. Chron. 26,* 294, 1972.

57. M.W. Hinds, *New Eng. J. Med. 291,* 741, 1974.

58. World Health Statistics Annual. 1960 Through 1970, W.H.O., Geneva.

59. Vital Statistics of the United States, Vol. 1, Natl. Ctr. for Health Stat., U.S. Dept. H.E.W., Washington, D.C., 1963-1968.

60. Monthly Vital Statistics Reports, Vol. 22-23, Natl. Ctr. for Health Stat.,

U.S. Dept. H.E.W., Washington, D.C., 1974.

61. Am. Med. Assoc. Ctr. for Health Services Research & Development, Distribution of Physicians in the U.S., Chicago, 1963-1973.

62. H.C. Chase and M.E. Byrnes, *Am. J. Pub. Health 60,* 1967, 1970.

63. N.J. Eastman, *Am. Practit. 1,* 343, 1947.

64. E. Oppenheimer, *Am. J. Pub. Health 51,* 208, 1961.

65. S. Schwartz and J.H. Vinyard, *Pub. Health Rep. 80,* 237, 1965.

66. M. Terris and M. Glasser, *Am. J. Pub. Health 64,* 869, 1974.

67. C.M.Drillien, *J. Obst. Gyn. Brit. Emp. 64,* 161, 1957.

68. M. Terris and E.M. Gold, *Am. J. Obst. Gyn. 103,* 358, 1969.

69. S.H. Kane, *Obst. & Gyn. 24,* 66, 1964.

70. B. Nold, R.A. Stallones and W. E. Reynolds, *Am. J. Epid. 83,* 481, 1966.

71. I. Rosenwaike, *Amer. J. Publ. Hlth. 62,* 186, 1972.

72. D. Rush, *Am. J. Dis. Child. 127,* 914, 1974.

73. L. Naggan and B. MacMahon, *New Eng. J. Med. 277,*1119, 1967.

74. N.L. Essex, D.A. Pyke, P.J. Watkins, J.M. Brudenell and H.R. Gamsu, *Brit. Med. J. 4,* 89, 1973.

75. K.R. Niswander, *Postgrad. Med. 48,* 123, 1970.

THE EFFECTS OF A LIBERALIZED ABORTION LAW ON PREGNANCY OUTCOME

Jonathan T. Lanman
Schuyler G. Kohl

A liberalized abortion law became effective in New York State on July 1, 1970. Before that date, elective abortion was permitted only for life-threatening indications in the mother at any time during pregnancy. After that date, the law permitted abortion up to the 24th week of pregnancy on agreement between the patient and her physician and a later time in pregnancy for life-threatening indications in the mother. When the new law became effective, striking changes occurred in both the obstetrical and pediatric services of a group of six Brooklyn, New York hospitals,[1] on comparing a period of 3½ years before the new law became effective (Period A: 1967– June, 1970) with one year after (Period B: July, 1970–June, 1971). During Period B extensive use of the right to abortion was made. We wondered whether the observed changes represented an initial surge which would abate with time or whether they would continue. Data now available for an additional year and a half (Period C: July, 1971–December 1972) show that most have continued.

Elective abortions in a predominantly non-white ward population at Kings County State University Hospital (KCH-SUH) rose from a negligible rate of 0.9 per 100 deliveries in Period A to a rate of 104/100 deliveries in Period B, and still further to a rate of 128/100 deliveries in Period C (Fig. 1). The rise affected all parity groups. Deliveries rose by 13% in Period B and fell by 14% in Period C. Spontaneous abortions, which occurred at a rate of 38 per 100 deliveries in Period A, fell to 27 per 100 in Period B and still further to 21 per 100 in Period C.

The rate of delivery of immature infants fell significantly in the non-white ward population of KCH-SUH from a rate of 20 per 1000 deliveries in Period A, to 9 in Period B and to 12 in Period C. Other patient groups at either KCH-SUH or its five affiliated Brooklyn hospitals (ABH) did not show similarly significant changes.

The rate at which unwanted infants were abandoned by their mothers

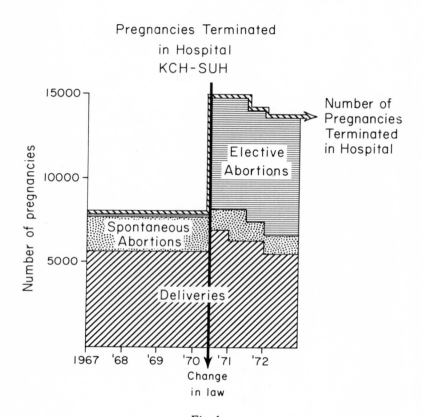

Fig. 1.

after delivery at KCH-SUH was lowered by 56% in Period B as compared with Period A. Unfortunately, because of failure to maintain records of in'fant placements in Period C, no additional data are available.

Among patients in five hospitals affiliated with KCH-SUH, in which there was a predominance of white private patients, changes were usually similar to those at KCH-SUH but less striking. The sharp rise in elective abortions from 1.0/100 deliveries in Period A to 34/100 deliveries in Period B was maintained at 32/100 deliveries in Period C but when white private patients were taken separately, the use of abortion declines more sharply in Period C. The number of deliveries followed a trend similar to that seen at KCH-SUH, with a more modest rise in Period B (+6%) and fall in Period C (-11%). However, spontaneous abortions, which fell slightly from 13 per 100 deliveries in Period A to 10 per 100 deliveries in Period B, failed to sustain the fall in Period C and instead returned to a level of 13 per 100 deliveries. The rates are far below those for spontaneous abortions among the predominantly non-white ward population of KCH-SUH.

These observations indicate that most of the changes occurring in the first year after the new abortion law became effective have continued in the following 18 months. The large number of elective abortions performed in hospitals after the change in the law, with no decrease of corresponding size in the number of deliveries, raises the question as to what happened previous to the change in that group seeking legal elective abortion. Examination of the various possibilities[1] leaves only one tenable explanation: that abortions were performed illegally before the change in the law about as frequently as they were legally after the change. We believe that the reduction in "spontaneous" abortions which occurred and has been sustained at KCH-SUH after the change in the law represented a decrease in women coming to the hospital for completion of an illegal abortion begun outside the hospital. We also believe that the reduction in the rate at which immature infants (of birth weight 500–999 gms) were delivered had a similar explanation.

Extensive use of the right to abortion continued to be made by all groups during Period C but the demand for abortion among the non-white private patients and continued to rise over the usage in Period B, as contrasted with a moderate fall among the white private patients. The contrast suggests a continuing and still unfilled need for contraceptive services and education among the economically deprived non-white population of Brooklyn.

REFERENCES

1. J.T. Lanman, S.G. Kohl and J.H. Bedell, *Am. J. Obstet. Gynec. 118,* 485, 1974.

THE RELATIONSHIP OF DEMOGRAPHIC FACTORS AND MEDICAL CARE TO ADVERSE PREGNANCY OUTCOME

Helen C. Chase

The relationships of demographic factors and medical care to adverse pregnancy outcome are many and complexly interrelated. Their consideration requires the simultaneous study of risk factors, utilization of medical care and outcome as gauged by survival, low birth weight or other indicators. One such recent study was conducted by the Institute of Medicine, National Academy of Sciences, in cooperation with the New York City Department of Health, with a view toward planning for health services. The study examined the interrelationships for a group of 142,017 infants born in New York City in 1968.[1,2] The population of that city is not representative of the country as a whole but the study is worth considering as a prototype for other areas.

The data were based on live birth and linked infant death certificates on permanent file with the New York City Department of Health. For those who are unfamiliar with the birth certificate form, it contains a lengthy supplemental confidential medical report which requires a considerable amount of demographic and clinical information.[1] An earlier paper examined the reporting of information on birth certificates, as reported by other investigators, and concluded that for the purpose of establishing classes of relative risk, the information was adequately reported.[1]

The information on the certificates was not used in detail but to enable the categorization of infants into maternal risk groups: *i.e.,* no reported risk, sociodemographic risk only, medical-obstetric risk only, both sociodemographic and medical-obstetric risks. Among the sociodemographic risks were illegitimate birth, age of mother/total birth order combinations with unfavorable outcomes and limited education of the mother. The most basic of the characteristics is the education of the mother. It encompasses an accumulation of her experience since the age of 6 years and her educational level at the time of the infant's birth. It is closely correlated with the education of the father and, in a general way, is an indicator of socioeconomic level. Mother's age, infant's total birth order and legitimacy status, on the other hand, pertain to a particular delivery, as do the medical-obstetric risks.

TABLE 1

Infant Mortality Rates by Race-Nativity Group and Age at Death:
New York City, 1968 Live Birth Cohort

Race of child and nativity of mother	Live births	Deaths			Mortality Rate		
		Infant	Neonatal	Post-neonatal	Infant	Neonatal	Post-neonatal
		Number			Rate per 1,000 live births		
Total	142,017	3,115	2,368	747	21.9	16.7	5.3
White							
Native-born	60,896	923	741	182	15.2	12.2	3.0
Foreign-born	18,959	291	235	56	15.3	12.4	3.0
Puerto Rican	22,505	572	430	142	25.4	19.1	6.3
Negro							
Native-born	32,051	1,143	815	328	35.7	25.4	10.2
Foreign-born	4,405	118	97	21	26.8	22.0	4.8
Puerto Rican	1,126	33	24	9	29.3	21.3	8.0
Chinese							
Native-born	125	1	1	—	(8.0)	(8.0)	(0.0)
Foreign-born	1,116	17	14	3	15.2	12.5	2.7
Puerto Rican	16	—	—	—	*	*	*
Japanese							
Native-born	30	1	1	—	*	*	*
Foreign-born	230	5	4	1	(21.7)	(17.4)	(4.3)
Puerto Rican	5	—	—	—	*	*	*
All Others	553	11	6	5	(19.9)	(10.9)	(9.0)

* Rate not computed; based on less than 100 live births.
( ) Rate based on 100-999 live births.

The designation of risk because of limited education was defined to be 8 years or less, which, at best, reflects approximately an elementary school education. The maternal age/total birth order risk combinations were as follows:

All under 15 years of age
15–19 years; second pregnancy or higher
20–24 years; fourth pregnancy or higher
25–29 years: fifth pregnancy or higher
30–34 years; first pregnancy, sixth or higher
35–39 years; first pregnancy, fifth or higher
All 40 years or over.

Among the medical-obstetric risks were previous fetal or infant loss, previous Cesarean section, cephalo-pelvic disproportion, maternal illnesses or conditions such as diabetes, syphilis, tuberculosis or narcotic addiction. The complete classification and the frequencies of occurrence of the detailed conditions are documented in an earlier publication.[1]

Infant death (under 1 year of age) was used as an outcome indicator to allow for some outcome effect in the last 11 months of the first year of life when socioeconomic factors predominate. Other outcomes which were examined were birth weight, Apgar scores and congenital malformations but the latter two proved of questionable utility.

Study Group

Because the population of New York City is so cosmopolitan, the data for the study were presented for population groups of particular relevance to that city (Table 1). Based on this table, white women were analyzed in three groups: those born in the United States, those born in Puerto Rico and those born elsewhere (foreign born); the Negro group, as a separate group, is limited to those women born in the United States; and the residual group consisted of all other women (5.4 percent of the total).

Risks

For 45.5 percent of the infants, there was no indication of risk as defined in the study (Table 2). More than half of the infants (54.5 percent) were associated with one or more risks. Almost two-fifths (39.9 percent) of infants were at sociodemographic risk and 28.9 percent at medical obstetric risk, with an overlap of 14.3 percent of infants with both types of risks. The distribution of risks according to ethnic group varied widely; some reported risk was present for 37.7 percent of white infants born to native born mothers and 73.3 percent of Negro infants. There were multiple risks for some infants and because of the size of the group with overlap another arrangement of risks and

141

TABLE 2

Percentage Distribution of Live Births by Risk Categories and Ethnic Group:
New York City, 1968 Live Birth Cohort

Risk Category	Total	White		Puerto Rican	Negro native born	All others
		native born	foreign born			
Number of live births	142,017	60,896	18,959	22,505	32,051	7,606
				Percent		
Total	100.0	100.0	100.0	100.0	100.0	100.0
Infants with no risk	45.5	62.3	44.7	29.1	26.7	40.7
All infants at risk	54.5	37.7	55.3	70.9	73.3	59.3
Infants with sociodemographic risks	39.9	19.6	40.0	60.4	63.2	43.7
Age of mother/birth order	19.8	13.0	16.7	27.6	28.9	19.6
Education of mother	13.2	2.3	26.0	36.7	8.5	19.2
Illegitimacy	18.5	6.2	5.1	24.9	45.3	18.8
Infants with medical-obstetrical risks	28.9	25.7	29.2	32.4	31.8	31.8
Identifiable at first prenatal visit	24.3	21.6	25.0	27.3	26.2	26.9
Identifiable during pregnancy	4.2	3.1	3.3	4.7	6.3	4.3
Identifiable at labor	5.5	5.5	6.1	6.4	4.4	5.6

categories, shown in Table 3, was used for most of the study.

The component risk sub-groups are presented in Table 4 and arranged according to their sequence in relation to the mother. This arrangement was an attempt by consultant obstetricians and pediatricians to identify the earliest times at which some preventive or corrective action might theoretically be introduced. In this table, once a mother was counted at risk (*e.g.,* because of limited education), she was not counted at risk again. For this particular population, the results indicated that limited education (as defined) was more pronounced among foreign born mothers of white infants and Puerto Rican mothers than among white or Negro native born mothers. Risks associated with age of mother/total birth order or illegitimacy were more highly concentrated among the Negro group. The elements of the medical-obstetric risks suggested that mothers newly identified at first prenatal visit represented about 12 percent of all live births. The proportion was highest for white native born women because fewer were identified through the sociodemographic risk characteristics, while the reverse was true of Negroes, for example. The table provides food for thought for health planners who may be contemplating preventive measures.

Medical Care

The available elements which could be included as indicators of medical care were the time of first prenatal visit and number of prenatal visits (both broadly grouped), type of hospital and private versus general (ward) service (Table 5). These are not refined indicators of medical care and obviously can not be regarded as specific indicators of the quality of medical care. In combination, they describe a gradation of participation in the medical care system. In this New York City population, mothers whose first prenatal visit came in the first 11 completed weeks of pregnancy, and who had 9 or more prenatal visits and who were delivered on private service included only about one-fifth of the total group. The percent increased from 5.9 to 44.4 percent with increasing level of education.

Two predominant patterns of medical care were evident: one for foreign born and native born white mothers and the other for the Puerto Rican and Negro groups. More of the former tended to begin prenatal care earlier and to have more visits. White foreign born mothers tended to delay the first prenatal visit and to have fewer visits, on the average, than white native.born mothers. Virtually all of the infants were born in the hospitals but there was wide variation in the type of hospital service used. For example, 83.6 percent of white native born mothers and 71.4 percent of foreign born white mothers made use of private hospitals and private service in voluntary hospitals. Almost the converse was true for the Puerto Rican and Negro groups; 83.6

TABLE 3

Percentage Distribution of Live Births by Risk Category and Ethnic Group:
New York City, 1968 Live Birth Cohort

Risk Category	Total	White		Puerto Rican	Negro native born	All others
		native born	foreign born			
Number of live births	142,017	60,896	18,959	22,505	32,051	7,606
			Percent			
Total	100.0	100.0	100.0	100.0	100.0	100.0
Infants not at risk	45.5	62.3	44.7	29.1	26.7	40.7
Infants at risk:	54.5	37.7	55.3	70.9	73.3	59.3
With sociodemographic risk only	25.6	12.1	26.1	38.5	41.5	27.5
With medical-obstetric risk only	14.6	18.1	15.3	10.5	10.1	15.6
With sociodemographic and medical-obstetric risk	14.3	7.6	13.9	21.9	21.7	16.2

144

TABLE 4

Sequential and Cumulative Percentage Distributions of Live Births by Risk Category
and Ethnic Group: New York City, 1968 Live Birth Cohort

| Risk Category | Total | White | | | Negro native born | All others |
		native born	foreign born	Puerto Rican		
			Percent			
Total	100.0	100.0	100.01	100.0	100.0	100.0
Infants not at risk	45.5	62.3	44.7	29.1	26.7	40.7
Infants at risk:	54.5	37.7	55.3	70.9	73.3	59.3
Sociodemographic risk	39.9	19.6	40.0	60.4	63.2	43.7
Education of mother	13.2	2.3	26.0	36.7	8.5	19.2
Age of mother/total-birth order	15.4	12.3	11.4	14.0	25.0	13.7
Illegitimacy	11.3	5.0	2.7	9.7	29.7	10.8
Medical-obstetric risk identifiable	14.6	18.1	15.3	10.5	10.1	15.6
At first prenatal visit	12.0	15.0	12.8	8.1	8.1	13.1
During pregnancy	1.4	1.5	1.1	1.4	1.4	1.4
At labor	1.2	1.5	1.4	1.0	0.6	1.0
			Cumulative percent			
Infants at sociodemographic risk	39.9	19.6	40.0	60.4	63.2	43.7
Infants at medical-obstetric risk	14.6	18.1	15.3	10.5	10.1	15.6
Infants at risk:	54.5	37.7	55.3	70.9	73.3	59.3
Education of mother	13.2	2.3	26.0	36.7	8.5	19.2
Age of mother/total-birth order	28.6	14.6	37.3	50.7	33.5	32.9
Illegitimacy	39.9	19.6	40.0	60.4	63.2	43.7
At first prenatal visit	51.9	34.7	52.8	68.5	71.3	56.8
During pregnancy	53.3	36.2	53.9	69.9	72.7	58.3
At labor	54.5	37.7	55.3	70.9	73.3	59.3

TABLE 5

Percentage Distribution of Live Births by Characteristics of Medical Care
and Ethnic Group: New York City, 1968 Live Birth Cohort

Characteristics of medical care	Total	White			Negro native born	All others
		native born	foreign born	Puerto Rican		
Number of live births	142,017	60,869	18,959	22,505	32,051	7,606
			Percent			
Prenatal care – Total	100.0	100.0	100.0	100.0	100.0	100.0
With prenatal care	91.1	94.7	94.8	87.4	84.6	90.1
Early care (less than 12 weeks)	33.3	52.0	39.9	12.0	11.2	23.3
Mid care (12–27 weeks)	44.7	35.6	44.8	57.0	51.7	51.7
Late care (28 weeks or later)	13.0	7.1	10.1	18.4	21.7	15.1
No prenatal care	3.3	1.5	1.7	5.3	6.4	3.5
Not stated	5.6	3.7	3.5	7.3	9.0	6.4
Number of prenatal visits – Total	100.0	100.0	100.0	100.0	100.0	100.0
9 or more visits	44.2	57.6	51.9	30.0	25.3	40.2
5–8 visits	32.7	29.5	33.3	37.2	34.7	34.6
1–4 visits	13.3	7.1	9.4	19.4	23.2	14.2
No visits	3.3	1.5	1.7	5.3	6.4	3.5
Not stated	6.4	4.3	3.8	8.1	10.4	7.5
Type of hospital – Total	100.0	100.0	100.0	100.0	100.0	100.0
Proprietary	9.5	13.7	16.3	2.3	3.5	4.9
Voluntary	69.6	80.9	73.0	57.9	55.0	67.4
Municipal	19.9	4.0	10.4	39.5	40.7	26.2
Other and non-hospital	1.0	1.5	0.4	0.2	0.9	1.5
Type of service – Total	100.0	100.0	100.0	100.0	100.0	100.0
Private service	53.9	83.6	71.4	14.5	17.4	43.6
General service	45.1	16.1	28.2	83.7	81.0	55.1
Non-hospital	0.9	0.3	0.4	1.8	1.6	1.2
Type of hospital and service – Total	100.0	100.0	100.0	100.0	100.0	100.0
Proprietary, private service	9.5	13.7	16.7	2.3	3.5	4.9
Voluntary, private service	44.3	69.9	55.1	12.1	13.2	38.4
Voluntary, general service	25.0	10.8	17.8	45.3	41.2	28.6
Municipal, general service	19.2	3.8	10.1	38.3	39.1	25.3
Other and non-hospital	2.0	1.8	0.8	2.0	3.1	2.9

146

percent of Puerto Rican and 80.3 percent of Negro women used general service in voluntary hospitals and municipal hospitals.

Infant Mortality

The cohort infant mortality rate for the total group of 142,017 infants was 21.9 per 1,000 live births, ranging from 15.2 and 15.3 for infants born to white native born and white foreign born mothers to 25.4 for the Puerto Rican and 35.7 for the Negro groups (Table 6). The level of infant mortality in relation to education level of the mother, and all that may imply, declined from 27.7 for those with at most an elementary school education to 11.0 for those with 4 or more years of college.

The differential in infant mortality according to weight at birth was 17-fold between infants who weighed 2,500 grams or less at birth (140.5 per 1,000) compared to the heavier infants (8.4). The proportion of low birth weight infants was comparatively low for white infants of foreign born mothers (6.5 percent) and highest (15.7 percent) for Negro infants whose mothers were born in the United States. Low birth weight was also inversely associated with education of mother but to a lesser degree than with ethnic group.

With regard to risk, infant mortality varied more than 3-fold, from 11.9 per 1,000 among those infants with no reported risk, to 41.6 among those with both types of risk (Table 7). The same kind of differential was observed for each ethnic group according to risk although at different levels. This may be an appropriate point at which to call attention to the white foreign born group. Despite their limited education, these mothers had a relatively high level of participation in the medical care system, relatively few low birth weight infants and low infant mortality. The Negro group, with higher average educational level than the Puerto Rican or the foreign born white group, with participation in the medical care system equal to the Puerto Rican group, with a higher proportion of low birth weight infants (15.7 percent for the Negroes and 10.3 percent for the Puerto Ricans), had the highest infant mortality of any of the ethnic groups in each of the risk categories.

Overview

Table 8 illustrates an attempt to bring together the various elements of the study, namely risks, medical care and outcome. This table was a late derivative of the study and in some ways differs from the tables previously presented. First, it is limited to infants who were at or near "full term", which for this table is defined as those liveborn infants who reached 36—43 completed weeks of gestation (88 percent of live births). Secondly, the dichotomies of medical care were defined more liberally. The dividing points were put at those with 5 or more prenatal visits and those who began prenatal

147

TABLE 6

Infant Mortality Rates by Birth Weight, Ethnic Group and Education of Mother:
New York City, 1968 Live Birth Cohort

Birth weight and ethnic group	Total	Education of Mother					
		None or elemen-tary school	High school		College		Not stated
			1–3 years	4 years	1–3 years	4 years or more	
			Rate per 1,000 live births				
Total	21.9	27.7	28.5	19.4	15.2	11.0	31.0
White, native born	15.2	32.8	21.8	14.7	11.6	9.4	23.5
White, foreign born	15.3	15.9	16.3	15.2	16.7	14.0	13.0
White, Puerto Rican	25.4	26.0	25.4	19.4	(16.6)	(9.6	45.5
Negro, native born	35.7	50.7	37.41	31.9	24.0	(29.1)	46.0
All others	24.5	29.5	29.6	22.1	(25.6)	(10.9)	(30.0)
2,500 grams or less	140.5	163.7	139.7	138.9	(119.4)	(96.2)	(179.2)
White, native born	116.7	(183.1)	(120.6)	120.7	(93.9)	(85.8)	(176.8)
White, foreign born	149.6	(150.5)	(161.8)	(155.8)	*	(139.1)	*
White, Puerto Rican	152.4	(151.9)	(139.9)	(155.1)	*	*	(234.3)
Negro, native born	150.5	(186.5)	139.7	151.5	(137.3)	*	(171.0)
All others	(178.2	(163.3	(229.7	(157.5	*	*	*
2,501 grams or more	8.4	11.8	11.6	7.0	5.4	4.6	10.4
White, native born	6.1	15.51	9.4	5.8	4.8	3.7	8.6
White, foreign born	5.9	7.6	5.3	5.2	6.7	5.0	4.4
White, Puerto Rican	10.5	11.3	10.8	7.2	(12.2)	*	16.6
Negro, native born	13.5	19.7	16.0	11.1	5.7	(16.0)	13.2
All others	7.7	13.0	5.0	7.1	(4.6)	(5.2)	(12.2)

* Rate is not computed because it is based on less than 100 live births.

( ) Rate is based on 100–999 live births.

TABLE 7

Percentage Distribution and Infant Mortality Rates by Risk Category and Ethnic Group: New York City, 1968 Live Birth Cohort

Risk Category	Total		Total	White		Puerto Rican	Negro native born	Other
	Number	Percent		native born	foreign born			
					Number			
Live births*	141,534	. . .	. . .	60,741	18,920	22,431	31,951	7,491
				Rate per 1,000 live births				
Total	141,534	100.0	21.6	14.9	15.2	25.2	35.1	23.8
No risk	66,447	45.5	11.9	9.4	9.2	17.4	19.8	17.2
Sociodemographic risk only	36,154	25.5	24.4	16.6	13.0	23.0	33.6	25.7
Medical-obstetric risk only	20,634	14.6	27.3	24.1	26.0	28.1	41.5	20.4
Sociodemographic and medical-obstetric risks	20,299	14.3	41.6	35.9	26.6	38.0	53.7	40.7

*Excludes 483 of 142,017 live births for which ethnic group, risk category, type of medical service or birth weight was unknown.

149

TABLE 8

Infant Mortality Rates by Risk Category and Elements of Medical Care: New York City, 1968 Live Birth Cohort

(Gestation Intervals of 36–43 Weeks Only)

| Risk category | Live births (number) | Total | Private service | | | | General service and all others | | | |
| | | | Early, mid care* | | Late care, no care not specified* | | Early, mid care* | | Late care, no care not specified* | |
			5 visits or more	Less than 5 visits, no visits, not stated	5 visits or more	Less than 5 visits, no visits, not stated	5 visits or more	Less than 5 visits, no visits, not stated	5 visits or more	Less than 5 visits, no visits, not stated
						Number				
Live births	124,732	...	61,556	4,007	2,683	2,819	30,083	4,680	6,324	12,580
					Rate per 1,000 live births					
Total	...	9.9	6.7	9.0	11.2	11.4	10.5	15.4	11.1	20.7
At risk	59,310	6.4	5.4	5.3	9.0	8.8	6.6	12.2	8.0	14.5
At some risk	65,422	13.0	8.9	13.8	13.7	14.2	12.5	16.4	12.2	22.5
Not at sociodemographic risk	77,636	7.4	6.0	6.6	10.6	11.1	7.9	13.0	10.7	17.4
All at sociodemographic risk	47,096	13.9	9.9	15.3	(12.6)	(11.9)	12.7	16.6	11.3	22.0
Not at medical-obstetric risk	89,657	8.3	5.8	7.4	10.1	9.4	8.1	13.7	9.0	18.6
All at medical-obstetrical risk	35,075	13.8	9.2	13.7	(14.4)	(17.3)	15.6	19.1	16.4	25.7
At no risk	59,310	6.4	5.4	5.3	9.0	8.8	6.6	12.2	8.0	14.5
At sociodemographic risk only	30,347	12.0	8.3	(14.0)	(12.8)	(10.9)	9.6	14.5	9.6	20.5
At medical-obstetric risk only	18,326	10.5	7.9	(11.2)	(15.6)	(19.2)	11.5	(15.3)	(19.3)	(27.3)
At sociodemographic and medical-obstetric risk	16,749	17.4	12.3	(17.5)	(12.1)	(14.4)	18.0	20.5	15.2	25.2

( ) Rate is based on 100–999 live births.

* First prenatal visit in following gestation intervals: early care (less than 12 weeks); mid care (12–27 weeks); late care (28 weeks or more).

150

care in approximately the first two trimesters of pregnancy. The table also attempts to encompass the type of hospital service, start of prenatal care and number of prenatal visits, as they relate to the various risk categories. The table is recommended for more leisurely study. I would, however, like to call attention to a few points.

For mothers on private service, if no risk was reported, the higher number of prenatal visits apparently was not associated with lower infant mortality. Nevertheless, in the same "no risk" group, the delayed onset of prenatal care was associated with higher infant mortality irrespective of number of visits. Among mothers on general service, despite the lack of reported risks, mortality was particularly high among infants whose mothers had few or no prenatal visits. For mothers with some reported risk, the difference between number of visits appeared more important.

If, for the moment, one were to regard the first column under Private service (Early or mid care, 5 or more visits) as an indicator of better partici- pation in medical care and the last column under General service (Late or no prenatal care, less than 5 visits) as the least desirable situation, the differentials in infant mortality persist, irrespective of the risk categories. When the rates were adjusted for birth weight distributions for the several ethnic groups, the range of rates was reduced but the differences were not completely eliminated.

Congenital Malformations

In view of the focus of this Symposium, it would be unfortunate not to comment on congenital malformations. The Certificate of Live Births con- tains an item for the recording of congenital abnormalities. The reporting of such conditions varies with the observer's ability to detect a specified abnor- mality at time of birth, the severity of the malformation and the completeness and accuracy of recorded information on the vital records. Several studies have compared the recording of congenital malformations on birth certificates and hospital records.[3-5] Each has reported incomplete recording on birth certificates of congenital malformations as a whole. The minor abnormalities such as birth marks, occur rather frequently, are relatively less severe and are often overlooked when the birth certificate is completed. However, malfor- mations such as those of the central nervous system or musculo-skeletal system are less frequent, more severe and are more completely recorded.

In the present study, the question regarding malformations was left unanswered in less than 1 percent of the certificates and malformations were reported on 1.4 percent of the certificates. According to ethnic group, the proportion with reported malformations was lowest (1.2 percent) for white infants of native born mothers and increased for white infants of foreign born mothers (1.4 percent), those with Puerto Rican mothers (1.6 percent) and

Negro mothers (1.7 percent). For the original purposes of the study, this level of occurrence was not high enough to make congenital malformations a useful terminal indicator.

Closing Remarks

The data, as presented, are indicative of associations between risks, medical care and outcome. As with other epidemiological studies of a demographic nature, there is the danger of over-simplifying the observations into a cause-and-effect relationship. For example, the tendency to delay the first prenatal visit by white foreign born women is not necessarily due to unavailability of medical care in the community, for such is not the case in New York City with 7 medical schools and 76 hospitals with organized maternity services. Instead, it probably reflects cultural patterns brought by these mothers from their homelands. Such cultural patterns resulted in a degree of self-selection which remained unmeasured. In this study, neither the close availability of medical care nor cultural attitudes toward pregnancy and childbirth was measured. Furthermore, although infants were classified into those with no reported risk and three risk classes, one can not assume that this was a foolproof classification. Some elements of unstated or misstated sociodemographic risk may remain in those infants categorized as at medical-obstetric risk only and *vice versa.*

The data have certain advantages which should also be noted. They refer to a real population and to that population in its totality and thus avoid the bias which is sometimes found in data from single hospitals. The population was large enough to permit the comparison of several ethnic groups and to permit the simultaneous subclassification of a number of other characteristics. And, although at times one would have wished for more data or more accurate data, one would be hard pressed to start a study of this magnitude *de novo* and expect the degree of cooperation required to reproduce the information represented by this group of vital records. Nor could a single hospital hope to duplicate a comparable data set in a number of years.

This study was based on the universe of live births in a given year (1968) in New York City. It is not purported to be a probability sample of the population of the United States nor any other universe. Some general similarities may be found in other large American cities but direct transfer of the statistical results should be avoided. The subcategories shown were not randomly drawn but were often the result of self-selection and this is particularly true with regard to the medical care items.

However, while the results must be interpreted with caution, they are not invalid or useless. The data gave insights into the inter-relationships of a number of characteristics. The results suggested directions for remedial action (for example, earlier education in health matters — including nutrition and perhaps even family planning) since 35.6 percent of the mothers had not completed 12 years of education (approximately high school graduation). The study also suggested that education is needed regarding the value and sources of early and regular prenatal care since many of the mothers postponed seeking such care. Another important consideration was the availability and use of medical care for women who may be unable to purchase it through their own resources. The data also reinforced the impact of sociodemographic characteristics as well as clinical considerations for certain subgroups of the population.

As far as I know, this study is the first time that this approach has been used with data of this kind. Since the generality of the results may be limited, it is important that the study be repeated elsewhere. It would, however, be important to select areas where the basic information is adequate to the problem at hand and to the study method used. The production of other data in a similar fashion will improve our ability to understand and plan for health services for the population.

REFERENCES

1.   H.C. Chase, *Amer. J. Pub. Health 63,* September Supplement, 1973.

2.   D. Kessner *et al.,* Infant Death: An Analysis of Maternal Risk and Health Care, Institute of Medicine, National Academy of Sciences, Washington, D.C., 1973.

3.   A.M. Lilienfeld *et al., Public Health Rep. 66,* 191, 1951.

4.   E. Oppenheimer *et al., Vital Statistics Special Reports 45,* 396, U.S. Dept. of H.E.W., 1957.

5.   M. Mackeprang *et al., H.S.M.H.A. Health Reports 87,* 43, 1972.

DISCUSSION

DR. HOOK: Dr. Emanuel, can one distinguish sociocultural effects frôm biological effects in an intergenerational hypothesis to explain congenital defects?   While   biological factors in childhood of females may affect size of organs at time of eventual pregnancy, may not behavior of mothers during pregnancy be affected by attitudes and viewpoints acquired during childhood? This might affect nutrition and other factors during pregnancy.   Are we not seeing cultural effect related to childhood experience, manifested by the roles these girls play when they become mothers later?

DR. EMANUEL: Since ASB forms early, I doubt that a sociocultural effect could manifest itself between the third and fourth week of embryonic development.   Alternatively, since there are common features operating in many of the health problems related to poverty, improper growth during childhood may have an effect on many organ systems.

JACK MILLER (Montreal Children's Hospital, Quebec, Canada): Dr. Lanman, have you comparisons of elective abortions between non-white ward and non-white private patients and, also white ward and white private patients?

DR. LANMAN: Yes.   The general trend is that the non-white ward patient has the most extensive use and the white private patient the least.   The other two groups are in a declining order.

CHARLES LAWRENCE: Dr. Lanman, at the hospitals you mentioned, was delivery capacity being used to the fullest or was there considerable excess capacity for deliveries?   This could help to explain that when the number of induced abortions increased, the number of deliveries increased.

DR. LANMAN: There was no excess capacity at the City Hospital. The slight increase was seen all over New York City. It lasted for about 6 months.

DR. LAWRENCE: Does that perhaps suggest that the number of deliveries in those particular hospitals is independent of induced abortions or is it more strongly related to the capacity for deliveries than any other variables?

DR. LANMAN: I don't know. We looked for these possibilities. The published figures that indicate a drop cover a different period; in corresponding periods the same thing happened all over the City.
Dr. Chase, if there were a difference between legitimate and illegitimate

155

births, was there a trend?

DR. CHASE: The rates were highest for the black group, second highest in the Puerto Rican group and lowest in the white, foreign-born group.

DR. LAMM: Dr. Lanman, in regard to your concern for the drops in the mortality rate for immature birth as a poor measure of the effect of the change in the abortion law, one might look at birth certificate data for the change on the incidence at birth at that weight group, rather than on mortality data.

DR. LANMAN: The point was that in the overall mortality rate, the number of babies contributed by the immature group was quite small.

DR. LAMM: Did the reduction in the number of children available for adoption, in addition to the drop in incidence of your very low birth weight, hold for the whole city as for Brooklyn?

DR. LANMAN: Not exactly. Our figures refer to the baby that was abandoned in the newborn nursery and not to those taken home and adopted later. Our problem of being crowded in the newborn nursery, with no room for newborn babies, disappeared.

DR. LAMM: Dr. Chase, have you specific data on children available for adoption in New York after the law change?

DR. CHASE: No. Jean Paxton's early observations suggested a drop in the number of illegitimate births for the City.

DR. EMANUEL: There are two sets of data that suggest there may be something hazardous to fetal well being in New York City: Dr. Chase's data of lower rates of low birth weight in white foreign-born women than in the native-born women, and Terrance and Gold's observation that rates of low birth weight in migrant black women increased with increasing residence in New York City.

DR. CHASE: I have no data on migrant black women. The groups which migrated into New York City in large numbers came mostly from the rural south and into a hospital atmosphere — mainly because the migrant black has little access at first to other organizations within the City. The white foreign-born women, on the other hand, may have brought the concept of unrestricted weight gain in pregnancy with them, as opposed to the restricted weight gain concept of native-born mothers.

DR. HOOK: Dr. Emanuel, it is difficult to see a consistent relationship between ASB, social class and nutrition in different countries as well as within a country. Even within the British Isles, the relationship is not clear.

DR. EMANUEL: Only the Birmingham study from the British Isles does not show a social class effect, perhaps because a relatively crude index was used — cost of rent per census tract. Social class measures are, of course, crude themselves. I think, however, that the socioeconomic gradient is the most constant and striking of the epidemiological relationships. Certainly it is more striking and constant than maternal age and parity. Dr. Naggan's study in Israel, based on occupation, also doesn't show much of a social class effect. If education or some other measure were used, social class effect might be seen.

SECTION IV

CIGARETTE SMOKING DURING PREGNANCY: THE RELATIONSHIP WITH DEPRESSED WEIGHT GAIN AND BIRTHWEIGHT. AN UPDATED REPORT*

David Rush

Smoking by the mother during pregnancy is associated with depressed fetal growth and increased perinatal mortality.[1] In a recent publication[2] it was noted that women who smoked during pregnancy gained less weight than those who did not smoke, that this was dose related and that depressed weight gain accounted for half or more of the association of smoking with depressed birthweight. The observations were of 162 mothers and their live born singleton infants who were the control group in a longitudinal study of nutritional supplementation in pregnancy, on whom data for the variables prepregnant weight, weight at final prenatal clinic visit, length of gestation, birthweight and number of cigarettes smoked per day at registration, were available. Since that time data have become available on an additional 59 mother-infant pairs and the updated data will be presented here.

In brief, there had been no prior systematic exploration of the possibility that cigarette smoking causes low birthweight by depressing maternal weight gain in pregnancy. Other postulated mechanisms have not adequately explained the relationship of cigarette smoking to depressed fetal growth, although there are suggestive effects in the experimental animal of hypoxia[3] and nicotine exposure.[5] Surprisingly, human placental blood flow has been reported to increase with smoking.[6]

A review of past human studies was not illuminating. A recent publication from Australia[7] reports height of mother for about 5,000 births and weight at delivery for a subgroup of about 3,400. Those smoking had, as expected, lighter infants. They were also taller than non-smokers but weighed significantly less at delivery, results consistent with those to be presented here. Miller and Hassanein[8] studying 241 (or 249) term, singleton pregnancies stated, "The weight gains of smoking and non-smoking mothers were not significantly

*This work was supported by NICHHD Contract No. 1-HD-9-2180.

TABLE 1

Correlation Matrix: Birthweight, Prepregnant Weight, Weight at Final Clinic Visit, Length of Gestation, and Number of Cigarettes per Day Smoked at Registration (n = 221)

	Prepregnant weight	Final weight	Gestation	No. of cigarettes per day
Birthweight	0.16	0.38	0.39	−0.21
Prepregnant weight		0.73	0.12	0.11
Final weight			0.19	0.08
Length of gestation			0.19	−0.09

$p < 0.05$ if $r \geq \pm$ .13

$p < 0.01$ if $r \geq \pm$ .17

different and were about 1 pound/week on the average." They did not report the actual magnitude of weight gains. They also stated that, "Maternal smoking tended to decrease birthweights (in all four groups of infants), but the decreases were not statistically significant."; however, calculating from their data for their entire study population, infants of smokers were, on average 128 grams lighter (t = 2.44, p < 0.01). Thus, their interpretation of weight gain patterns may, in part, be a function of how statistical tests were applied and it would be valuable to be able to study the actual data.

Methods

We have been engaged for several years in a randomized controlled trial of nutritional supplementation in pregnancy in a poor urban black population. The details of the study design have been described elsewhere.[9,10] As part of this project, some of the pregnant women were randomly allocated to a group who were closely observed but whose obstetric care and nutritional supplementation continued identical to that of all other patients in the clinic. The outcome for all 221 women from this group who delivered a singleton liveborn infant, for whom there are data available for each variable used in Tables 1 and 2 and for whom there was at least eight weeks between the initial and final measurement of maternal weight, are reported here. All women were primarily English speaking, were without known medical problems (diabetes, hypertension, urinary infection, alcohol or drug addiction, etc.) thought to be determinants of fetal growth, were registered prior to 30 weeks gestation and had a history of preconception weight under 140 pounds. In order to be invited into the project, they also had to meet one of the following additional criteria: had a prior low birthweight infant; had low weight gain during pregnancy at the point of registration (as judged by past experience for this population); had a reported preconception weight of under 110 pounds; or had a protein intake of less than 50 grams (as judged by quantitative dietary recall) for the 24 hours prior to registration. Prior to random allocation to one of two groups receiving additional nutritional supplementation, or to a third group continuing regular clinic care, all agreed to participate in the study, with the knowledge that they might or might not be receiving nutritional supplementation beyond that prescribed for all clinic registrants.

Average weekly weight gain was derived by subtracting the maternal weight at registration (measured with light clothing, without shoes) from that at the last clinic visit and dividing by the time between the two measurements. This variable was calculated differently for the prior publication[2] where the increment in weight was divided by the time between registration and term; the current variable is thus somewhat more precise. Height was measured at registration. The preconception weight was that reported by the women.

163

TABLE 2
Multiple Regression Analysis on Birthweight (n = 221)

	Cumulative R^2	Increment in R^2	$F_{I_{R^2}}$	B (g)
SEQUENCE 1				
Prepregnant weight (pounds)	0.026	0.026	5.90	− 7.5
Cigarettes/day (No.)	0.081	0.054	12.87	− 9.4
Duration of gestation (weeks)	0.205	0.125	34.11	64.7
Final weight (pounds)	0.291	0.085	25.94	13.8
SEQUENCE 1a				
Cigarettes/day	0.046	0.046	10.58	
Prepregnant weight	0.081	0.034	8.16	
SEQUENCE 2				
Prepregnant weight	0.026	0.026	5.90	
Duration of gestation	0.168	0.141	37.03	
Final weight	0.275	0.108	32.28	
Cigarettes/day	0.291	0.015	4.63	
SEQUENCE 3				
Duration of gestation	0.154	0.154	39.99	
Prepregnant weight	0.168	0.01	3.46	
Cigarettes/day	0.205	0.038	10.32	
Final weight	0.291	0.085	25.94	
SEQUENCE 3a				
Duration of gestation	0.154	0.154	39.99	
Cigarettes/day	0.187	0.032	8.64	
Prepregnant weight	0.205	0.019	5.13	
Final weight	0.291	0.085	25.94	
SEQUENCE 4				
Duration of gestation	0.154	0.154	39.99	
Prepregnant weight	0.168	0.013	3.46	
Final weight	0.275	0.108	32.28	
Cigarettes/day	0.290	0.015	4.63	

$p = 0.05$, for $F \cong 3.88$

$p = 0.01$, for $F \cong 6.74$

(See text for interpretation of column headings)

Final weight was the weight reported at the last clinic visit. The smoking status at registration was what the women reported to be their current smoking behavior. Postpartum, the participant was asked whether she had continued smoking up to delivery. Length of gestation was calculated from the first day of the reported last menstrual period.

Results

Those reporting cigarette smoking at registration had significantly lower subsequent mean weight gain. (.91 versus 1.02 pounds per week, t=1.89, d.f.=220, p < .05) (Table 3). There was a strong and highly significant decreasing gradient of weekly weight gain with the amount of reported smoking (0.13 fewer pounds per week gained per additional cigarette smoked; F=10.25, d.f.=1 and 220, p < .005). Only for those who were initially smoking 10 or more cigarettes per day was there an association of stopping of smoking with increased weight gain; however, there were only four such women.

Birthweight had the expected relationship with smoking (Table 4) (3107 vs. 2834 grams; t=3.89, p < .001). The gradient of decreasing birthweight with amount reported smoked at registration, although not as regular as for weight gain, was highly significant (15.7 fewer grams of birthweight per additional cigarette smoked, F=10.60, d.f.=1 and 220, p < .005). Although those who stopped smoking before delivery had infants of considerably higher birthweight (199 grams), the difference was not statistically significant (t=1.56, d.f.=79, p < .10).

The gestation of smokers was 0.5 weeks less than non-smokers (Table 5). This difference was not significant nor was the slope of the regression of shortened gestation with increased smoking (.23 fewer days of gestation per additional cigarette smoked; F=1.84, d.f.=1 and 220, p < .10). There was no association of gestation with whether smoking was continued to the time of delivery. Past research has suggested that there is only a minimal relationship of maternal smoking with gestation.[11]

Smokers and non-smokers had many different characteristics (Table 6). Smokers were significantly taller (160.2 cm vs. 158.5 cm; t=2.40, p < .01). None of these attributes accounted for the marked differences in weight gain or birthweight. Indeed, since smokers were taller they would be likely, if all things were equal, to have heavier babies. The mean prepregnant weights of smokers and non-smokers were nearly identical.

In order to quantitate the association of birthweight, cigarette smoking, weight change and gestation, multiple regression analyses were performed with birthweight the dependent variable. The correlation matrix among birthweight, prepregnant weight, weight at last clinic visit, length of gestation and number

165

TABLE 3

Mean ($\pm$ SD) of Weekly Weight Gain (Pounds) While Under Study Observation, by Amount Smoked at Registration

	Cigarettes/day at registration					All those smoking at registration	Total
	0	< 5	5–9	10–14	15+		
	1.02 ± 0.41 (n = 137)	1.04 ± 0.44 (n = 22)	0.97 ± 0.37 (n = 23)	0.89 ± 0.40 (n = 23)	0.66 ± 0.35 (n = 16)	0.91 ± 0.42 (n = 84)	0.97 ± 0.42 (n = 221)

166

TABLE 4

Mean ($\pm$ SD) of Birthweight (in g.), by Amount Smoked at Registration

	Cigarettes/day at registration				All those smoking at registration	Total
0	<5	5–9	10–14	15+		
3107 $\pm$ 508 (n = 137)	2795 $\pm$ 410 (n = 22)	2825 $\pm$ 396 (n = 23)	3014 $\pm$ 512 (n = 23)	2641 $\pm$ 418 (n = 16)	2834 $\pm$ 457 (n = 84)	3003 $\pm$ 507 (n = 221)

TABLE 5

Mean ($\pm$ SD) Duration of Gestation (Weeks) by Amount Smoked at Registration

	Cigarettes/day at registration				All those smoking at registration	Total
0	< 5	5–9	10–14	15+		
39.0 $\pm$ 2.4 (n = 137)	38.4 $\pm$ 2.6 (n = 22)	38.9 $\pm$ 2.5 (n = 23)	38.8 $\pm$ 3.1 (n = 23)	37.9 $\pm$ 2.3 (n = 16)	38.5 $\pm$ 2.7 (n = 84)	38.8 $\pm$ 2.5 (n = 221)

TABLE 6

Age, Prepregnant Weight, Height, Marital Status, Primiparity and Amount of Schooling, by Amount Smoked at Registration

		Cigarettes/day at registration				All those smoked at registration	Total
	0	< 5	5–9	10–14	15+		
Age (years) Mean ±SD	22.5 ± 4.9	19.4 ± 4.1	21.0 ± 4.7	21.3 ± 4.1	25.0 ± 4.8	21.4 ± 4.8	21.1 ± 4.9
Prepregnant weight (pounds) Mean ±SD	116.2 ±12.8	115.5 ±16.3	116.5 ±11.9	113.7 ±11.1	121.6 ±12.5	116.4 ±13.4	116.3 ± 13.0
Height (cm) Mean ±SD	158.5 ± 6.4	162.7 ± 5.5	159.4 ± 5.3	160.0 ± 6.4	160.2 ± 5.7	160.6 ± 5.9	159.3 ± 6.3
Married at registration (percent)	36.5	18.2	21.7	26.1	43.8	26.2	32.6
First pregnency (percent)	48.2	81.9	43.5	43.5	25.0	50.0	48.9
11 or more years of school (percent)	66.4	50.0	69.6	56.5	56.3	58.3	63.3
n	137	22	23	23	16	84	221

of cigarettes smoked per day at registration is presented in Table 1 and several different sequences of regression analysis are presented in Table 2.

The meaning of the column headings in Table 2 are as follows: *Cumulative* R^2 is the total variance of birthweight accounted for by the (linear components) of all independent variables so far entered into the regression analysis; *Increment in* R^2 is the amount of variance of birthweight uniquely accounted for by the independent variable just entered, controlling for the variables previously entered; F_{IR}^2 is the F ratio for the significance of the increment in R^2 (it has 1, [220 minus the number of variables so far entered] d.f.); *B(grams)* is the regression coefficient in the final regression equation, expressed as the amount of change (in grams) of birthweight, associated with one unit of change in the independent variable, controlling for the other three independent variables.

Analyses using average weekly weight gain, rather than final weight, gave parallel results but at somewhat lower levels of association. Weekly weight gain was preferable in the bivariate analysis (Table 3) because it is free of confounding from differing lengths of gestation. Controlling for gestation is more efficiently done in the regression analyses by using a sequence of independent variables in which length of gestation precedes final weight; this procedure also allows for pregnancy weight gain prior to registration to function in the analyses.

These different sequences help to allocate to the several independent variables their shared and their unique contributions to the variance of birthweight. Analyses were performed assuming both that the relationship between smoking and length of gestation may have been a chance finding, and thus to be controlled away, and also assuming it might be other than chance. One analysis assumed that smoking status, even though ascertained during pregnancy, would be contributory to prepregnant weight and thus should take precedence in a causal sequence.

Sequence 1 shows that the variable, "Number of cigarettes per day at registration", accounts for an additional 5.4 percent of the variance in birthweight when entered into the analysis after prepregnant weight (which by itself accounted for 2.6 percent). When the order of these variables was reversed (Sequence 1a), "Number of cigarettes" accounted for 4.6 percent of the variance, and prepregnant weight an additional 3.4 percent. If the number of cigarettes per day is entered after gestation, prepregnant and final weight (Sequence 2), it then accounts for only 1.5 percent of the variance in birthweight (with an F value which is weakly significant). This 1.5 percent is the unique contribution of smoking to birthweight, after controlling for gestation and maternal weight and weight change; thus, two-thirds or more of the initial association of smoking with birthweight is jointly shared with weight gain (and gestation). Sequences 3, 3a and 4 assumed that the present finding of shorter gestation with smoking was due to chance. Therefore, gestation is controlled first. In these sequences, "Number of cigarettes per day" alone contributes 3.2 percent of the variance of birthweight but this contribution is more than halved, if the weight status during pregnancy is first controlled (Sequence 4). Thus, the greatest part of the variance of birthweight associated with cigarette smoking is jointly shared with the change in maternal weight in pregnancy.

Discussion

For the population under study, the greatest part of the association of cigarette smoking with lowered birthweight is shared with lowered maternal weight gain. The gradient of lowered weight gain with increased smoking was regular, steep and highly significant. The mechanisms for the presumed causal effect of smoking on birthweight is thus likely to be, in large part, nutritional. There is no obvious reason why other postulated mechanisms by which smoking might retard fetal growth, such as direct toxicity of tobacco products, changes in vascular supply or increased circulating levels of carbon monoxide, should be associated with decreased maternal weight gain. The magnitude, specificity and coherence of this presumably nutritional association strongly suggests that it is more than association and that the decreased weight gain and probable caloric restriction associated with increased cigarette smoking in pregnancy is probably the most important mechanism for the effect of cigarette smoking on depressed fetal growth.

Smokers and non-smokers differed in several characteristics (smokers were taller). None of these differences, however, could explain away the weight gain or birthweight differences.

ACKNOWLEDGMENTS

I am indebted to Mervyn Susser and Zena Stein for their help, to Joseph Fleiss for review of the manuscript and for statistical advice and to Hillard David for help in data analysis.

REFERENCES

1.   D. Rush, *Am. J. Epidemiol. 96,* 183, 1972.

2.   D. Rush, *J. Obstet. Gynaecol. Br. Commonw. 81,* 746, 1974.

3.   P. Astrup, D. Trolle, H.M. Olsen and K. Kjeldsen, *Arch. Environ. Health 30,* 15, 1975.

4. P. Astrup, D. Trolle, K. Kjeldsen *et al.*, *Lancet 2*, 1220, 1972.

5. K. Suzuki, T. Horiguchi, A.C. Comas-Urrutia *et al.*, *Am. J. Obstet. Gynecol. 111,* 1092, 1971.

6. S.E. Cloeren, T.H. Lippert and R. Fridrich, *Arch. Gynaekol. 216,* 15, 1974.

7. I. Cope, P. Lancaster and L. Stevens, *Med. J. Aust. 1,* 673, 1973.

8. H.C. Miller and K. Hassanein, *Pediatr. Res. 8,* 960, 1974.

9. D. Rush, Z. Stein and M.W. Susser, *Nutritional Reports International, 7,* 547, 1973.

10. D. Rush, Z. Stein, G. Christakis and M.W. Susser, *in* Nutrition and Fetal Development, M. Winick (Ed.), John Wiley and Sons, New York, p. 95, 1974.

11. C.R. Buncher, *Am. J. Obstet. Gynecol. 103,* 942, 1969.

CHANGES IN TOBACCO SMOKING AND INGESTION OF ALCOHOL AND CAFFEINATED BEVERAGES DURING EARLY PREGNANCY: ARE THESE CONSEQUENCES, IN PART, OF FETO-PROTECTIVE MECHANISMS DIMINISHING MATERNAL EXPOSURE TO EMBRYOTOXINS?*

Ernest B. Hook

Introduction – Nausea and Vomiting in Pregnancy

It has been estimated that nausea and vomiting (NVP) of some degree occur early in the gestation of about 75% of all pregnancies.[1] Of these, about two-thirds, 50% of all pregnant women, may manifest overt vomiting and the remainder just "subjective" nausea.[2] Yet, despite the fact that this ubiquitous symptom complex occurs so frequently, rather little is known of the factors that cause it or are associated with it, nor its effects, both direct and indirect, upon the fetus.[3]

A good deal has been written, however, about hyperemesis gravidarum (HEG), an infrequent but extreme manifestation of NVP, which may be defined operationally as vomiting of degree sufficient to jeopardize the health of the mother and warrant admission to the hospital.[4] The reported incidence of HEG varies markedly from locality to locality, depending on the precise criteria for severity, over a range from about one to 15 per 1,000 pregnancies. In some areas at least, it appears to be diminishing in recent years.[5] Many reports in the literature on "nausea and vomiting in pregnancy", in fact, discuss only HEG. Nowhere in the literature could we find a single paper reporting the effects of NVP (as distinguished from HEG) upon maternal diet or other habits during pregnancy that could be of significance to the fetus.

Studies that have appeared, however, indicate that the occurrence of NVP is, in general, a favorable prognostic sign.[6–9,1,10] The evidence from these studies indicates that mothers carrying singleton infants who have NVP are (a) less likely to have an abortion prior to the 20th week of pregnancy and

*This work was supported in part by a grant from the National Institute of Child Health and Human Development (HD 05755) and a grant from the American Medical Association – Educational and Research Foundation.

TABLE 1

Abortion Rates Reported in the Literature in Those With and Without NVP (NVP+ and NVP−)

Senior Author and Year of Publication	Abortion Rate	
	NVP+	NVP−
Irving, 1940	6/225 = 2.7%	16–20%*
Speert, 1954	8/166 = 4.8%	52/119 = 43.7%
Medalie, 1957	0/52 = 0	11/48 = 22.9%**
Walford, 1963	8/331 = 2.4%***	97/954 = 10.2%
Yerushalmy, 1965****	$\dfrac{104}{2740} = 3.8\%$	$\dfrac{116}{1113} = 10.4\%$
Brandes, 1967	2.8%*****	6.6%*****

*Expected rate estimated by author.
**Mild NVP pooled with no NVP by author.
***NVP+ = those treated for symptoms.
****Numerators are calculated from the rates and denominators given in the reference. Data here are on those entering in first 12 weeks.
*****Calculated from rates given on 7027 singletons (72.0% NVP+) and 84 multiple births (86.9% NVP+).

174

TABLE 2

Pregnancy Outcomes Other than Abortion in Those With and Without NVP (NVP+ and NVP−)

Senior Author and Year of Publication	Outcomes			
Yerushalmy, 1965*	Stillbirths:	NVP+ = 2.16%	NVP− = 2.21%	Entry 1st 12 wks.
	Neonatal Deaths:	NVP+ = 1.01%	NVP− = 1.95%	NVP+ = 2,740
	Perinatal Deaths:	NVP+ = 3.15%	NVP− = 4.11%	NVP− = 1,113
	Severe Anomalies:	NVP+ = 1.20%	NVP− = 3.30%	
Brandes, 1967**	Stillbirth:	NVP+ = 2.05%	NVP− = 2.00%	
	Neonatal Deaths:	NVP+ = 1.25%	NVP− = 1.72%	
	Birthweight ◀ 2500 gm.:	NVP+ = 5.6%	NVP− = 7.9%	**
	Gestation ≤ 36 weeks:	NVP+ = 0.6%	NVP− = 11.6%	
Tylden, 1968	Perinatal Deaths:	NVP+ = 8.1%	NVP− = 5.0%	NVP+ = 159
	Birthweight ◀8 lbs.	NVP+ = 66.0%	NVP− = 71.9%	NVP− = 317

*Those entering study in 1st 12 weeks. Data on those in the entire study are provided only for meclizine exposure and cannot be separated out by symptom complex. If meclizine administration is used as a "marker" for NVP+ in entire group, the same trends for all outcomes are seen as were observed in those entering in the 1st 12 weeks, with the exception of severe anomalies.

** Birthweight data are on 6,667. Gestation data are for 20 to 36 weeks vs over 36 weeks and are on 6,729 individuals. The other two outcomes are on 6,756 pregnancies not ending in abortion of which 145 resulted in stillbirths. Approximately 75% in the groups are NVP+.

175

TABLE 3

Reason for Change in Smoking Habits in First Trimester

Total population interviewed	3,743
Non-smokers	1,858
Women who smoked in previous year	1,885
Number diminishing in first trimester	444
Number increasing in first trimester	80

Reported Reason for Decrease **,***

Sickness or nausea in response to cigarettes	162
Loss of urge (NVP not specifically cited)	55
Concern for infant	157
Doctor's orders or other reasons related to health or comfort of mother	38
Other****	32
Total:	444***

Reported Reason for Increase **,***

Increased anxiety	34
Increased urge	20
Other	26
Total:	80***

* The total number of deliveries in the hospitals surveyed in this period was 3,930. See text for exclusion.

** The "Decrease" and "Increase" categories are exclusive. Four women decreased because of NVP but then increased when symptoms diminished. They are coded only in the "Decrease" category. Similarly, two women who increased because of anxiety, but then went down, are coded only in the "Increase" category.

*** Less than 10% of women who changed patterns cited two or more reasons for the change. Those who did were further queried as to the *main* reason, which was the only one included in the tabulations here.

**** Includes 13 who cited social pressures.

(b) if they have a livebirth are more likely to have had a longer gestation and infant of higher birthweight. (See Tables 1 and 2, a summary of evidence from the literature.) Evidence concerning a diminished risk of birth defect in liveborn infants of mothers experiencing nausea and vomiting is suggestive but still equivocal.[9] (See Table 2.)

There is a small subgroup in whom NVP may be associated with less favorable "outcome". These are women who (a) are carrying twins, (b) have a hydatidiform mole and/or (c) have severe hyperemesis. Such women are relatively infrequent and so their occurrence does not significantly diminish the much more favorable prognosis for the entire group afflicted with NVP.

One study of drug treatment found in control groups that NVP can have an onset as early as the 2nd or 3rd week of gestation but the modal week of onset is the 5th week. At the 12th week, all (untreated) mothers who had NVP during pregnancy manifested this symptom but NVP began to diminish in this group after this point and afflicted only about 90% at the 14th week, 50% by about the 19th week, 10% by about the 23rd week and none by about the 27th week.[11]

The causes of NVP are completely unknown. Some have suggested that high levels of human chorionic gonadotrophins (HCG) are responsible, since these are elevated in early pregnancy, and higher in mothers carrying twins or hydatidiform moles in which the frequency of NVP is higher. Others have reported, however, that HCG levels do not correlate well with the severity of vomiting in early pregnancy and, in fact, are even higher in normal subjects than in those with hyperemesis.[12] Some have attributed the effects to estrogen production, because similar symptoms occur following estrogen administration to non-pregnant women, although even when large doses of estrogen are used, as in treatment of cancer patients, vomiting lasts no longer than two weeks.[13] It seems likely that some hormone or breakdown product associated with formation of trophoblast tissue in the early developing fetus is responsible for NVP, but the responsible compounds have not been identified.[4]

The Study

The results reported here arose from an investigation of smoking habits during pregnancy of mothers, who were interviewed shortly after delivery of ostensibly normal infants.[14] It was discovered, unexpectedly, that a fraction of mothers reported diminishing smoking in early pregnancy. The protocol was then revised and mothers were queried (in an unstructured interview) concerning their reasons for change (Table 3). Many reported the drop was attributable to NVP which led to rejection of cigarettes, while another fraction just reported a 'loss of urge' in early gestation without identifying NVP as the specific cause. Others report 'concern for the infant' as the cause for the drop.

The results noted in Table 3 depend, of course, upon the accuracy of recall and reporting of this particular population. But, if anything, they appear likely to be underestimates of the true fraction who decreased exposure because they found smoking less pleasurable. "Concern" for the infant or similar health related factors are more socially acceptable reasons that appear more likely to be provided to an interviewer.

These observations, in any event, strongly suggest NVP or associated physiological events diminish smoking in early pregnancy. They also suggest that NVP is a variable for which adjustment may be required in studies of the association of smoking and fetal wastage. NVP is known to occur less frequently during pregnancies resulting in abortion, so such mothers would tend to smoke more in any event. Thus, the reported association of smoking and abortion may be (at least partially) confounded by the presence of NVP. Alternatively, NVP may be associated with a more favorable prognosis regarding fetal wastage, at least in part, because it reduces tobacco smoking.

The results of our interviews, obtained at the end of pregnancy, also indicated that ingestion of coffee and alcoholic beverages tend to be diminished for reasons similar to those cited for smoking (Tables 4—6). Little has also noted trends similar to those discussed here for these beverages.[15,16]

Our own study, because it was designed with other goals in mind, involved interviews right after delivery only of mothers who had given birth to an ostensibly normal liveborn infant. Thus, by necessity, we have an unrepresentative sample of all conceptuses, even of those surviving to 12 weeks of gestation and, of course, no way of evaluating a possible negative association of NVP with abortion. We did find, however, no association of increased birthweight with the presence of vomiting in pregnancy in the non-smokers in our population; i.e., those who had not smoked for one year prior to delivery.

Discussion — Evolutionary Implications

An outstanding question is why NVP is so frequent. It appears plausible that any trait affecting such a large proportion of women during gestation would appear to have or have had some selective value. Certainly, as discussed above, NVP appears to be associated with factors that are feto-protective in most studies to date.

It could be argued that NVP is a deleterious manifestation of hormonal changes accompanying pregnancy — certainly it is an uncomfortable one — and the beneficial effects of these physiological factors outweigh any deleterious effects of the symptom complex. But as natural selection acts upon the entire

TABLE 4

Change in Beverage Ingestion in Early Pregnancy

| | Total number interviewed = 295 | | | | | | | |
	Coffee	Tea	Milk	Colas	Beer	Wine	"Other Spirits"
Number (and percent) reported regularly drinking the beverage at start of pregnancy**	205 (69.5%)	240 (81.3%)	166* (91.7%)*	251 (85.1%)	123 (41.7%)	167 (56.6%)	190 (64.4%)
Number (and percent) of those who drank beverage who decreased in first trimester	70 (34.1%)	21 (8.8%)	15 (9.0%)	47 (18.7%)	35 (28.4%)	37 (22.3%)	49 (25.8%)
Number (and percent) of those 295 interviewed who increased in first trimester	11 (3.7%)	30 (10.2%)	153 (51.9%)	26 (8.8%)	2 (0.7%)	4 (1.4%)	3 (1.0%)

*Only 181 were asked specifically if they drank milk at start of pregnancy but all were asked if they increased or decreased. Since a decrease can only occur in those who drank at least some milk at the start of pregnancy, percentages in this column concerning *decrease* are only in those 166 of 181 (91.7%).

**With the exception of milk (see footnote above) a specific query concerning ingestion at the start of pregnancy was made for each of the other beverages in all 295.

179

TABLE 5

Distribution of Reasons Cited for Decrease in Beverage Consumption*****

Reasons cited for decrease (NVP)	Coffee	Tea	Milk***	Cola	Beer	Wine	"Other Spirits"
Nausea stimulated by beverage	38 (18.5%)	9 (3.8%)	10 (6.0%)	4 (1.6%)	7 (5.7%)	9 (5.4%)	14 (7.4%)
Loss of urge	16 (7.8%)	10 (4.2%)	1 (0.6%)	7 (2.8%)	14 (11.4%)	7 (4.2%)	6 (3.2%)
Concern for infant	1 (0.5%)	0	0	5 (2.0%)	3 (2.4%)	9 (5.4%)	13 (6.8%)
Doctor's orders	0	0	0	5 (2.0%)	0	0	0
Peer influences	1 (0.5%)	0	0	0	1 (0.8%)	0	2 (1.1%)
Economic reasons	0	0	0	3 (1.2%)	0	0	0
Dieting	1 (0.5%)	0	1 (0.6%)	8 (3.2%)	3 (2.4%)	1 (0.6%)	2 (1.1%)
Other health (e.g., "nerves", "indigestion")	13 (6.3%)	2 (0.8%)	3 (1.8%)	15 (6.0%)	6 (4.9%)	7 (4.2%)	5 (2.6%)
Greater susceptibility to alcoholic beverages	0	0	0	0	1 (0.8%)	4 (2.4%)	7 (3.7%)
Total decreasing	70 (34.1%)	21 (8.8%)	15 (9.0%)	47 (18.7%)	35 (28.4%)	37 (22.2%)	49 (25.8%)
Total who drank beverage in question at time of onset of pregnancy	205	240	166***	251	123	167	190

* Very few (< 5% here) reported more than one reason. Those that did were tabulated by the main reason provided.
** I.e., the taste was now less appealing.
*** Out of 181 specifically queried concerning the amount of this beverage drunk at start of pregnancy. See footnotes to preceding table.
**** All percentages listed are of the total who drank the beverage at onset of pregnancy.

180

TABLE 6

Distribution of Reasons Cited for Increase in Beverage Consumption*

	Coffee	Tea	Milk	Cola	Beer	Wine	"Other Spirits"
Reason cited in 295 interviewed							
Increase in urge**	5	17	45	10	0	0	0
Social reasons	1	0	0	0	1	1	1
Concern for infant	0	0	77	0	0	0	0
Doctor's orders	0	0	12	0	0	0	0
Other reasons***	2	3	9	9	1	3	0
In response to nausea****	0	7	5	5	0	0	0
No reason given	3	3	5	2	0	0	0
Total and	11	30	153	26	2	4	1
Percent of total interviewed	(2.7%)	(10.2%)	(51.9%)	(8.8)	(0.7%)	(1.4%)	(0.4%)

* As with Tables 3 and 5, if two reasons were cited ($<$ 5% of respondents here), only the main reason was coded.

** I.e., its taste was now more appealing.

*** I.e., in response to increased thirst, or because beverage relieved "heartburn" or "cramps".

**** I.e., because the beverage relieved symptoms.

181

phenotype, if the symptoms themselves were deleterious in balance, one would expect the emergence of symptomatic resistance to the causal physiological factors.

The observations reported here provide a rationale for the hypothesis that NVP (and other symptoms affecting diet) in early pregnancy evolved as a spectrum of response to environmental factors which are selectively toxic (or beneficial) to the fetus. They may have emerged during that time in evolution when marked changes in the human diet occurred, perhaps during the introduction of agriculture. Certainly, one aspect of human evolution that would accompany increase of intelligence is a marked increase in the variety of foodstuffs that would be sampled and introduced on a large scale if found palatable. (To my knowledge, NVP has not been described in lower animals, even higher primates, although a systematic search may not have been undertaken, and anecdotal observations may not have been thought worthy of formal report. Hyperemesis has been said to complicate only the pregnancies of humans.[4])

If this view is correct, then changes in diet in early pregnancy may not be haphazard and arbitrary responses to the state of pregnancy, but rather signals of a homeostatic mechanism protecting the fetus. Foods diminished in early pregnancy would appear to merit investigation for adverse fetal effects, and conversely, those for which cravings appear are plausible candidates for investigation as possible beneficial factors. The hypothesis thus provides a rationale for ordering priorities in investigation of effects of specific nutritional factors upon pregnancy outcome.

In our investigation of beverage consumption, for instance, (Tables 4–6), it is of interest that 153 of 295 (51.9%) women interviewed increased milk consumption in the first trimester and 45 reported doing so because of an increased craving for milk, and not because of a doctor's recommendation or 'concern'. Only 9% diminished. With regard to caffeinated beverages, however, 3.7% increased coffee, 10.2% increased tea and 8.8 increased colas, but 34.1% of coffee drinkers, 8.8% of tea drinkers and 18.7% of cola beverage drinkers reported decreasing intake in the first trimester. Over half of those diminishing coffee ingestion (38/70 = 54.3%) specifically cited nausea stimulated by the beverage, while the remainder cited primarily other intolerances to the beverage which appeared or were accentuated in early pregnancy (13/70 = 18.6%), or simply a loss of taste for the beverage (16/70 = 22.9%). Thus, on the basis of the hypothesis proposed here, coffee would appear a prime factor for investigation as a potentially adverse agent.

ACKNOWLEDGMENTS

The interviews were carried out by G. Conway, M. Aldrich, K. Westendorf, S. Carey and J. Garvey. N. Reiss and M. Aldrich assisted with the tabulation of the data.

182

REFERENCES

1. J.M. Brandes, *Obst. Gynecol. 30,* 427, 1967.

2. V.V. Sterk, R. Prywes, A.M. Davies, P. Ever-Hadani and P. Lilos, *Isr. J. Med. Sci. 7,* 1248, 1971.

3. A. Midwinter, *The Practitioner 206,* 743, 1971.

4. D.V.I. Fairweather, *Am. J. Obs. Gynecol. 102,* 135, 1968.

5. W. Barr, *in* Practical Obstetric Problems, I. Donald (Ed.), Lloyd-Luke, London, pp. 202–211, 1969.

6. H. Speert and A.F. Guttmacher, *J.A.M.A. 155,* 712, 1954.

7. J.H. Medalie, *Lancet 2,* 117, 1957.

8. P.A. Walford, *Lancet 2,* 298, 1963.

9. J. Yerushalmy and L. Milkovich, *Am. J. Obstet. Gynecol. 93,* 553, 1965.

10. E. Tylden, *J. Psychom. Res. 12,* 86, 1968.

11. P.L.C. Diggory and J.S. Tomkinson, *Lancet 2,* 370, 1962.

12. D.V.I. Fairweather and T.A. Loraine, *Brit. Med. J. 1,* 666, 1962.

13. E.B. Astwood, *in* Pharmacological Basis of Therapeutics, L.S. Goodman and A. Gilman (Eds.), The MacMillan Company, New York, 1538–1565, 1970.

14. E.B. Hook, *in* Birth Defects, Monitoring and Environment—The Problem of Surveillance, E.B. Hook *et al.* (Eds.), Academic Press, New York, 177–192, 1971.

15. R.E. Little, Personal communication, 1974.

16. R.E. Little and F.A. Schultze, *Proc. N.Am. Congr. Alcohol and Drug Problems* (in press).

17. Irving, F.C., *Virg. Med. Month. 67,* 717, 1940.

STRATEGIES IN EVALUATION OF UNCERTAIN CLAIMS OF ENVIRONMENTAL CAUSES OF BIRTH DEFECTS

Godfrey P. Oakley, Jr.

As a society, we are becoming more and more conscious of diseases that can be caused by environmental agents. We know about rubella and thalidomide embryopathy. More recently, we have learned that *in utero* exposure to diethylstilbestrol can lead to carcinoma of the vagina in girls and young women and that certain occupational exposures to polyvinyl chloride can cause sarcoma of the liver.

With our new awareness has come a shift in attitude. We are more suspicious of environmental agents. For example, there are few marketed drugs that have had adequate testing for human teratogenesis. When asked if an incompletely tested drug caused a birth defect, we used to say a teratogenic effect is not known. Now, we say that the safety of the drug for use in pregnancy has not been established.

We look back on episodes of environmentally caused disease hoping to learn lessons that will help us find unrecognized environmental diseases and prevent such new diseases. Thalidomide showed us that if the side-effect was serious and appeared in the majority of those exposed, a small study of infants exposed *in utero* could identify the problem. The 1962 amendments to the Food and Drug Act required clinical trials of drugs prior to marketing in an attempt to find serious adverse effects before use became widespread.

It is difficult if not impossible, however, to assemble cohorts of pregnant women who have been exposed to all the environmental agents to which each of us is exposed. If an agent becomes widespread and causes a serious birth defect in the majority of embryos exposed to it, one would expect the incidence of birth defects to rise. In 1970 a whole symposium was based on monitoring the environment through surveillance and monitoring systems. The New York State Health Department has been monitoring birth defect incidence from its birth certificates since 1962. We have monitored birth defect incidence by regular visitations to Atlanta hospitals since 1967. We, in collaboration with the National Institute of Child Health, the National Foundation-March of Dimes and the Commission on Professional and Hospital

Activities, have just begun to use hospital discharge summaries for newborns to monitor the incidence of birth defects in one-third of the nation's births. Monitoring systems exist in several countries. The World Health Organization and the National Foundation-March of Dimes are working concurrently to facilitate communications among various groups that monitor for birth defects.

These communications will facilitate the interpretation of minor increases in incidence that one surveillance system might note. An increase that we might notice in the Atlanta data would become much more believable if it were also noted in the National data, the New York State data or one of the Canadian registries.

Clinical observations, however, first led to the suspicion that rubella and thalidomide were teratogenic. The American Academy of Pediatrics sponsors a program called "The Alert Practitioner". The idea is to encourage clinicians to look for unusual associations of environmental exposure with pediatric diseases. When an alert practitioner notes the association of an *in utero* exposure and the birth of a child with a birth defect, he is usually left with a dilemma. Has he just made the first observation that the agent causes a birth defect or has he merely observed the chance association of the factor and the birth defect? If the former alternative is the correct one, there is every reason to spread the news of the observations widely and quickly.

When such observations are made, there usually is not enough information available to know if the association is causal or due to chance. In our desire to eliminate all environmental diseases, one approach to take in the face of minimal data is to suggest that exposure be stopped, no matter how flimsy the data implicating the agent are. There is, however, risk associated with such an approach. The major problem is that the majority of the observations will be due to chance. Repeated cries of "wolf" will make it more difficult to deal effectively with a real problem.

Widespread publicity about a false-positive association is a special risk for exposed, pregnant women. They will be anxious about their pregnancy. This anxiety often leads to consideration of abortion. Some women will decide for abortion and expose themselves and their fetuses to unnecessary risk.

Although associations are made daily, few are reported in a way that produce great anxiety. I should like to discuss two of them and report some work done at the Center for Disease Control that was done rather promptly and provided a better perspective on the question of the teratogenicity of the agents concerned.

A little over two years ago, Dr. William McBride reported seeing three Australian children with reduction deformities whose mothers had ingested one or another of the tricyclic antidepressants.[1] At the time the observation was made, people were worried that this was to be another thalidomide-type epidemic. It was on the front pages of newspapers. Let me describe to you the epidemiologic approaches that were used to evaluate this situation. First of all, the incidence of this kind of birth defect associated with McBride's report, namely reduction deformities, was reviewed in Atlanta and Los Angeles. There was no recent increase. It was conceivable, however, that the drug was used so infrequently that no increase could be noted; therefore, case investigations were done. From 101 cases in the Atlanta registry, 43 chidren with the most severe reduction deformities were selected. Clinic and private obstetrical records of all the Atlanta cases were reviewed. None of the records had any indication that the drug had been used. An attempt was made to interview 18 of the mothers whose children had been born most recently in Atlanta. Twelve were personally interviewed and shown 16 different dosage forms of 6 tricyclic compounds. None recognized any of the samples and all denied using the drugs. Five similar cases were reviewed in Los Angeles and no positive history of using the drug could be found.[2] Similar results were found in Canada.[3] This particular approach, while not proving that the drugs were safe, did give some indication that they were not likely to be causing an epidemic and reassured women who were pregnant at the time and had to decide for or against abortion. More than 2 years have now passed and no other data implicating this class of drugs have been published.

In the summer of 1973, the Consumer Product Safety Commission received a report from an Oklahoma City physician linking exposure to spray adhesives with birth defects. The physician reported 2 children with multiple birth defects who had an increased number of chromosomal breaks in metaphase plates of cultural lymphocytes. The only defect common to the 2 was arthrogryposis. The parents of one of the children were involved during pregnancy in a "foiling" hobby that resulted in the exposure to spray adhesives. The parents of the other children had exposure to spray adhesives before, but not after, conception. All parents had an increased number of breaks in the metaphase plates. Four friends of the parents who had been involved in the use of sprays had an increased breakage rate, too. All together, there were 10 exposed individuals (9.0% of their metaphase plates had breaks). In the control group of 12, the breakage rate was 1.6%. The Commission was unable to locate study data suggesting that exposure to spray adhesives was safe for animals or humans. On August 17, 1973, it announced its intention to ban 13 sprays. This announcement led many pregnant women who had used sprays to seek counseling regarding the advisability of therapeutic abortion. We undertook epidemiologic studies in an attempt to rapidly gather information that could be of help to these counselors and their patients.

We thought there were 3 questions at that time: (1) Do adhesive sprays

TRENDS IN BIRTH DEFECT INCIDENCE AND SPRAY
ADHESIVE SALES, METROPOLITAN ATLANTA, 1969-1973

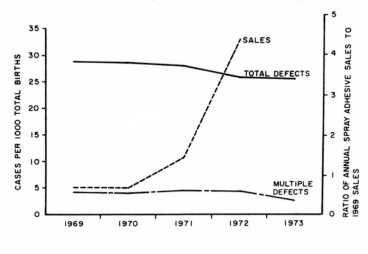

Fig. 1

TRENDS IN BIRTH DEFECT INCIDENCE AND SPRAY
ADHESIVE SALES, OKLAHOMA COUNTY, 1969-1973

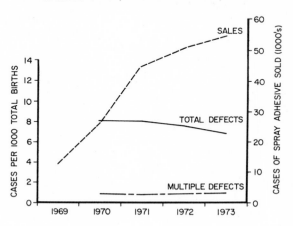

Fig. 2.

188

cause chromosome breaks? (2) Do adhesive sprays cause birth defects? (3) Do adhesive sprays cause chromosome breaks which cause birth defects? We decided to look at the question of: "Do adhesive sprays cause birth defects?"

We looked at the incidence of birth defects in the Atlanta registry for the previous 4 years. We saw no increase in multiple defects or in arthrogryposis, the defect that was common to each patient. We next looked at sales of spray adhesives in Atlanta and found sales had increased over the past 3 years (Fig. 1). With the State Health Department and the University of Oklahoma, we looked at birth defects on birth certificates from Oklahoma County for recent increases in birth defects. There had been none but there had been a dramatic increase in the sale of the spray adhexive (Fig. 2).

We were still left with the question of whether pregnant women were using the products. Eight of 173 (or 4.6%) women who had recently given birth to babies in Metropolitan Atlanta claimed that they had been exposed sometime in their lives to the sprays (3 of the 8, during their pregnancies). This allowed us to make certain calculations by assuming that 1,500 (or 5%) of the 30,000 births in Atlanta were to exposed women. If all those women produced babies with the birth defect in question, there would be 1,500 cases of the defect. If that attack rate was as low as 5%, then there would be 75 new cases in Atlanta in a year. To put this in some perspective, let me point out that 98% of the birth defect categories monitored in Atlanta occur with an incidence of 1 in 1,000 or less, which means that almost all birth defects occur with a frequency of no more than 30 cases per year. Thus, if the attack rate were 5%, we would have seen 105 infants in a given birth defect category in a year. This incidence of a defect would have been obvious to us. We therefore felt that if there was any risk to exposed women, the maximum risk was 5% and was probably less than that. Most women do not have an abortion when they learn that the risk for an affected fetus is 5% or less, rather than 25%, 50% or 100%.[4]

In summary, we have seen that the public announcement that an agent is thought to cause birth defects leads many exposed pregnant women to consider abortion. Acute epdiemiologic studies in such situations can rapidly test the hypothesis at issue. If they fail to confirm the hypothesis, they may be able to suggest the maximum risk to the embryo. In this spray adhesive hypothesis, we have seen that the epidemiologic studies did not confirm the hypothesis and suggested that the maximum possible risk of birth defects from exposure was less than that usually considered to be a fetal indication for abortion.

Deciding that there is enough evidence to identify a new teratogen can be difficult for a clinician, a university professor, an epidemiologist, a journal editor or a government official to make regulatory decisions. Early on, some real teratogens will be judged to be safe and agents without teratogenic properties will be declared teratogenic. Our goal must be to reduce the occurrence of each type of error as much as possible. I would like to offer some suggestions that I believe will help. They are concerned mainly with early communication to rapidly generate extra data when needed.

First, epidemiologists who note changes in incidence should communicate with others looking for confirmation. Once it is felt that a real increase in the incidence of a birth defect has occurred, this should be widely published. Meanwhile, epidemiologists and others can begin the search for the etiologic agent.

Second, if epidemiologists or clinicians associate an exposure with a birth defect, they should notify the appropriate government agency, which should have a panel of appropriate consultants to review the data quickly and offer suggestions on the plan of attack.

Third, the people monitoring for birth defects should also be reached. The status of the secular trends of the incidence of that birth defect in many locations around the world can be determined within a matter of days.

Fourth, a search should be made for existing sources of data that might shed light on the appropriate hypothesis. For example, the Collaborative Perinatal Study may be an invaluable source of such data. Drs. Slone, Heinonen and Shapiro have been analyzing these data looking for drugs that might be teratogenic. Certainly, one would not publicly release data suggesting that a drug is teratogenic for humans without consulting this data set. The data set may, in fact, be able to refute or support a hypothesis within a matter of days.

Fifth, if enough data are not available from existing sources, then priority should be given to testing the hypothesis that the agent is associated with the disease through case-control or retrospective cohort studies.

Sixth, when the results of these studies are ready for distribution, the release of data should be coordinated. Practicing physicians, in particular, should be notified so they can offer appropriate counseling to patients who call. A commendable example of such coordination has occurred recently when it was announced that an unusual association had been observed between reserpine and carcinoma of the breast. The hypothesis was raised by the Boston Drug Surveillance Group in December 1973. The Boston group notified colleagues of their observations and two sets of investigators conducted epidemiologic studies to test the hypothesis. Recently they confirmed the association.[5-7] The commissioner of the Food and Drug Administration notified practicing physicians of the findings and his interpretations as the 3 articles were being published. I hope that the next time an agent is seriously suspected of being

190

teratogenic that those of us interested in birth defects can coordinate our efforts and communications so that unnecessary anxiety can be kept to a minimum.

REFERENCES

1. W.G. McBride, *Med. J. Aust. 1*, 492, 1972.

2. G.S. Rachelefsky, J.W. Flynt, Jr., A.J. Ebbin and M.G. Wilson, *Lancet 1*, 838, 1972.

3. P. Banister, C. Dafoe, E.S.O. Smith and J. Miller, *Lancet 1*, 838, 1972.

4. Center for Disease Control, *Morbidity and Mortality Weekly Rep. 22 (44)*, 365, 9 Nov. 1973.

5. H. Jick, D. Slone and S. Shapiro, *Lancet 2*, 669, 1974.

6. A. Armstrong, N. Stevens and R. Doll, *Lancet 2*, 672, 1974.

7. O.P. Heinonen, S. Shapiro, L. Tuominen and M.I. Turunen, *Lancet 2*, 675, 1974.

CHROMOSOME BREAKAGE: THE IMPLICATIONS FOR HUMAN POPULATIONS *

Arthur D. Bloom

Certain chemical and physical agents in the environment may have adverse effects on health. The immediate problems are carcinogenesis and teratogenesis; the longer term risk is mutagenicity. Recent evidence of a relationship between chromosome aberrations and the teratogenic and carcinogenic effects of a given agent reinforces our earlier concept that chromosomal breakage should be avoided if possible.[1]

RECENT ADVANCES IN CYTOGENETIC TECHNIQUES

Two rapidly developing approaches to the study of human chromosomes promise to change our fundamental views of the breakage phenomenon — banding techniques and electron microscopy.

The recent electron microscopic studies of Brinkley[2] and Comings[3] clearly reveal the multistranded nature of the chromosome arm, which appears relatively homogenous with the standard giemsa stain. They support the view that achromatic regions (gaps) and half-chromatid lesions may represent a true breakage of chromatin fibers, despite earlier misconceptions of their significance as aberrations. Thus, electron microscopy can be used selectively for accurate estimates of the frequencies of induced aberrations.

The new banding methods [quinacrine (Q), modified giemsa (G), reverse giemsa (R) and constitutive chromatin (C)], including the Hoechst procedure of Latt,[4] provide us with finer tools for investigating the questions of specific "break sites" of chromosomes and of hidden exchanges between sister chromatids, as indicated by observations made with the Latt technique and documented in Bloom's syndrome cells.[5]

---

*Supported by grants from the National Institute of General Medical Sciences (GM 22052–01) and the Environmental Protection Agency (EPA-68 -02-1738).

Banding and EM methods, clearly, are powerful tools for probing the nature of chromosome structure and relating it to the molecular and physical nature of breaks.

CHROMOSOME BREAKAGE AND CANCER

Indirect epidemiologic evidence, based mainly on studies of radiation-exposed populations, including the atomic bomb survivors and radiation workers, suggests that human populations exposed to chromosome-breaking agents have an increased risk of neoplastic disease. Furthermore, cells with certain kinds of chromosomal aberrations have provided direct evidence for increased oncogenic virus sensitivity,[6] and several studies of the so-called "chromosomal breakage" syndromes, i.e., ataxia telangiectasia, Bloom's syndrome, Fanconi's anemia and xeroderma pigmentosum, have revealed an association between chromosomal instability and the development of cancer.

Patients with these disorders have a predisposition to tumor formation, in addition to extensive chromosomal breakage in several kinds of cells. Patients with ataxia, Fanconi's and Bloom's, furthermore, have other pathological similarities, e.g., cutaneous lesions, immunological deficiencies and retarded growth. Bloom's syndrome and ataxia telangiectasia, in particular, will serve as models of the biology of the breakage syndromes.

1. Bloom's syndrome

Patients with Bloom's have a telangiectatic, sun-sensitive, facial rash. They are small at birth and thereafter. IgA and IgM are reduced, and cell mediated immunity mechanisms are impaired.

Fifty patients are under surveillance for cancer.[7] Of the first 48 observed through 1971, 8 have developed cancer: 4 with leukemias, 3 with gastrointestinal tumors and 1 with carcinoma of the tongue. While the chromosome number and basic karyotype are normal, the proportion of skin, peripheral blood and bone marrow cells with abnormal configurations is increased. The major abnormalities include abnormal monocentric chromosomes, quadriradial figures, which are the most common and the aberration seen in all patients with Bloom's syndrome, and occasional dicentrics. Up to 14% of PHA-stimulated lymphocytes of patients with Bloom's syndrome may have aberrations, up to 10% of fibroblasts, compared to 1–2% of control fibroblast cultures, and those of the obligate carriers, have an intermediate proportion, 5–7%. German's observations of bone marrow cells suggest that the aberrations represent an in vivo phenomenon rather than in vitro instability.[8]

2. Ataxia Telangiectasia (AT)

Patients with AT become ataxic early in life and develop telangiectatic lesions of, first, the bulbar conjunctivae and, later, the face, neck, hands and legs. IgA and IgE levels are low and, again, cell mediated immunity is impaired. The neoplasias of AT are usually reticuloendothelial, including lymphomas, lymphosarcomas and leukemias.

The chromosome aberrations of AT lymphocytes include fragments, dicentrics and involvement of chromosome 14. The observations of Harnden,[9] Hecht[10] and others, that chromosome 14 is frequently involved in translocations in lymphocytes which form clones, is of related interest. Furthermore, breakage occurs in the cells of obligate carriers.

3. Mechanisms of Cancer Formation

The mechanism by which cancers arise in Bloom's syndrome and ataxia telangiectasia are apparently associated with immune mechanisms. The increased incidence of tumors in immunologically deficient patients[11] suggests that immunologic surveillance mechanisms are at fault or that their cells are predisposed to neoplastic transformation *in vivo* by radiation, chemicals or viruses, as they are *in vitro*. The tendency of AT lymphocytes to form clones is our best evidence that thay have an unusual potential for proliferation.

The lymphocyte clones of AT involve the D group chromosomes, in particular, the long arm of chromosome 14. Clonal evolution has been documented by serial observations of the patient's cells. The percentage of cells with a 14/14 translocation in McCaw and Hecht's patient, increased from 1−2 percent initially to 78 percent after 3.5 years. The evolution of the AT clone is analogous to that in chronic myelogenous leukemia, in which both cytogenetic evidence (Ph′ chromosome and 22/q translocation) and biochemical data (G6PD) support the thesis for a clonal origin of cancerous cells. Porokeratosis of Mibelli may involve the same clonal phenomenon.[12] A dominantly inherited disorder of later childhood, the clinical signs consist of multiple skin eruptions (cornoid lamella) on the limbs. The foci extend peripherally, with central areas of epidermal atrophy or hyperplasia. Sixteen epitheliomata have been described, originating from clones of single epidermal cells, provoked, perhaps, by external environmental agents.

It is reasonable to assume, therefore, that some tumors arise from precursor cells which are cytogenetically abnormal and that certain persons, those immunologically deficient, perhaps, are at risk when exposed to chromosome-altering agents.

FETAL IMPLICATIONS

The problems related to the effects of chromosome-breaking agents on the developing fetus are complex. The properties of chromosome-breaking and induction of malformations are clearly associated, in some instances, as, for example, the effects of drugs (amethopterin and methotrexate), viruses (rubella), radiations (x-rays, high energy gamma rays and neutrons) and environmental contaminants (mercury). While chromosome breakage may not be at the root of developmental anomalies, the association is frequent enough for us to suspect that agents which produce chromosome damage may produce teratogenic effects. On the other hand, the teratogen thalidomide has little cytogenetic effect.

One must also consider the possible carcinogenic effect of chromosomolytic agents on the fetus. Stewart and colleagues' observations suggest that intra-uterine, low doses of x-ray, received during pelvimetry, may cause a significant increase in leukemia during the first 10 years of childhood. Similar exposure to unknown environmental agents may also be important in the etiology of other neoplasias of childhood.

MONITORING BY THE FEDERAL GOVERNMENT

The evidence suggests that we formulate plans to protect the fetus and sensitive adult from the clinical effects of agents which damage human chromosomes. The federal government is in the best position to establish committees with responsibilities for developing and overseeing genetic evaluations of pharmaceuticals, food additives and environmental contaminants. Although several systems of laboratory analysis are available, systematic screening of human cell lines for cytogenetic abnormalities after exposure to known concentrations of the agents in question would be well worthwhile, as would screening cell lines for a limited number of biochemical mutations.

In time, screening of fetal tissue by amniocentesis for chromosome breakage may prove a feasible means of assessing the results of exposure to putative teratogens.

REFERENCES

1. M.M. Cohen and A.D. Bloom, *in* Monitoring, Birth Defects and Environment: The Problem of Surveillance, E.B. Hook, D.T. Janerich and I.H. Porter (Eds.), Academic Press, New York, pp. 249–272, 1971.

2. B.R. Brinkley and M.W. Shaw, *in* Genetic Concepts and Neoplasia, Williams and Wilkins, Baltimore, pp. 313–345, 1970.

3. D.E. Comings, *in* Advances in Human Genetics, H. Harris and K. Hirsch-

horn (Eds.), Vol. 3, Plenum Press, New York, pp. 237–431, 1972.

4.   S. A. Latt, *Proc. Nat. Acad. Sci. USA 70*, 3395, 1973.

5.   R.S.K. Chaganti, S. Schonberg and J. German, *Ibid. 71*, 4508, 1974.

6.   A.D. Bloom, *J. Pediat. 81*,1, 1972.

7.   A.D. Bloom, *in* Advances in Human Genetics, H. Harris and K. Hirsch-horn (Eds.), Vol. 3, Plenum Press, New York, pp. 99–172, 1972.

8.   J. German, *in* Chromosomes and Cancer, J. German (Ed.), Wiley, New York, pp. 601–617, 1974.

9.   D.G. Harnden, *Ibid.,* 619–636, 1974.

10.   F. Hecht, B.K. McCaw and R.D. Koler, *N. Engl. J. Med. 289,* 286, 1973.

11.   R.D.A. Peterson, W.D. Kelly and R.A. Good, *Lancet 1,* 1189, 1964.

12.   A.M.R. Raylor, D.G. Harnden and E.A. Fairburn, *J. Natl. Cancer Inst. 51,* 371, 1973.

DISCUSSION

LAWRENCE SHAPIRO: Dr. Bloom, are simple chromosome breaks or gaps significant in studies of potentially harmful agents? Are rearrangements and complex breaks weighed differently from simple breaks?

DR. BLOOM: It's quantitative. One can't really distinguish between the significance of complex breaks because the number of breaks necessary to induce them, i.e., dicentric or ring formation, is perhaps greater than the number of breaks required to produce simple chromatin deletions or simple chromatin breaks. Since the dicentric and ring are easier to see, they are a more objective measure. One should regard both kinds, however, with appropriate respect.

DR. HOOK: The early data of an increase in the simple break between 48 and 72 hours of culture suggested it was an artifact. The Scottish investigators, furthermore, found that the distance the drop of cell suspension fell on the slide affected the number of simple breaks. Certainly, the most complex breaks and rearrangements are more likely evidence of harmful agents since they are less likely to be artifactual.

DR. BLOOM: Strong and consistent base line data from your own laboratory are helpful in deciding whether simple breaks are significant. Radiation workers have used this simple kind of break as a valid indicator of chromatin disturbances as well as the more complex rearrangements. The more complex aberration is easier to find and, therefore, more useful in screening.

DR. LAMM: Dr. Oakley, what is the epidemiological and scientific evidence for a relationship of marijuana to breaks and defects?

DR. OAKLEY: We have not confirmed that exposure to this particular agent is the cause of birth defects. Although not yet implicated as dangerous, the drug is not known to be safe and, therefore, exposure before and during pregnancy should be avoided.

DR. BLOOM: Although the possibility exists that some individuals who use drugs have a tendency for chromosome breakage, the breakage in those individuals is not necessarily produced by marijuana.

MASON BARR (University of Michigan, Ann Arbor, Michigan): Dr. Hook, I might point out that nausea and vomiting of pregnancy (NVP) is not all that

199

innocuous. When the pregnant mother goes to the well-meaning physician he may give her something rather disasterous like thalidomide. Have you examined your data for the effects of treatment with the question of what drugs are given for nausea and vomiting? We are constantly being asked questions as to whether this or that is teratogenic.

DR. HOOK: No. I believe that there are published data on the possible teratogenicity of antiemetics in routine use. Thalidomide was used more as a tranquilizer and sedative than as an antiemetic. The published data on antiemetics suggested that they were not teratogenic. Most of the investigations of antiemetics have been accepted as being non-teratogenic. We may be suppressing an important symptom. In other words, it may not be a drug effect; we may be missing it because mothers who are taking the drug are likely to have benign outcomes because they may be reverting to the status of those who have no symptoms at all.

HAROLD KALTER (Children's Hospital Research Foundation, Cincinnati, Ohio): A few years ago we found a poor correlation between the prenatal induction of chemical teratogens or abnormalities and their chromosome aberration-producing tendencies in fetuses. You mentioned thalidomide as being a proven teratogen and a rather poor chromosome damager. The same is true of various other compounds examined in the laboratory. To draw inferences and apply it to man might be dangerous. Conversely, the human carcinogen — x-radiation — *protects* some animals from tumor formation. In our laboratories, for example, we've given a transplacental carcinogen to pregnant animals and those fetuses that had been irradiated a day or so before treatment of the mothers developed fewer tumors in postnatal life than those not irradiated. Again, an odd situation, but one that warns us against glib generalizations and easy transferences from one species to another.

There may not be much improvement in the tests you mention — somatic cells grown *in vitro*, for example. They, too, will have their complications and will require modifications to make them applicable.

RICHARD G. SKALKO (Birth Defects Institute, New York State Health Department, Albany, New York): This type of teratogenic interference also causes maternal hypoxia in gamma radiation — a type of interference of two noxious elements.

DR. BLOOM: I think that there are more examples of positive correlation between mutagenic agents, chromosome breakage and carcinogens than of negative, despite the exceptions. We should be able to prove that a compound is or is not teratogenic or carcinogenic if it damages chromosomes. Many compounds are capable of doing all three and should not go on the market without being tested properly. The risk of teratogenicity is there if it breaks chromosomes. The drug companies should prove that the agents which damage chromosomes do not also produce fetal damage. That is not saying, however, that every agent that produces chromosome damage will be teratogenic.

Fibroblast cells are a good source of human material. They lend themselves readily to the kind of systematic study that could be carried out appropriately by regulatory agencies.

PHILIP L. TOWNES (University of Rochester, Rochester, New York): Dr. Bloom, how can we establish whether a given drug has a significant breaking potential? I am sure that any drug at any given dose will be a "breaker", like caffeine. How can we ever decide this issue?

DR. BLOOM: The technique must establish in the *in vitro* system the likely *in vivo* level. One must also weigh the potential advantages of the drug against the potential risk. If one can choose among drugs, as one can in treating congestive heart failure, one might choose the non-chromosome breaking rather than the chromosome breaking one. On the other hand, if the drug is lifesaving for the patient, its potential teratogenicity is of secondary importance. When safer drugs are available, there is no need, for example, to continue proliferating compounds, like thalidomide, which may be potentially dangerous.

DR. HOOK: A distinction should be made between *in vivo* and *in vitro* observations. *In vitro* observations are far less informative of the actual problem than studies of populations known to be exposed to a suspect agent, like LSD and marijuana, matched with control groups.

DR. OAKLEY: Although *in vitro* systems have their value in studying teratogenic potential, there are apparently no instances of a causal relationship between chromosome breakage and the mechanism producing birth defects. Fanconi's anemia, in which breakage occurs *in utero*, a reduction deformity occurs which is always the same, and the gene product may be missing. If the defect were due to chromosome breakage, a variety of birth defects would develop.

ALLEN BREGNAN (State University of New York, New Paltz, New York): Dr. Oakley, what is the FDA's policy on brand names or substances containing vinyl chloride?

DR. OAKLEY: Apparently the FDA or other regulatory agencies can't release "proprietary information" because of a legal issue. On the other hand, the companies themselves might list their products.

SECTION V

MATERNAL STARVATION AND BIRTH DEFECTS *

Zena Stein
Mervyn Susser

In spite of the attention given to the influence of malnutrition on mental performance and on birth defects in recent years, in human beings it has proved difficult to demonstrate effects of undernutrition and even starvation on the developing brain. Studies of intrauterine development of the fetus have not succeeded in proving such effects. The problem of specifying and assessing nutritional intake in free-living human populations has not been solved. It is equally difficult to separate the experience of malnutrition from the poverty with which it is usually associated. There are also several theoretical problems which may have contributed to the difficulty; e.g., the prenatal growth phase may not be a large enough part of the growth period for malnutrition to exhaust brain reserves. Above a threshold level of malnutrition, the fetus may be buffered by maternal stores. In the study discussed by David Rush, we devised an experimental approach to the problem.[1]

The authors, with Gerhart Saenger and Francis Marolla, report a study in the Netherlands[2,3] in which the experience of a six-month period of famine and its after-effects could be isolated from the wider environment. The circumstances of the famine in the Netherlands, from October, 1944 to May, 1945, enabled us to relate maternal starvation during pregnancy to fertility and the course of the pregnancy, to birth weight, to mortality during early and later years, and to health status and mental performance in young men.

The Dutch famine was remarkable in three respects:

First, a famine has seldom occurred where extensive, reliable and valid data have been available to document the vital and health statistics of the population. We were able to find records of births and deaths, details of pregnancies and births from certain teaching maternity hospitals and complete records from the military induction process of all young men at 19 years.

---

*This work has been supported by the National Institutes of Health Grants: HD04454-02, HD06751 and HD00322.

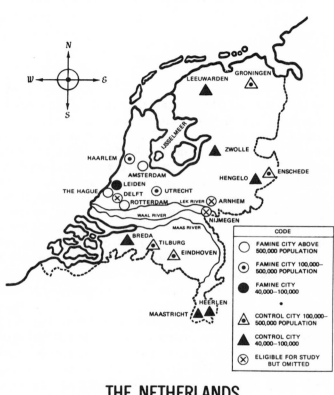

THE NETHERLANDS

N.Y. STATE DEP'T OF HEALTH

MARCH 1975

Fig. 1. Map of the Netherlands: cities selected for study.
Source: Stein, Susser, Saenger and Marolla.[3]

Second, the famine was sharply circumscribed in time and place. Usually, the onset and termination of famine is gradual but the Dutch famine started and ended abruptly. On September 17, 1944, British paratroops landed at Arnhem in an attempt to force a bridgehead across the Rhine (Fig. 1). In response to a call from the London-based Dutch government in exile, the Dutch railway workers went on strike to support the paratroop landings, an heroic effort since they knew what the consequences would be if the Allied attempt on the bridgehead should fail, as indeed it did. In reprisal, the Nazis imposed a transport embargo on Western Holland and a severe winter froze the barges in the canals and no food reached the large cities. Thus, we can date the onset of the famine to the latter part of September and the beginning of October, 1944. The relief occurred with the arrival of the liberating armies, on May 6, 1945.

The famine was also circumscribed in place: it affected the western part of Holland and it was principally the cities, Amsterdam, Rotterdam, Leiden, The Hague, Utrecht and Delft, and not the rural areas, which were affected.

The third unusual feature of the famine was that the nutritional deprivation was rather precisely described. The official food rations (which covered all aspects of the diet from 1942 onwards) could be analyzed in some detail. Of course, the rations did not comprise the whole diet and not all people could buy them.

Unquestionably, the famine was truly severe. At the worst times, official rations were four or five hundred calories *per day*. Calories declined gradually through November, the famine grew severe in December and reached its height in February, March and April. On May 6, 1945, the Allied army entered the cities of Holland and brought relief. A nutrition relief team accompanied the troops and documented the anguish of the starving population. They estimated the numbers who had died of starvation, the weakness and apathy of those lying helpless in their homes and the numbers with acute hunger edema lying in hospital beds waiting to die.

Our task was to document the effects of exposure to maternal starvation during intrauterine life. Briefly, we created an historical cohort design (Fig. 3). and we argued that if there are adverse effects of intrauterine exposure to maternal starvation, then the phase at which the maternal starvation took place is likely to be important. We assumed that those born in a particular month would have been conceived 280 days earlier. Next, we defined certain birth cohorts as time controls; namely, those born *before* (A1, A2) and *after* (E1, E2) the event of the famine. For cohorts exposed during gestation, we distinguished B1, B2 and C cohorts as those exposed during the third trimester (with B2 having maximum exposure during the height of the famine). Cohort C and D1 were exposed during the second trimester; D1 and especially D2

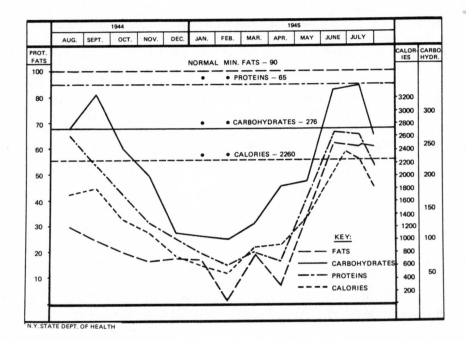

Fig. 2. Course of the rationing in average quarterly figures of the food-stuffs distributed to persons with a normal consumption of food, expressed in the quantities of calories by means of protein, fats and carbohydrates, supplied to the western parts of the Netherlands during the years 1941 up to 1945 inclusive. Derived from data supplied by the Board of Agriculture, Fishery and Food Supply, Directorate of the Food Supply. Section Statistics.

Source: reproduced from Malnutrition and Starvation in Western Netherlands, Berger, Drummond and Sandstead, 1948, Part 1, p. 6.

Desired norms, according to Dr. N. v. Eekelen and Prof. Dr. B.C.P. Jansen (*Journal of Nutrition,* 1-15, October, 1929).

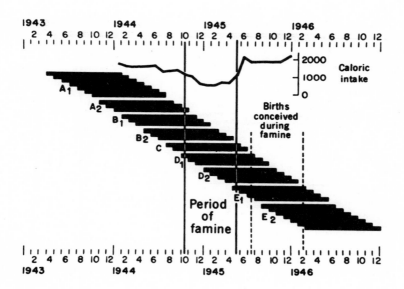

Fig. 3. Design of Study. Cohorts by month of conception and month of birth in the Netherlands, 1943 through 1946, related to calories in the rations of famine cities. Solid vertical lines bracket the period of famine and broken vertical lines bracket the period of births conceived during famine.

Source: Stein Susser, Saenger and Marolla.[2]

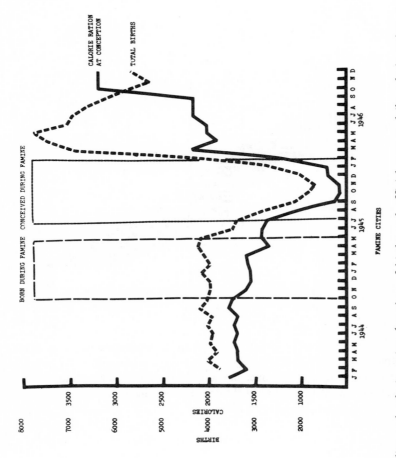

Fig. 4. Fertility and calorie ration (number of births and official average daily caloric ration at estimated time of conception for the period June 1944 to December 1946 inclusive in (A) famine cities, (B) Northern control cities and (C) Southern control cities. Source: Stein, Susser, Saenger and Marolla.[3]

210

were exposed to maternal starvation early in pregnancy. The cohort design thus provides time controls. We also allowed for *place* controls by selecting comparison populations from birth cohorts in the cities unaffected by the famine, matched with the famine cohorts for date of birth.

In order to examine the hypothesis that early starvation during pregnancy can affect the developing nervous system, let us consider some findings relating to various times in the course of development.

The first stage is the effect of the famine on fertility. Briefly, the birth rate nine months after the most acute period of the famine (February, March and April, 1945) was seriously affected (Fig. 4). There was a period of severe infertility. For many of those who were conceived during this period, early gestation occurred at a time when their parents were almost certainly starving. For many other couples at that time, fertility was impossible.

The information about the course of pregnancy is taken from five teaching hospitals. Three are from the famine cities of Rotterdam, Amsterdam, Leiden; one, Heerlen, is a non-famine city from the south; and one, Groningen, a non-famine city from the north. We have analyzed extant records of these hospitals. First, we analyzed birth weight (Fig. 5). The mean birth weight declined for those exposed to the famine during the third trimester. Our interest is in the D2 cohort, exposed to the famine early in pregnancy. The mean birth weight of this cohort was not low in any of the three areas. Hence, the birth weight recovered if the mother was exposed to starvation early in pregnancy but was given adequate food in the second and third trimesters. In spite of these reassuring results, however, the standard deviation for birth weight was higher in the D2 cohort than in any other cohort. This increase in SD was accounted for by a higher proportion of babies with birth weights less than 2500 grams in the maternity hospitals. In this cohort in the famine area we expected 25 babies of low birth weight and we observed 35. This number does not reach statistical significance but it was the highest proportion of low birth weight babies among the cohorts in famine or control areas.

Next, the duration of the gestation apparently is not influenced by famine exposure in the third trimester (Fig. 6) but in the D2 cohort exposed to famine early in gestation, there is a tendency for a decline in mean length of gestation. Again, this decline is not statistically significant but, again, the standard deviation for duration of gestation in the D2 cohort is higher than in the other cohorts.

The slightly higher proportion of babies with very low birth weight and perhaps reduced length of gestation, while not statistically significant, might reflect true biological differences in this cohort. We were concerned, however, that our assignment of a date of conception from the date of birth might have distorted the results. Therefore, we reanalyzed the data by using the reported

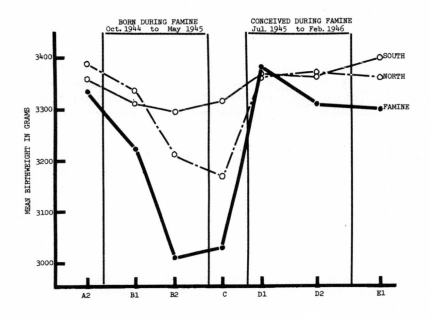

Fig. 5. Birth weight by time and place (mean birth weight in grams for births in maternity hospitals for seven birth cohorts: famine, Northern control and Southern control areas compared for the period August 1944 to March 1946 inclusive).

Source: stein, Susser, Saenger and Marolla.[3]

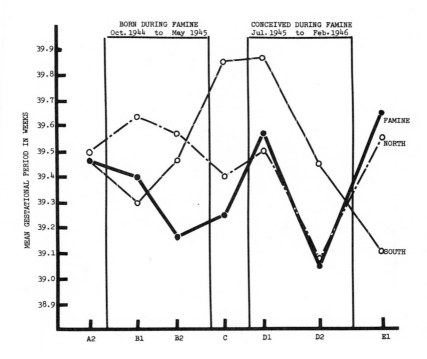

Fig. 6. Length of gestation by time and place (mean weeks of gestation for births in maternity hospitals, for seven birth cohorts, Northern control and Southern control areas compared for the period August 1944 to March 1946 inclusive).

Source: Stein, Susser, Saenger and Marolla.[3]

213

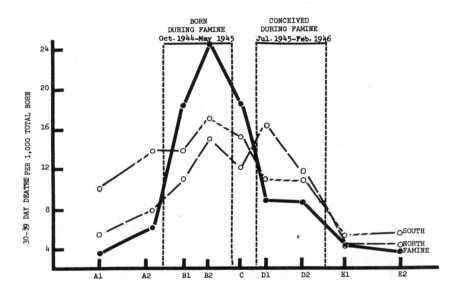

Fig. 7. Deaths at 30 to 89 days by time and place (deaths at 30 to 89 days per 1,000 total births: famine, Northern control and Southern control areas by cohort for births January 1944 to December 1946.

Source: Stein, Susser, Saenger and Marolla.[3]

214

last menstrual period to assign date of conception. The reanalysis confirmed the results for birth weight and length of gestation. For those mothers with LMP at the height of the famine, there were 9% of infants weighing less than 2500 grams, when 5% were expected.

Next, we considered mortality. The year 1945 was a period of extraordinarily high infant mortality in the Netherlands. We went to great pains to describe this mortality and to see if it could be attributed to the experience of intrauterine maternal starvation. Although exposure to third trimester maternal starvation (that is, cohorts B1, B2 and C) was associated with a lower birth weight, the stillbirth rate was not raised. The death rate during the first week was slightly raised; however, there was an enormous increase in deaths from 30 to 89 days (Fig. 7). This high death rate was much in excess of any rise in control areas for the same cohorts; the excess can be attributed to intrauterine starvation in the third trimester.

The cohort conceived during the famine (the D2 cohort), did not experience high post neonatal mortality. When we examine the stillbirth rate, however, there is a sharp peak for those conceived during the starvation period and this is also true for deaths during the first week (Fig. 8). Although these effects also occur, to some extent, in other parts of the country, the rise is more marked for the famine area. We are, therefore, inclined to attribute at least part of this raised stillbirth and first week mortality to intrauterine starvation during the first trimester. The fact that there was a rise, although a lesser one, in control areas suggests the presence of interaction between famine exposure and some other prenatal factor.

With regard to the cause of death, one category, "prematurity", is interesting because it is rather specific in the international classification of diseases of that time. Prematurity is a cause of death limited by definition to babies whose birth weight is less than 2500 grams. Here there is a contrast between the birth cohorts (Fig. 9). The babies of low birth weight exposed late in pregnancy (B1, B2, C cohorts) had a two-fold risk of deaths assigned to prematurity, and the excess deaths for that cause occurred *after* the first week of life and up to three months of age. Those exposed early in pregnancy (the D2 cohort), however, had a risk of death assigned to prematurity that was increased five-fold within the first week of life, and not later. So, even within the crude ICD categories of cause of death, we can distinguish two different syndromes of low birth weight: one syndrome occurred in those exposed to intrauterine starvation early in pregnancy, probably with premature delivery and very low birth weight; it resulted in an excess of stillbirths and of deaths during the first week. Another syndrome occurred in infants exposed during the third trimester of pregnancy, without a reduction in length of gestation but with lowered mean birth weight; they

215

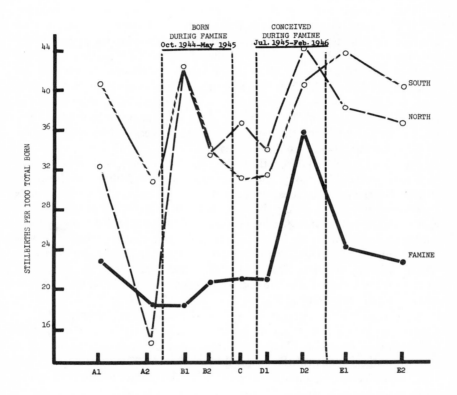

Fig. 8. Stillbirths by time and place (stillbirths per 1,000 total births: famine, Northern control and Southern control areas by cohort for births January 1944 to December 1946.

Source: Stein, Susser, Saenger and Marolla.[3]

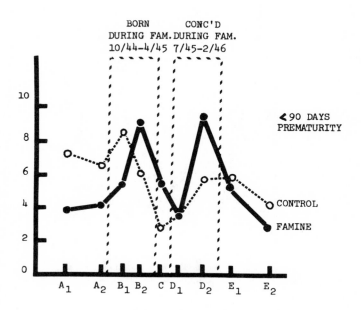

Fig. 9. Cohort deaths by cause and area: Prematurity.
Source: Stein, Susser, Saenger and Marolla.[3]

217

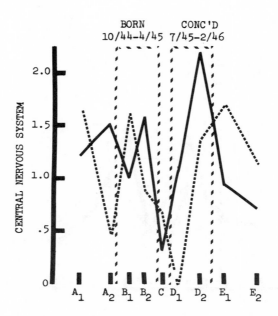

Fig. 10.   Congenital Anomalies of the Central Nervous System (ICD 751-753): ICD code assigned at military induction examinations in rates per 1,000 for nine successive cohorts in famine cities and in northern and southern control cities combined.

Source: Stein, Susser, Saenger and Marolla.[3]

suffered an excess of deaths assigned to "prematurity" only after the first week of life; many other deaths assigned to other causes probably belong to the same syndrome, since they, too, were associated with fetal growth retardation.

For deaths between one and 18 years, the single finding that related to famine exposure occurred in the D2 cohort exposed early in pregnancy. In that cohort, there is a rise in the death rate due to diseases of the central nervous system (but not to congenital anomalies). Most of these deaths were listed as meningitis. This may be a chance finding. On the other hand, it may be a secondary cause of death hiding information about underlying central nervous system anomalies. A result from the data on the military induction examination gives grounds for this suspicion.

We have standard records on all Dutch men called up in their nineteenth year for psychological, medical and physical examination. Unlike the American draft, in which a man may be exempted before examination, in the Netherlands, a man must be examined. Each disorder discovered is classified according to the ICD code (1948). Forty percent of all men were assigned a coded diagnosis. We have analyzed the incidence of various diagnoses, in relation to intrauterine famine exposure (Fig. 10). There is only one group of conditions (central nervous system anomalies) that shows any relationship at all to famine exposure and only one cohort was affected; namely the group exposed to severe famine early in gestation (D2). Four cases of spina bifida and hydrocephalus were expected and eight cases were found. The excess is significant at the five percent level. The relative risk is two. The attributable risk is, of course, small.

In conclusion, we have carried out extensive studies of the effects of maternal starvation in a large population of young men. With one exception, we demonstrated no detectable effects of exposure to famine on various measures of mental performance, physical stature or disorders of health in this investigation. Of the many outcomes measured in this adult population, the one which varied in frequency with prenatal exposure to famine was the incidence of congenital disorders of the central nervous system diagnosed at military induction. The time relations as well as the process of development require that this outcome was determined early in gestation. The numbers affected are small. Those born in the cohort in the famine area were not large (3600 men) because they were conceived during a phase of infertility and the disorders are rare.

We have noted several other effects on the D2 cohort, which was exposed to the height of the famine early in gestation. Each effect was not remarkable in magnitude and some were not statistically significant but, taken together, they form the elements of a plausible sequence: this begins with nutritional deprivation of the mother, which interferes with the development of the central nervous system during the first trimester of pregnancy, leads to premature birth with low birth weight and ends either with perinatal death or with death from meningitis at later ages (perhaps complicating spina bifida or hydrocephalus) or with survival into adulthood, despite the presence of central nervous system anomalies. It is likely that nutritional deprivation did not act alone to produce this sequence of events. We noted, in particular, that the stillbirth and death rates during the first week, raised in the D2 cohort, were raised in control areas as well as in the total famine cohorts, if to a lesser degree. On the other hand, the excess of early deaths from prematurity and congenital central nervous system anomalies in the D2 cohort and also the excess of congenital CNS disorders in surviving adults are special to the famine area.

The population born of this cohort was of average birth weight and dimensions, was healthy intellectually and physically and was of higher social class than those born before or after. The phenomena we have described affected a small number of individuals among the large cohorts studied. It is possible that most of the affected fetuses did not survive and the survivors represent only a small residual group that is left to tell the tale.

Lastly, the Dutch famine induced acute and shortlived maternal starvation. Effects of chronic malnutrition may not be the same. Thus, chronic malnutrition has no clear effect on fertility, while it almost certainly does have an effect on adult stature, and it is possible that it may affect mental performance. In the Dutch famine, unequivocal effects were, on the one hand, those of third trimester exposure on fetal growth and early infant mortality, and on the other hand, those of first trimester exposure on gestation, perinatal mortality and development of the central nervous system.

REFERENCES

1. D. Rush, Z.A. Stein, G. Christakis and M. Susser, Proceedings of the Symposium on Nutrition and Fetal Development, M. Winick (Ed.), Wiley, New York, 1972.

2. Z.A. Stein, M. Susser, G. Saenger and F. Marolla, *Science 178*, 708, 1972.

3. Z.A. Stein, M.W. Susser, G. Saenger and F.A. Marolla, Famine and Human Development: The Dutch Hunger Winter of 1944/45, Oxford University Press, New York, 1975.

RISK FACTORS FOR CONGENITAL HEART DISEASE
A PROSPECTIVE STUDY*

Olli P. Heinonen

INTRODUCTION

In general, congenital anomalies are thought to account for about 75%[1] of all heart disease in childhood, and cardiovascular lesions have been estimated as being present in about 0.8% of all births.[2]

Genetic factors,[3] chromosomal aberrations — particularly trisomy 21,[4] maternal rubella and diabetes[5] and exposure to thalidomide during pregnancy[6] — are all well established risk factors for congenital heart disease in man. In animals, hypoxia[7] and azo dyes[8] have been shown experimentally to cause cardiac malformations. Most of these factors have been linked with more than one specific congenital defect.

Close observation of the cardiovascular system in newborn babies and in children during the early years of life, together with examination of the backgrounds of these children represents one approach to the problem of multifactorial etiology in humans. Basic requirements of such an approach include proper selection of persons for study and collection of carefully documented observations in sufficiently large groups of mothers and their children, followed from the time of conception to an age when virtually all cardiovascular malformations will have been diagnosed. Unfortunately, in the context of day-to-day clinical practice, it is seldom possible to achieve these objectives. However, when they are feasible, analyses of non-experimental follow-up materials by modern techniques may well yield clues for further research. Such clues may result in better understanding and, possibly, ultimate control of at least some of the factors leading to cardiovascular malformations.

*Supported by a contract (NO1-NS-2-2322) with the National Institute of Neurological Diseases and Stroke, U.S. Public Health Service; a contract (NO1-GM-4-2148) with the National Institute of General Medical Sciences, U.S. Public Health Service and by the Food and Drug Administration.

TABLE 1

Background of the Study Cohort

	No of Mother-Child Pairs
Pregnant women seen in participating hospitals: 1959–1965	132,560
Women registered into the study, including special groups	58,828
Women registered in accordance with the universal sampling scheme	55,908
Mother-child pairs followed	52,931
Cohort, omitting abortions and ectopic pregnancies	51,977
Study cohort after exclusions	50,282

This presentation describes, among 50,282 mother-child pairs, the background of 404 children in whom the cardiovascular system was found to be defective.

PARTICIPANTS AND METHODS

The data used in the analyses presented here are part of the Collaborative Perinatal Project.[9]

Twelve university medical centers participated in the collection of data on pregnant women selected for study during a period of seven years, from January 2, 1959 to December 31, 1965. These medical centers also collected data on the outcomes of pregnancies. The offspring have been followed to school age and follow-up is continuing. Fourteen hospitals affiliated with the universities were involved, and in Boston and Philadelphia, separate obstetric and pediatric hospitals participated.

Selection of the Participants

The participants in the study were selected from the obstetric patients admitted to collaborating hospital clinics. The selection procedures were not uniform in all hospitals; they were modified because of considerations such as the capacity of each center to commit its resources to the study for one-and-a-half decades, the degree of interference with the different routines of the maternity clinics and the individual interests of researchers in each institution.

In all hospitals, for women to be eligible for acceptance into the sampling frame, certain constraints were imposed. Common disqualifications were a woman's intentions to leave the area; certain geographic areas of residence; and delivery on the same day as first registration into the study — so-called "walk-in" cases. With these predefined limitations, there were 132,560 gravidas in the sampling frame available for study before the local selection scheme for entry was applied (Table 1).

In two of the hospitals, all presenting gravidas in the sampling frame were entered into the study; in nine hospitals systematic selection was based upon the terminal digit of the patient number, or the woman's day of birth or on some similar selection device; and in one hospital random selection was used. If a woman had more than one pregnancy at a collaborating hospital during the time interval for recruitment to the study, she could be admitted as a participant more than once.

Depending on the special interests of individual centers, it was permissible, to an agreed extent, to enroll and collect data as a routine part of the study, for certain distinct groups. For example, one special group consisted of all gravidas under 16 years of age seen at Johns Hopkins. For gravidas registered according to the principal scheme of the study, the sampling ratio was approximately 2 out of 5 eligible pregnancies at this hospital.

In all, 58,828 pregnancies were registered in the study (Table 1). Of these, 2,622 were members of special groups, 198 were "walk-ins", while 55,908 registrants conformed strictly with the selection rules. The correctly selected proportion of women registered into the study in each hospital ranged from 14% to 100% of those initially available for recruitment in the sampling frame. In each of the participating institutions, the sample correctly enrolled in the study did not differ with regard to age, ethnic group, marital status, or weeks of gestation at admission, as compared with the total group of women who initially formed the sampling frame.[9]

Certain correctly selected registrants could not be followed: in most of these instances, the gravida refused to participate or she moved and could not be traced; or sometimes, for one or another reason, no information concerning labor, delivery or the offspring could be obtained. In all, this loss to follow-up affected 2,977 mother-child pairs (5.3%) and reduced the sample from 55,908 to 52,931 mother-child pairs. While there were no statistically significant differences between the non-responders and responders with regard to age, ethnic group, marital status and weeks of gestation at registration, the non-responders were, overall, slightly more commonly well-educated, married and over the age of 35 years than the responders. However, these differences were not consistent by the hospital.

There were 954 pregnancies (1.7%) that terminated in spontaneous abortion before the 20th week after the last menstrual period, or in therapeutic abortion, ectopic pregnancy or hydatidiform mole. This reduced the study cohort to 51,977 mother-child pairs (Table 1).

Finally, for purposes of this report, certain exclusions, representing a total of 1,695 pregnancies (3.3%), were stipulated for the following overlapping reasons: twin and triplet pregnancies (1.2%); mother's ethnic group other than White, Black or Puerto Rican (1.0%); important pertinent data (e.g., diseases and/or obstetric complications prior to delivery; sex of child not available (1.0%); and clinically evident maternal rubella during pregnancy and/or congenital rubella syndrome in the offspring (0.2%). Thus, 50,282 mother-child pairs in which the pregnancy lasted five lunar months or longer, including children who survived or died during the follow-up period, were ultimately available for analysis.

Data Collection

For the general purposes of the study, information on the prospective mother's social and medical background, co-existing diseases and complications of pregnancy was recorded in a systematic and standardized manner. Similarly, data concerning the child's birth, development, any diseases that occurred and any congenital defects that were noted were also collected, according to systematic design, up to the eighth birthday. Information on the child's siblings, father and other relatives was obtained.

This presentation is based on data concerning cardiovascular malformations identified during an average follow-up period of four years after birth. The data also include cardiovascular defects found at autopsy in non-survivors from twenty weeks of gestation up to the fourth birthday in the entire cohort. In addition, autopsy data in a segment of the cohort registered during the earlier years of the study have been included if the child died after the fourth birthday and was found to have a cardiovascular defect. Overall, autopsy was carried out in 81% of those children who died.

On entry to the study, usually while visiting the participating clinic the first time during the pregnancy, each woman was interviewed by a specially trained examiner to obtain medical, genetic and social data. A medication history covering the time from the last menstrual period was also obtained. Detailed, structured forms were used and the data collection procedure was guided by use of extensive manuals (available on request from the Perinatal Research Branch, NINDS, NIH, Bethesda, Maryland 20014). Initially, at monthly visits to the clinic and then at shorter intervals during the last trimester. Interviewers and obstetricians continued to collect standardized data. The completed study forms were then reviewed and compared with the hospital records for completeness by another person. If the women had received medical attention before entry into the study, further information on events taking place prior to registration was acquired from "non-study" physicians and from hospitals partly to complement and partly to verify certain items of interview data. Completed forms were once more edited in the study hospital, this time by attending medical personnel. The assembled material was then sent to a central facility where it was processed into computer files. Once again, various precautionary measures were taken to prevent coding and punching errors in the massive flow of data. In addition, certain computer procedures were routinely used to identify and correct obvious mistakes in the original computer files.

Information on the offspring was collected from birth and processed in a similar manner. The first period of systematic data collection covered the baby's stay in the hospital. Among other things, the baby was examined by a pediatrician every day during the first week after delivery or weekly if the child remained in the hospital longer. In addition to the detailed forms, a summary for this period was produced locally.

The mother was interviewed for what was termed an "interval history" when the child was 4, 8, 12, 18 and 24 months old and thereafter, annually. If, in the interim, there had been visits to physician or hospital, further data about the child's illness were acquired from these sources. An extensive, standardized pediatric examination was performed on all participants at the age of one year. The response rate for the one-year examination was 91% of the surviving children. For most of the remaining children, an interval history was available.

The method of ascertaining cardiovascular defects was somewhat different from that used to obtain data on other congenital anomalies recorded in the study. Before the one-year follow-up had been completed for all surviving children, the existing computer files, interim reports and records of children known to have died were searched for diagnoses of definite or possible congenital heart disease. In each participating institution, searches were organized under the personal supervision of one physician. Local study personnel scanned forms that were still awaiting processing and a pediatric cardiologist reviewed records of cardiac clinics and other records in an attempt to find every child even suspected of having a cardiovascular defect. When all the potential cases identified from the above sources were listed, about 90% of the surviving children were re-examined. In addition, all autopsy protocols were reviewed: 35% of the preserved hearts were re-examined by an independent pathologist and additional confirmation of the diagnosed lesions was sought by the reviewing pathologist personally interviewing the pathologist who had originally performed the autopsy.

The thoroughness of the methods of ascertainment is reflected in the fact that a diagnosis of cardiovascular defect was based, in more than half of the cases, on either autopsy, cardiac surgery or cardiac catheterization. In over 90% of the remaining cases, a pediatric cardiologist confirmed the diagnosis after personally examining the patient. Even among the small number of children who were not re-examined by a cardiologist, the evidence for a cardiovascular birth defect was considered to be firm.

After the extensive exploration to find cardiovascular defects was completed, further follow-up material was subsequently computerized. Search of the files revealed a few cases not previously suspected of having cardiovascular defects. The original records of these children were reviewed and those found to have definite diagnoses were included into the outcome group with cardiovascular defects.

Malformation other than those affecting the cardiovascular system were considered to be sufficiently accurate when an individual diagnosis was recorded in at least two of the following independent computer files: nursery period summary; summary of the period after discharge from the nursery up to one year of age and the autopsy file. Alternatively, when the diagnoses were not identical in the various files or when they were recorded in only one of them, the original case records were reviewed by hand and the diagnosed

226

malformation was only considered acceptable if the record was unequivocal in terms of predetermined criteria. Certain malformations were ignored because they were considered trivial: for example, accessory nipples, which showed extremely variable rates by hospital, were not considered.

Preparation of the Data for Analysis

For the specific purposes of the present study, in order to gain maximal efficiency in data retrieval and analysis, all cardiovascular diagnoses were re-coded to allow immediate access to classifications in terms of broad embryologic entities (*e.g.,* conus arteriosus syndrome),[10] clinical syndromes (*e.g.,* Fallot's tetralogy) and specific lesions (*e.g.,* pulmonic valvular stenosis).

Each coded cardiovascular entity was evaluated for variability by hospital and by ethnic group. Overall, the total cardiovascular malformation rate showed a fairly uniform distribution in the 12 hospitals and in the three ethnic groups, with one exception: isolated ventricular septal defect was diagnosed more commonly in the Children's Hospital, University of Buffalo, than elsewhere. The excess was partly accounted for by children with definite openings in the ventricular septum at birth followed by definite spontaneous closure. As expected, atrial septal defects, while less common, showed conaiderable variability in rates between the hospitals.

Among the large array of recorded factors for each mother-child pair, all maternal diseases present during pregnancy were selected for analysis. In addition, other factors were selected. Some of these were chosen on the basis of existing suspicion in the medical literature of an adverse effect on normal embryogenesis (*e.g.,* smoking status); others were chosen because of biological similarities with reported risk factors. For example, since hypoxia is believed to interfere with the normal development of the fetal heart, complications of pregnancy, such as vena cava syndrome, that may intermittently stimulate this condition, were considered. Certain factors were chosen for their intrinsic interest (*e.g.,* social class) and some were chosen for technical reasons (*e.g.,* hospital).

For each item, distributions of the recorded values (*e.g.,* maternal age, birthweight) were scrutinized. In addition, data were checked for internal consistency. Questionable or conflicting values were checked in the original source documents and, if necessary, corrected accordingly. For most data items it was only necessary to check and correct a small proportion of the material and the corrections were mostly of minor importance. Nevertheless, the total number of records that had to be processed increased as the number of factors under scrutiny increased. However, in contrast to other data items, all data related to dates, such as duration of pregnancy, showed both considerable variability and inconsistency with, for example, birthweight. About 10% of the entire

227

material had to be examined in order to check the dates and more than half of these had to be corrected. Erroneous dates showed clear concentration around the New Year.

In multivariate analysis, missing information gives rise to difficulties and proper analytical treatment is generally costly. A considerable effort was therefore made to ensure the greatest possible completeness of the data. Often, data on the same or on a similar item was available from more than one source. For example, the genetic history obtained for each child contained information on stillborn siblings and half-siblings: this information could be used to substitute for missing information in the mother's reproductive history. An additional method used to minimize the amount of missing information was to examine successive data in women who registered into the study during more than one pregnancy. For example, if, during the current pregnancy, the gravida did not have a recorded smoking history, but was known from a later pregnancy never to have smoked, this was considered to apply to all pregnancies: likewise, if the mother's height was only recorded once, this variable was applied to all of the registered pregnancies.

Generally, missing information was randomly distributed but there were some exceptions. Placental weight and the number of umbilical arteries were unknown during the earlier years because routine registration of these variables was only introduced after the study had been in progress for some time. Thus, unknown values of these variables were clearly not random with respect to time of entry. To give another example, there were some women accepted into the study because their gestation period exceeded twenty weeks, but who in clinical terms, had spontaneous abortions often only a day or two after registration. Understandably, it was quite common for a large proportion of the data items concerning these pregnancies to be missing. However, as mentioned earlier, it was unusual for crucial information to be missing and only 484 mother-child pairs to whom this applied were excluded from analysis.

The analytical pathways utilized in this study required that the values of all variables be classified in categories. Maternal age, for example, was classified by half decade from below the age of 15 years to 45 years and over. In general, extreme values were considered to be of particular interest and were kept in separate categories; otherwise, relatively broad categories were created.

Certain variables concerned recorded symptoms and signs in the mother. Some of these were relatively easy to categorize (e.g., various signs and symptoms of urinary tract infection with concomitant fever) while others were more difficult. For example, certain signs and symptoms are generally regarded as forming the poorly defined complex of toxemia: these signs and symptoms were categorized according to hierarchical classification based on severity.

All categories were created without knowledge of how the cardiovascular defects, or other defects, distributed in each of them.

Data Analysis

Children with cardiovascular defects were considered to be sufficiently evenly distributed in the participating hospitals to justify combining the data in the analysis.

Every maternal disease present during pregnancy was evaluated to determine whether it was related to the risk of giving birth to a child with a cardiovascular defect. The cardiovascular malformation rate in children born to mothers having the disease was compared with the rate in children born to those mothers who did not. If the ratio of the two rates was close to unity (relative risk approximately 1.0), this indicated lack of association between the disease in question and cardiovascular malformations, and such a disease did not have to be considered further.

Over fifty factors, other than maternal diseases, previously selected for analysis without knowledge of whether they were related to cardiovascular defects, were examined. Most of the factors were divided into several categories. To compute the relative risk, the category that was considered normal on medical grounds or, alternatively, the category that was closest to the median, was selected as the reference. For example, since the median duration of gestation fell in the range of nine to ten lunar months, the relative risks for children born to mothers in other duration categories were derived accordingly.

The above-mentioned sets of comparisons between rates were, in all instances, carried out separately within each ethnic group and a summary relative risk estimate, using a maximum likelihood method, was computed. The approximate 95% confidence limits for the relative risk were estimated.

Factors that were associated, after adjustment for the influence of ethnic group, with cardiovascular defects in the children — *i.e.,* covariates of defects — were identified and selected for further analysis. When the covariates of congenital heart disease had been isolated in this way, the categories were combined to reduce their number, as much as possible, whenever rates were reasonably similar. Ordinal scaling was applied only if the rate of congenital heart disease was monotonically related to ordered categories of a given variable (*e.g.,* values of 0, 1 and 3 were assigned to decreasing ranges of birthweight). In all other circumstances, binary scaling (0, 1) was used.

The variables, re-coded in this way, were subjected to Fisher's linear discriminant function analysis. Certain variables were highly correlated with each other: in the presence of their covariates, some of these variables showed no discriminating ability between children with and without cardiovascular defects (increasing relative weight of the mother, for example, failed to discriminate in the presence of its covariate, advancing age). Such factors were eliminated and the discriminant function analysis was then repeated retaining only variables not eliminated in this way.

Finally, in order to derive relative risk estimates of congenital heart disease for the relevant factors in this cohort, another mathematical model was applied. For this purpose, a multiple logistic risk function model was selected. This model was first developed for epidemiologic research by Cornfield[11] and has since been utilized with certain computational modifications[12-14] to meet the needs of a variety of study objectives. The multiple logistic risk function computes, for each study unit, the probability of an event (such as congenital heart disease) conditional on the values of its covariates $(x_1, x_2, ..., x_k)$ associated with that study unit (*e.g.*, the "profile" or set of k variable-values for a mother-child pair), as

$$p(x_1, x_2, ..., x_k) = (1 + \exp[-\beta_0 - \sum_{i=1}^{K} \beta_i x_i])^{-1}$$

Unknown coefficients, β_0, β_1, ..., β_K, were estimated by a maximum likelihood method. A detailed description of the computations has been recently published.[15] The coding of the variables used in the discriminant function analysis was maintained in multiple logistic risk function analysis using the same ordinal values or binary scaling. To assist in finding initial estimates for solution of the maximum likelihood equations for β_i, the results of the linear discriminant function were used.[12] However, discriminant function coefficients with large absolute values were trimmed — often to half or less — in order to improve convergence. Four to five cycles were needed for the final results.

To check the adequacy of the multiple logistic model, the probability of giving birth to a child with congenital heart disease was computed for each mother-child pair. Within two percentile strata, and within each decile of estimated risk in the entire material, the observed number of children with cardiovascular defects was compared with the expected value.

In the present context, for most of the mother-child pairs, the probability of giving birth to a child with a cardiovascular defect was small. Consequently, for the ith factor, the estimated coefficient, β_1, approximated the natural logarithm of relative risk (or more accurately, the relative odds, which is an acceptable estimator of relative risk for the rare outcomes studied here) — and with due allowance for the other factors in the risk function. The exponential of β_1 was then the standardized relative risk estimate. When a factor was assigned more than two ordinal values, to derive the relative risk estimate for the extreme category, the estimated coefficient was multiplied by the largest assigned value and the exponential was taken.

RESULTS

The 50,282 gravidas (or more precisely, the pregnancies from which the children in the study cohort were born) included 11,811 Whites, 24,030 Blacks and 3,441 Puerto Ricans. Their mean age was 24.1 years overall: 24.7 years in Whites, 23.7 years in Blacks and 23.6 years in Puerto Ricans. The mean socioeconomic index[16] was 4.7 (5.7, 3.8 and 3.8). The proportion of nulliparous women was 30% (32, 28 and 30). The mean time of registration into the study was 21.6 weeks from the first day of the last menstrual period (approximately 19 to 20 weeks from conception) and the mean duration of the entire pregnancy from the last menstrual period was 276 days (279, 272 and 275). While the mother-child pairs represented 50,282 children, some mothers had more than one pregnancy in the study and the total number of mothers was 41,796: 84% of the women had one pregnancy registered in the study; 5,467 women were registered twice; 1,154 three times; 188 four times; 33 five times; and 3 six times.

The average weight at birth was 3,131 g (3,521, 3,019, 3,114) and 50.8% of the children were males. At the end of the postnatal observation period, 95.5% of the children were alive; there were 798 stillbirths (1.6%), 806 neonatal deaths (1.6%), 384 infant deaths (0.8%) and 239 childhood deaths (0.5%).

Cardiovascular Malformations

The array of anomalies that together constituted this group was large and markedly heterogeneous. In addition, 26% of cardiovascular malformations were multiple. Any satisfactory classification is thus a complex matter. Full details will not be presented here but Table 2 gives a broad classification based on embryological considerations; Table 3 gives data on a variety of clinical syndromes; and Table 4 gives data on rare malformations.

The overall cardiovascular malformation rate was 8 per 1,000 births. This rate is somewhat higher than that noted by others.[2] Isolated ventricular septal defect, considered together with isolated single ventricle (one case) was the most common malformation (2 per 1,000). Defects of the conus arteriosus (principally transposition of the great arteries and Fallot's tetralogy) had a rate of slightly under 1 per 1,000; endocardial cushion defects and isolated sucundum atrial septal defects had rates of between 0.6 and 0.7 per 1,000.

The relative frequencies of the various syndromes, and isolated cardiovascular defects, in this cohort of children correspond closely with those observed in other bodies of data. It should be noted, however, that Fallot's tetralogy usually accounts for a considerably greater proportion of all cases of congenital heart disease in reports based on clinical practice in cardiac centers.

TABLE 2

Major Developmental Defects of the Cardiovascular System in 50,282 Children

Embryologic Entity	No.	Rate/1,000
Isolated ventricular septal defect and single ventricle	110	2.19
Conus arteriosus syndrome*	44	0.87
Endocardial cushion defect**	34	0.68
Isolated atrial septal defect (secundum)	28	0.56
Hypoplastic left heart syndrome***	24	0.48
Other defects	164	3.26
Total	404	8.04

*tetralogy of Fallot, Eisenmenger, transposition of great arteries, truncus arteriosus, double outlet right ventricle

**atrial septal defect (primum), atrioventricular canal, cleft mitral value

***aortic and mitral valve atresia, hypoplastic left heart

TABLE 3

Cardiovascular Malformations According to Ethnic Group (Rates per 1,000)

	White (22,811)		Black (24,030)		Puerto Rican (3,441)		Total (50,282)	
	No.	Rate	No.	Rate	No.	Rate	No.	Rate
Ventricular septal defect*	48	2.10	52	2.16	9	2.62	109	2.17
Atrial septal defect*	17	0.74	16	0.67	4	1.16	37	0.73
Pulmonic stenosis*	15	0.66	17	0.71	2	0.58	34	0.68
Patent ductus arteriosus*	8	0.35	18	0.75	3	0.87	29	0.58
Coarctation of aorta*	10	0.44	9	0.37	0		19	0.38
Tetralogy of Fallot*	9	0.40	3	0.13	1	0.29	13	0.26
Ventricular septal defect and pulmonic stenosis*	2	0.09	7	0.29	1	0.29	10	0.20
Atrioventricular canal*	9	0.40	2	0.08	1	0.29	12	0.24
Aortic and mitral valve atresia*	4	0.18	7	0.29	1	0.29	12	0.24
Aortic stenosis*	6	0.26	5	0.21	0		11	0.22
Endocardial fibroelastosis*	3	0.13	7	0.29	1	0.29	11	0.22
Other isolated cardiovascular malformations**	26	1.14	12	0.50	0		38	0.76
Other multiple cardiovascular malformations***	40	1.75	25	1.04	4	1.16	69	1.37
Any cardiovascular malformation	197	8.64	180	7.49	27	7.85	404	8.04

*no other cardiovascular anomalies

**see Table 3

***see text

TABLE 4

Rare Isolated Cardiovascular Malformations According to Ethnic Group
(Rates per 1,000)

	White (22,811)	Black (24,030)	Total (50,282)*	
	No.	No.	No.	Rate
Right subclavian artery	3	1	4	0.08
Vascular ring	1	2	3	0.06
Anomalous coronary artery	2	1	3	0.06
Wolff-Parkinson-White syndrome	3	0	3	0.06
Mitral insufficiency	1	1	2	0.04
Truncus arteriosus	2	0	2	0.04
Double outlet right ventricle	0	2	2	0.04
Endomyocardial fibrosis	1	1	2	0.04
Aortic insufficiency	2	0	2	0.04
Absent mitral valve	1	0	1	0.04
Ebstein's anomaly	1	0	1	0.02
Tricuspid valve atresia	0	1	1	0.02
Pulmonary atresia	1	0	1	0.02
Hypoplastic pulmonary artery	0	1	1	0.02
Single pulmonary artery and vein	1	0	1	0.02
Absent pulmonary vein	1	0	1	0.02
Transposition of great arteries	1	0	1	0.02
Single ventricle	1	0	1	0.02
Hypoplastic heart	0	1	1	0.02
Hypoplastic left atrium	1	0	1	0.02
Anomalous renal artery and vein	1	0	1	0.02
Anomalous origin of renal artery	0	1	1	0.02
Vena azygos	1	0	1	0.02
Stenosis ductus venosus	1	0	1	0.02
Total	26	12	38	0.76

*none of these anomalies occurred in 3,441 Puerto Ricans

In Table 3 the most common combinations of individual defects are shown for 104 children who had more than one specific lesion. In the remaining 69 children who had "other multiple" anomalies of the cardiovascular system, there was a large variety of combinations. The most common specific components diagnosed in this group of children were: ventricular septal defect in 39 cases; coarctation of the aorta (all preductal), 17; patent ductus arteriosus, 16; transposition of the great arteries, 16; atrial septal defect of any type, 15; pulmonary atresia, 10; malformations of the tricuspid valve, 8; vascular ring, 6; single ventricle, 5; and aortic stenosis, 5.

Relationships between Cardiovascular and Other Malformations

In the same way as multiple malformations within a given anatomical system tend to occur more frequently than would be expected on the basis of chance, a malformation within one anatomical system tends to be accompanied by one or more malformations affecting other organ systems.

In this presentation, 404 children who had cardiovascular defects will be evaluated in relation to other malformations, syndromes or tumors. There were 1,989 children who had other malformations, either alone or in combination with cardiovascular defects. This latter number includes only children with malformations whose rates showed random inter-hospital variability. Certain malformations have been ignored because the rates between hospitals were variable, probably because there was a large subjective component to their diagnosis. This applied, for example, to conditions such as inguinal hernia, clubfoot and cleft gum (but not other clefts). Details concerning non-cardiac malformations will be reported elsewhere.[7]

In this study, on the basis of chance, cardiovascular malformations occurring in combination with malformations elsewhere would have been expected in 16 children; 116 were observed. Thus, 29% of the 404 children with cardiovascular malformations also had malformations elsewhere. Table 5 gives the observed and expected figures according to the principal classes in which the other malformations were classified. Consistently, the observed numbers are well in excess of the expected numbers. It is worth noting that among 176 children with various syndromes, 61 had Down's syndrome. As expected, the latter condition was strongly associated with cardiac malformations; 25 affected (41%) had congenital heart disease. In addition, eight of the 25 children (32%) had malformations in other anatomical systems. In this small sample, the co-existence of cardiac defects and other defects was as common as it was in the cohort as a whole.

Administrative Factors

As already mentioned, fluctuations in the rates of cardiovascular defects

TABLE 5

Observed and Expected Numbers of Children Having Cardiovascular Malformations Together with Other Malformations, Syndromes or Tumors

	Cardiovascular with Other Malformations		Percentage among Children with Cardiovascular Malformation
	Observed No.	Expected No.	
Central Nervous System	22	2.1	5.5
Musculoskeletal	26	5.8	6.4
Respiratory	32	1.8	7.9
Gastrointestinal	42	2.4	10.4
Genitourinary	34	2.9	8.4
Eye and/or Ear	10	1.0	2.5
Syndromes (including Down's syndrome)	48	1.4	11.9
Tumors	4	1.3	1.0
Any malformation, syndrome or tumor	116	16.0	28.7

between the hospitals were minor. For present purposes, the study centers were combined and the sample of children with cardiovascular defects was taken to be reasonably uniform.

Since it was possible for the same woman to give birth to more than one child in the study center within the seven-year enrollment period, and since increasing age is believed to be a risk factor for congenital heart disease, it was anticipated that cardiovascular birth defects would have been more common with an increasing number of enrollments. Table 6 shows that the reverse was actually observed: congenital heart disease was 7% more common (relative risk, (1.4) in children born to women with a first, or only, pregnancy registered into the study; the remaining children born to successive study pregnancies had lower rates. The reason for this difference may well be self-selection: congenital heart disease is known to aggregate in families and it is possible that mothers with affected children may have delayed their subsequent pregnancies for longer than did mothers of normal children. There are suggestive data in favor of this possibility: when the first child did not have congenital heart disease, 16% of the mothers were again enrolled into the study; however, when the first child was affected, only 13% of the mothers were again enrolled for a subsequent pregnancy. Malformations other than those affecting the cardiovascular system did not have any influence on repeat entries.

Among 6,845 sibships born in the study to mothers who registered during more than one pregnancy, the probability that more than one sibling would have congenital heart disease within a sibship was 0.7. One such instance was, in fact, observed: one child had isolated pulmonic stenosis and the other childhad patent ductus arteriosus.

In 1,091 children born to mothers who registered during the first two lunar months of pregnancy, only three had congenital heart disease, 8.9 were expected.

Cardiovascular defects were slightly more common when the mother attended for less than ten antenatal visits (Table 7).

When the data were analyzed by calendar month of the last menstrual period, no seasonal trend was apparent. It should be noted that this method more closely approximates the time of origin of cardiovascular defects than does the time of birth since the duration of pregnancy can fluctuate widely. There were only random differences in the cardiovascular malformation rates according to the year of entry into the study.

Personal Characteristics of the Mother

Tables 2, 3 and 4 indicate that the cardiovascular malformation rates were similar in White, Black and Puerto Rican children. To the best of one's knowledge, the data concerning the latter ethnic group are the first to be

OLLI P. HEINONEN

TABLE 6

Distribution of Children with Cardiovascular Malformations by
Mother's Ordinal Number of Entry to the Study Cohort

Mother's Ordinal Number of Entry	No. of Children	Cardiovascular Malformation No.	Rate/1,000	Relative Risk
First	41,796	352	8.4	1.4
Other	8,486	52	6.1	1.0*

*reference category

TABLE 7

Distribution of Children with Cardiovascular Malformations by Number of
Antenatal Visits

No. of Antenatal Visits	No. of Children	Cardiovascular Malformation No.	Rate/1,000	Relative Risk
1–9	29,588	254	8.6	1.2
≥ 10	20,694	150	7.3	1.0*

*reference category

238

reported.

Maternal age was a strong determinant of the cardiovascular malformations (Table 8) and this effect was evident within each ethnic group. As already pointed out, however, 25 affected children had Down's syndrome; this, in large part, accounts for the apparent effect of maternal age. Because there was a monotonic trend by decade of maternal age, ordinal scaling was applied in further analysis.

Socioeconomic status did not relate to the cardiovascular malformation rate in any of the ethnic groups. Overall, the rate was 8.5 per 1,000 in classes I and II (19,620 mother-child pairs) and 7.8 per 1,000 in classes III and IV.

There were 34 affected children born to 3,326 separated mothers and the relative risk was 1.3 compared with the remainder.

Religion was recorded in the study as Protestant, Roman Catholic and other. There were 1,441 White women whose religion was recorded as "other": the bulk of them were probably Jewish. The offspring in this group had a cardiovascular malformation rate of 12.5 per 1,000 giving a risk of 1.5 relative to White Protestants and Roman Catholics. In Blacks and Puerto Ricans, no association between religion and cardiovascular defects was noted.

On average, Puerto Rican mothers were a little shorter (155 cm) than Whites (161 cm) or Blacks (161 cm). Although maternal height was not related to the cardiovascular malformation rate, a high relative body weight was. The relative body weight was estimated by computing the ponderal index (prepregnancy weight in kilograms x 1,000/height in centimeters^2). Cardiovascular defects were 1.5 times more common in children both to mothers with an index value of 3.0 or over than in the remainder (Table 9). Quite commonly, pre-pregnant weight was not recorded and the malformation rate was also increased when the ponderal index was unknown. In further analyses, high and unknown ponderal indices were combined because the malformation rates were closely similar.

Characteristics and Survival of the Child

The cardiovascular malformation rate was 8.3 per 1,000 in males and 7.8 per 1,000 in females. However, the sex-specific rates varied in each ethnic group: the rate was higher in White males (males, 9.5; females, 7.7); there was virtually no difference in Blacks (males, 7.4; females, 7.6); and Puerto Rican males had a lower rate (males, 5.7; females, 10.0). The latter difference could be due to sampling variation since there were only 10 male and 17 Puerto Rican children with congenital heart disease.

Table 10 shows that in each ethnic group, in children weighing less than 2,500 g at birth, there was a monotonic increase in the frequency of cardiovascular malformations with decreasing birthweight. By contrast, in the

TABLE 8

Race-Specific Distribution of Children with Cardiovascular Malformations by Mother's Age at Registration

Mother's Age (years)	No. of Children	Cardiovascular Malformation		Relative Risk
		No.	Rate/1,000	
White				
⩽ 19	4,074	22	5.4	1.0*
20 – 29	14,220	110	7.7	1.4
30 – 39	4,131	54	13.1	2.4
⩾ 40	386	11	28.5	5.3
Black				
⩽ 19	6,978	45	6.5	1.0*
20 – 29	12,747	97	7.6	1.2
30 – 39	3,953	32	8.1	1.3
⩾ 40	352	6	17.1	2.6
Puerto Rican				
⩽ 19	852	6	7.0	1.0*
20 – 29	2,100	18	8.6	1.2
30 – 39	455	3	6.6	0.9
⩾ 40	34	0	0.0	—

*reference category

240

TABLE 9

Cardiovascular Malformations According to the Ponderal Index of the Mother

Ponderal Index*	No. of Children	Cardiovascular Malformation		Relative Risk
		No.	Rate/1,000	
⩽ 3.0	44,381	335	7.6	1.0**
⩾ 3.0	3,106	36	11.6	1.5
Unknown	2,795	33	11.8	1.6

*(prepregnant weight in kilograms x 1,000) / (height in centimeters)^2

**reference category

TABLE 10

Race-Specific Distribution of Children with Cardiovascular Malformations by Birthweight

Birthweight (grams)		No. of Children	Cardiovascular Malformation		Relative Risk
			No.	Rate/1,000	
White					
	≤ 1,499	357	12	33.6	4.7
1,500	– 1,999	288	8	27.8	3.9
2,000	– 2,499	1,201	28	23.3	3.3
	≥ 2,500	20,965	149	7.1	1.0*
Black					
	≤ 1,499	602	8	13.3	2.3
1,500	– 1,999	606	15	24.8	4.3
2,000	– 2,499	2,259	39	17.3	3.0
	≥ 2,500	20,563	118	5.7	1.0*
Puerto Rican					
	≤ 1,499	57	1	17.5	3.0
1,500	– 1,999	66	4	30.3	5.2
2,000	– 2,499	244	6	24.6	4.2
	≥ 2,500	3,074	18	5.9	1.0*

*reference category

242

birthweight categories, the cardiovascular malformation rates were similar In the multivariate analyses, ordinal scaling of birthweight was used.

Table 11 gives the cardiovascular malformation frequencies according to the birth order of the child. Relative to the first three children, the rates were higher for fourth to seventh children and for children ranking eighth or higher, the rate was more than doubled. In later analyses, ordinal scaling was therefore used.

Of the 404 children with cardiovascular malformations, 164 (41%) were either stillborn or they died during the four to seven-year follow-up period. The cardiovascular malformation rate was increased about 15-fold in non-survivors. Table 12 gives more detailed data according to age at death in each ethnic group. Among those who did not survive, the cardiovascular malformation rate was lower in Black children. Overall, the proportion of Black children who did not survive was 32% higher than in White children. This may partly explain why cardiovascular malformations were less common in Black children who died.

Autopsy reports were available in 79% of White and in 83% of Black children who did not survive. In both ethnic groups, congenital heart disease was diagnosed about twice as commonly at autopsy.

Death can be considered a consequence rather than a cause of congenital heart disease and will not be further analyzed with other factors. However, no effort has been made to determine how often death was, in fact, attributable to cardiac causes and how often death and congenital heart disease were unrelated coincidental phenomena.

Reproductive History of the Mother

A history of prior abortion was associated with an increased cardiovascular malformation rate (Table 13). This increase was only slight when there was one prior abortion (relative risk, 1.2) and more convincing when there had been repeated abortions (relative risk, 1.7). In further analyses, the categories of one and no prior abortions were combined.

Histories of prior stillbirth (relative risk, 1.4) and prior siblings who died within 28 days of birth (relative risk, 1.6) were also associated with cardiovascular malformations.

On the other hand, histories of prior premature birth and of dysmenorrhea (recorded as slight, moderate or severe) were not associated with congenital heart disease.

Gestation and its Complications

Birthweight was somewhat lower in non-White children. Table 14 shows that the cardiovascular malformation rates in each ethnic group were increased

TABLE 11

Distribution of Children with Cardiovascular Malformations by Birth Order of Child

Birth Order (liveborn and stillborn)	No. of Children	Cardiovascular Malformation		Relative Risk
		No.	Rate/1,000	
1	15,166	110	7.3	1.0*
2–3	19,729	137	6.9	1.0
4–7	13,294	124	9.3	1.3
≥ 8	2,093	33	15.8	2.2

*reference category

TABLE 12

Race-Specific Distribution of Children with Cardiovascular Malformations by Survival of the Child

		No. of Children	Cardiovascular Malformation		Relative Risk
			No.	Rate/1,000	
White	Stillbirth	327	20	61.2	11.9
	Neonatal death	302	36	119.2	23.1
	Infant death	130	18	138.5	26.9
	Childhood death	91	10	109.9	21.4
	Survived	21,961	113	5.2	1.0*
Black	Stillbirth	407	10	24.6	5.0
	Neonatal death	450	30	66.7	13.5
	Infant death	229	19	83.0	16.9
	Childhood death	134	9	67.2	13.7
	Survived	22,810	112	4.9	1.0*
Puerto Rican	Stillbirth	64	4	62.5	13.7
	Neonatal death	54	6	111.1	24.3
	Infant death	25	2	80.0	17.5
	Childhood death	14	0	—	—
	Survived	3,284	15	4.6	1.0*

*reference category

245

TABLE 13

Distribution of Children with Cardiovascular Malformations by History
of Prior Fetal or Neonatal Loss

Mother's Reproductive History	No. of Children	Cardiovascular Malformation		Relative Risk
		No.	Rate/1,000	
Two or more prior abortions	2,504	33	13.2	1.7
One prior abortion	6,631	60	9.1	1.2
No prior abortion**	26,979	212	7.9	1.0*
No prior pregnancy	14,168	99	7.0	0.9
Prior stillbirth	2,837	33	11.6	1.4
No prior stillbirth***	32,280	261	8.1	1.0*
No prior pregnancies 20 weeks or over	15,165	110	7.3	0.9
Prior neonatal death	2,174	28	12.9	1.6
No prior neonatal death****	32,554	262	8.1	1.0*
No prior liveborn	15,554	114	7.3	0.9

*reference category
**includes 108 unknowns
***includes 179 unknowns
****includes 947 unknowns

TABLE 14

Race-Specific Distribution of Children with Cardiovascular Malformations by Duration of Pregnancy

Length of Gestation (lunar months)	No. of Children	Cardiovascular Malformation		Relative Risk
		No.	Rate/1,000	
White				
5–6	178	3	16.9	2.2
7–8	896	21	23.4	3.0
9–10	21,293	164	7.7	1.0*
11	444	9	20.3	2.6
Black				
5–6	354	2	5.7	0.8
7–8	2,147	30	14.0	2.1
9–10	21,068	140	6.7	1.0*
11	461	8	17.4	2.6
Puerto Rican				
5–6	27	0	—	—
7–8	249	3	12.1	1.7
9–10	3,075	22	7.2	1.0*
11	90	2	22.2	3.1

*reference category

247

when the pregnancies lasted less than nine lunar months or longer than ten lunar months. In each instance, the cardiovascular malformation rates were two to three-fold higher. In further analyses, abnormally short and abnormally long gestation periods were classified as separate binary variables.

In parallel with birthweight, placental weight tended to be lower in non-White children. As shown in Table 15, low placental weight was associated with cardiovascular malformations. However, in White children the rate began to rise as the placental weight dropped below 400 g, while in Black children a trend only became evident at placental weights of less than 300 g. In further analyses, separate cutting points were used for the two ethnic groups and two variables, placental weight in White and in non-White children, were used.

Toxemia, in one form or another, is one of the principal complications of pregnancy. Table 16 gives a hierarchical classification of what might be termed the toxemia syndrome. By "hierarchical" it is meant that if, say, a mother had both edema and an associated late rise in blood pressure (systolic greater than 160 mmHg and/or diastolic greater than 110 mmHg, she was classified in the latter category. With the exception of eclampsia, of which there were only 22 pregnancies, the table shows a steady monotonic decrease in the relative risk estimates from 3.0 down to 0.8, corresponding with decreasing degrees of severity until generalized edema (without other features of toxemia) gave no evidence of being a risk factor for cardiovascular malformations. In further analyses, the seven categories in Table 16 were coalesced to form three: the top three categories together were given an ordinal scaling of 2; blood pressure 160/100 occurring only after the sixth lunar month was given an ordinal scaling of 1 and the lowest three categories were given an ordinal scaling of 0.

Table 17 lists seven further complications of pregnancy that were found to be related to cardiovascular malformations in this study. For single umbilical artery the relationship is well known. However, a point estimate of relative risk of 7.2 is noteworthy. There were 99 pregnancies complicated by hemorrhagic shock (due to placenta previa and/or abruptio placentae in two-thirds, and other causes in the remainder). There were five children with cardiovascular malformations born to this group, giving a five-fold increase in risk. For total or partial placenta previa overall, the increase risk was about four-fold. Other complications associated with congenital heart disease were: hydramnios, vena cava syndrome, weight loss during pregnancy and abruptio placentae; the increases in relative risk varied from 1.5 to 3.3.

In contrast to the above complications, the following were not associated with congenital heart disease: true cord knot (relative risk, 0.9), vomiting during pregnancy (relative risk, 0.9), hyperemesis gravidarum (relative risk,

TABLE 15

Race-Specific Distribution of Children with Cardiovascular Malformations by Placental Weight

Placental Weight (grams)	No. of Children	Cardiovascular Malformation		Relative Risk
		No.	Rate/1,000	
White				
≤ 299	864	21	24.3	3.6
300–399	5,377	65	12.1	1.8
≥ 400**	16,570	111	6.7	1.0*
Non-White				
≤ 299	1,619	20	12.4	1.6
300–399	7,738	49	6.3	0.8
≥ 400***	18,114	138	7.6	1.0*

*reference category

**include 2,644 unknown values

***include 3,770 unknown values

249

TABLE 16

Distribution of Children with Cardiovascular Malformations by Eclampsia
and Signs of Toxemia During Pregnancy

	No. of Children	Cardiovascular Malformation		Relative Risk
		No.	Rate/1,000	
Eclampsia	22	0	—	—
Chronic hypertension and BP ⩾ 160/110 after LM 6 without eclampsia	283	7	24.7	3.0
Chronic hypertension without either BP 160/110 after LM 6 or eclampsia	386	7	18.1	2.2
BP ⩾ 160/110 after LM 6 without either chronic hypertension or eclampsia	930	11	11.8	1.4
Proteinuria without hypertension	1,213	10	8.2	1.0
Generalized edema without other signs	11,425	74	6.5	0.8
None	36,023	295	8.2	1.0*

*reference category

TABLE 17

Distribution of Children with Cardiovascular Malformations by
Complications of Pregnancy Other than Toxemia

	No. of Children	Cardiovascular Malformation		Relative Risk*
		No.	Rate/1,000	
Single umbilical artery	341	19	55.7	7.2
Hemorrhagic shock	99	4	40.4	5.1
Total or partial placenta previa	131	4	30.5	3.8
Hydramnios	694	18	25.9	3.3
Vena cava syndrome	144	3	20.8	2.6
Weight loss (without weight gain)	741	12	16.2	2.1
Abruptio placentae	1,030	12	11.7	1.5

*For each disease or complication the reference category consists of those
without that complication.

0.7), incompetent cervix (relative risk, 1.4 — but there were only two cases of cardiovascular malformations), vaginal bleeding not associated with placenta previa, abruptio placentae or hemorrhagic shock (relative risk, 1.0), large placental infarcts with a diameter of 3 cm or more (relative risk, 1.3 — but based on a small number of cases and no evidence of association in Whites) and marginal sinus rupture (relative risk, 1.4) — but based on observed and expected numbers of only 7 and 5.1 children with cardiovascular malformations).

Table 18 documents a well known relationship: the cardiovascular malformation rates were considerably elevated in the offspring of diabetic mothers. Although there may have been a great deal of sampling variation due to small numbers, the table also suggests that the risk is increased, the greater the severity of the diabetes and the longer its duration. In further analyses, untreated diabetics were combined with those who did not have diabetes. Ordinal scaling was used for the remaining categories.

The relative risk was 3.5 for 144 pregnancies complicated by thrombophlebitis. However, this relationship was based on very small numbers (Table 19).

There were 11,761 gravidae who had a clinical diagnosis of anemia (Table 19). For this group, the observed and expected numbers of children with congenital heart disease were 82 and 98, respectively, giving a relative risk of 0.8. This was the only instance, based on substantial numbers, where a "disease" showed a "protective" effect. The factor, anemia, was included in the subsequent multivariate analyses.

Endocrine disorders other than diabetes or malfunction of the thyroid gland were recorded in 1,537 mothers and the relative risk was 1.3 (Table 19).

Urinary tract infection with concomitant fever was recorded in 709 gravidae. The cardiovascular malformation rate given this condition was 12.7 per 1,000 and the relative risk was 1.6 (Table 19). Hematuria (15 or more red cells per high power field) showed much the same effect: for 1,052 pregnancies, the cardiovascular malformation rate was 14.2 per 1,000, giving an estimated relative risk of 1.8 (Table 19).

Unexpectedly, bacterial infection recorded after the first trimester (899 pregnancies) was associated with congenital heart disease. For this condition, the relative risk was 2.0 (Table 19).

All of the factors listed in Table 19 were taken into account in the multivariate analyses.

Of the large number of additional disorders that were recorded in the study, none was associated with congenital heart disease to any meaningful extent.

Cigarettes, X-rays and Rubella Exposure
Cigarette smoking was not associated with congenital heart disease in this

TABLE 18

Distribution of Children with Cardiovascular Malformations by Maternal
Diabetes Mellitus

Maternal Disease	No. of Children	Cardiovascular Malformation		Relative Risk
		No.	Rate/1,000	
Diabetes for 5 years or more	98	6	61.2	7.8
Diabetes with insulin and/or oral antidiabetic drug	96	3	31.3	4.0
Diabetes mellitus without insulin or oral antidiabetic drug	142	1	7.1	0.9
No diabetes	49,946	394	7.9	1.0*

*reference category

TABLE 19

Distribution of Children with Cardiovascular Malformations by
Selected Diseases of the Mother During Pregnancy

Maternal Disease	No. of Children	Cardiovascular Malformation		Relative Risk*
		No.	Rate/1,000	
Thrombophlebitis	144	4	27.8	3.5
Anemia	11,761	82	7.0	0.8
Endocrine disorder other than diabetes, hypo- thyroidism, or hyper- thyroidism	1,537	16	10.4	1.3
Urinary tract infection with fever ($\geq$ 100.4°)	709	9	12.7	1.6
Hematuria (15 RBC/HPF or over)	1,059	15	14.2	1.8
Bacteria infection during 2nd and/or 3rd trimester	899	14	15.6	2.0

*For each disease the reference category consists of those without that disease.

study. There were 7,076 gravidae who smoked 15 to 20 cigarettes per day and 1,785 who smoked 30 or more cigarettes per day. Compared with non-smokers, the relative risks for congenital heart disease were 0.9 and 0.7, respectively.

Table 20 shows that among 11,400 pregnancies exposed to pelvic and/or abdominal x-rays, the cardiovascular malformation rate was increased by 30%.

As already mentioned, clinically evident rubella during pregnancy, or the congenital rubella syndrome in the child, was a criterion for exclusion in the present study. Nevertheless, it is still possible that some cases of congenital heart disease in the presented material could have been due to rubella. Table 21 gives the cardiovascular malformation rates for early and late pregnancy according to exposure to rubella. Among 1,404 early exposures, the rate was 12.1 per 1,000 (relative risk, 1.5), while there was no evidence of an effect in late pregnancy.

Genetic and Teratologic History

Table 22 shows that there was some increase in the cardiovascular malformation rate in offspring of 690 fathers recorded as having a physical birth defect (relative risk, 1.6). Congenital defects were recorded in 1,225 gravidae. However, there was only a very modest increase in the cardiovascular malformation rate in the offspring of affected mothers. In further analyses, congenital physical defects in either the mother or the father (in three instances, both parents were affected) were considered together.

In contrast to a parental history of congenital defects, a variety of malformations in prior siblings were more consistently related to a high cardiovascular malformation rate. While the rates in Table 22 have not been adjusted for the size of the sibship, it is of interest that having a prior sibling with congenital heart disease trebled the risk. Having prior siblings with malformations affecting the head and/or spine (relative risk, 2.8) or the fingers and/or toes (relative risk, 2.1), also appeared to increase the risk of congenital heart disease. To a certain extent, even the less accurately defined category of prior siblings with other miscellaneous malformations appeared to be associated with an increased risk (relative risk, 1.6).

The study recorded whether the parents or maternal grandparents of the child were related. Marriages between second half-cousins, or closer relatives, in either generation were rare: 98 of the parental couples and 115 couples (0.2%) who were parents of the mothers were related. In the former instance, there was one and, in the latter instance, two children with congenital heart disease (expected, 0.8 and 0.9). Thus, the sample was far too small to evaluate the effect of consanguinity on the cardiovascular malformation rate. It does serve to make the point, however, that, in America, the proportion of

TABLE 20

Distribution of Children with Cardiovascular Malformations by Maternal
Exposure to X-radiation During Pregnancy

Pelvic and/or Abdominal X-ray Exposure	No. of Children	Cardiovascular Malformation		Relative Risk
		No.	Rate/1,000	
Yes	11,400	111	9.7	1.3
No	38,882	293	7.5	1.0*

*reference category

TABLE 21

Distribution of Children with Cardiovascular Malformations by Maternal
Exposure to Rubella Infection During Pregnancy

Time of Exposure	No. of Children	Cardiovascular Malformation		Relative Risk
		No.	Rate/1,000	
First and/or second trimester	1,404	17	12.1	1.5
Third trimester	583	2	3.4	0.4
None	48,295	385	8.0	1.0*

*reference category

TABLE 22

Distribution of Children with Cardiovascular Malformations by a
Family Malformation History

	No. of Children	Cardiovascular Malformation		Relative Risk*
		No.	Rate/1,000	
Congenital malformation in child's father*	690	9	13.0	1.6
Congenital malformation in child's mother	1,225	11	9.0	1.1
Congenital heart disease in a prior sibling	662	15	22.7	2.9
Malformation of head and/or spine in a prior sibling	597	13	21.8	2.8
Malformation of finger and/or toe in a prior sibling	474	8	16.9	2.1
Miscellaneous other malformations in a prior sibling**	1,797	22	12.2	1.6

*The reference category consists of those without malformation and those with unknown malformation history.

**excluding siblings with cleft lip and/or palate and clubfoot.

congenital heart disease attributable to consanguinity must be very small indeed.

ABO and Rh Blood Groups and Incompatibility

ABO and Rh typing was recorded in 92% and 94% of the mother-child pairs, respectively. To analyze the relation of blood groups to cardiovascular malformations, a single-mother-child pair was selected at random in all instances when the mother registered into the study more than once. No evidence of association between blood type and cardiovascular malformations was noted.

Definite and possible erythroblastosis fetalis due to Rh incompatibility was recorded in 266 and 40 children, respectively. Three of the children had congenital heart disease (expected, 2.4). Rh incompatibility was recorded in 3,286 mother-child pairs. The cardiovascular malformation rates for incompatible and compatible pairs were similar, being 6.7 and 7.9 per 1,000, respectively.

Neither erythroblastosis nor different degrees of severity of ABO incompatibility had any influence on the rate of congenital heart disease.

Multivariate Linear Discriminant Function Analysis

One of the major difficulties in a univariate approach to the background of congenital heart disease is the widely acknowledged problem that there may be interrelationships between the factors that require evaluation. That this is a real problem is illustrated by the fact that no less than 15 of the 39 variables, initially found on univariate analysis to be associated with cardiovascular malformations, were no longer associated when multivariate linear discriminant function analysis was completed. One or more of the 24 factors retained for further evaluation were covariates for each of the 15 factors that were eliminated. The eliminated factors were: less than two prenatal visits, ethnic group, child born to a separated mother, high relative weight, history of abortion, stillbirth or neonatal death, short gestation, abruptio placentae, anemia, endocrine disorder, urinary tract infection, abdominal or pelvic x-ray exposure, prenatal history of malformations and history of miscellaneous birth defects in siblings (histories of more specific defects in siblings were not eliminated).

For most of the eliminated variables, the reason for disappearance of the association with the dependent variable, in the presence of other variables, was quite obvious. For example, short gestation was strongly correlated with low birthweight. However, in some instances, a factor had many covariates, none of them being self-evident prior to linear discriminant function analysis.

In the present context, discriminant function analysis was used as a

258

multivariate screening device to eliminate factors that were not relevant. The next step in the analytical process was to estimate the adjusted relative risk for each retained factor, while making due allowance for the influence of the other factors under consideration.

Multiple Logistic Risk Function Analysis

The 24 variables not eliminated by multiple linear discriminant function analysis were subjected to multiple logistic risk function analysis, and risk functions for cardiovascular deformities were computed.

Table 23 summarizes the contribution of each variable, in turn, to the risk of cardiovascular malformations, when each of the 23 remaining variables were simultaneously taken into account. The factors have been arranged in descending order of "standardized" relative risk estimates. Three types of factors are listed in the table: biological factors associated with congenital heart disease in terms of meeting formal requirements for statistical significance; biological factors that could be of interest, despite absence of formal statistical significance but showing strong associations in terms of relative risk; and lastly (and of lesser interest), administrative factors that had to be retained in the analysis because of technical considerations. In interpreting the table, it is generally accepted that when the risk function coefficient is greater than twice (or more exactly, 1.96 times) its standard error, the association is unlikely to be due to chance. This criterion applies, for example, to the first factor listed in Table 23, i.e., single umbilical artery. This factor, therefore, remained a powerful predictor, having an estimated relative risk of 5.1 even when all other factors in the table were controlled. By the same token, low placental weight in non-Whites (last on the list), although showing a relative risk of 1.6 on univariate analysis, not only ceased to be a risk factor, but the relative risk was reduced to 0.8, and the ratio of the coefficient to its standard error was so low that the relative risk could have differed from 1.0 by chance. While placental weight had different relationships with cardiovascular malformations in each ethnic group, it is obvious that conditional on the other factors considered here (particularly birthweight), placental weight was not a risk factor.

Single umbilical artery, low birthweight, maternal diabetes, congenital heart disease and malformations of head and spine in siblings, thrombophlebitis and hydramnios were all associated with at least doubling of the risk of cardiovascular malformation, even when other factors were taken into account, and none of these associations are likely to have been due to chance. Other associations of a lower order of magnitude, but consistent with statistical significance, included hematuria in pregnancy; religion other than Protestant or Roman Catholic in White women; advanced maternal age; first

259

TABLE 23

Factors Related to the Risk of Cardiovascular Malformations Based Upon Multiple Logistic Risk Function Analysis

	Estimated Risk Function Coefficient	Standard Error of Coefficient	Estimated Standardized Relative Risk
Single umbilical artery	1.63	0.25	5.1
Birthweight less than 2,000 grams	1.29	0.13	3.6
Maternal diabetes, duration 5 years or more	1.19	0.44	3.3
Thrombophlebitis during pregnancy	1.14	0.52	3.1
Vena cava syndrome (positional shock)	1.01	0.60	2.7
Hydramnios	0.86	0.26	2.4
Congenital heart disease in prior sibling	0.81	0.27	2.2
Malformation of finger and/or toe in prior sibling	0.71	0.36	2.0
Malformation of head and/or spine in prior sibling	0.71	0.30	2.0
Bacterial infection in 2nd and/or 3rd trimester	0.57	0.28	1.8
Hematuria (15 RBC/HPF or over) during pregnancy	0.55	0.27	1.7
White and religion other than Protestant or Roman Catholic	0.54	0.25	1.7
Age of mother 40 years or greater	0.53	0.21	1.7
Hemorrhagic shock during pregnancy	0.53	0.58	1.7
Placenta previa	0.50	0.55	1.7
Chronic hypertension and/or eclampsia	0.46	0.27	1.6
Weight loss (without weight gain) during pregnancy	0.43	0.30	1.5
First entry to the study	0.43	0.15	1.5
Birth order 8th or higher	0.40	0.19	1.5
Exposure to rubella in 1st and/or 2nd trimester*	0.39	0.25	1.5
Duration of gestation 11 lunar months or more	0.11	0.02	1.1
Entry to the study during the first three lunar months	−0.11	0.06	0.9
White and placental weight less than 400 grams	0.38	0.13	1.5
Non-White and placental weight less than 300 grams	−0.29	0.25	0.8

Estimated constant term − 6.09
*Cases of clinically evident rubella have been excluded.

260

entry into the study; and high birth order ranking. Then again, there were some factors that could have been associated with cardiovascular malformations by chance but which had increased relative risks. These included positional shock; hemorrhagic shock; placenta previa; the more severe degrees of toxemia; weight loss or failure to gain weight during pregnancy; and exposure to rubella (as distinct from clinically evident rubella).

One point should again be stressed: 41% of the children with Down's syndrome had cardiovascular malformations and this accounted, in large part, for the association with advanced maternal age.

Table 24 evaluates the adequacy of the model as fitted to the data. The observed and expected numbers of malformed children with each decile of risk scores are similar. In addition, the separation between the highest and lowest decile of risk suggests that the model is efficient in separating high and low risk groups. It must be pointed out, however, that the model is not really effective in predicting the risk for any individual pregnancy — a great deal still has to be learned if prediction is to be made accurate in this context. This is also attested by the relatively high constant term in Table 23.

Comments

In a relatively large follow-up study, it has been shown that a large number of factors proved to be related to the risk of cardiovascular malformations when univariate analyses were performed. Well over half of these factors remained associated after a two-stage set of multivariate analyses was carried out. One multivariate analysis was used to reduce the number of variables and the other was used for direct estimation of adjusted relative risks for each variable retained in the final analysis.

After selection of factors on the basis of univariate analysis, the two-stage multivariate analysis had certain advantages. Given a large number of variables, linear discriminant function analysis was less costly than multiple logistic risk function analysis and could be used to reduce the number of factors that need to be considered. In addition, the estimated coefficients derived from the linear discriminant function analysis could be used as initial estimates of the coefficients in the logistic model, thereby further improving efficiency.

While the data represented registrations during more than one pregnancy for certain mothers, lack of independence of the observed values of the factors selected for analysis did not prove to be a problem because there was only one instance of the same woman giving birth to a child with congenital heart disease during two study pregnancies. However, while no pregnancy is identical in all respects to any other pregnancy, there was, nevertheless, some loss of independence. This is likely to have been less serious than would have been the loss of information if repeat pregnancies had been excluded.

261

TABLE 24

Distribution of Observed and Expected Numbers of Children with
Cardiovascular Malformations by Multiple Logistic Risk Function Scores

| Percentile* | Cardiovascular Malformation | |
	Observed No.	Expected No.
99–100	60	55.4
97–98	22	26.4
95–96	18	21.0
93–94	17	18.0
91–92	16	15.7
Subtotal (91–100)	133	136.5
81–90	64	61.4
71–80	37	42.9
61–70	42	33.8
51–60	28	29.3
41–50	28	25.6
31–40	19	21.9
21–30	23	20.8
11–20	21	17.9
1–10	9	14.0
Total	404	404.0

*Each decile contains 5,025 mother-child pairs, except the lowest which contains 5,067 mother-child pairs.

Most of the known risk factors for cardiovascular malformations were also found to be risk factors in the present study. However, when some of them (*e.g.,* vaginal bleeding) were subjected to multivariate analysis, they were not found to be risk factors and were better explained by their covariates.

For some of the factors, reasonably stable estimates of relative risk of cardiovascular malformations were obtained. Other factors have been presented here, not as established risk factors, but more in the spirit of suggesting the need for further research.

SUMMARY

The occurrence of congenital cardiovascular defects has been related to a number of factors, hereditary and environmental, both in humans and in animals. At present, however, in the vast majority of affected children the origin of these birth defects remains obscure. Most studies have focused on a single factor, and very few attempts have been made to elucidate the role of several factors acting simultaneously, even though there is unanimity about the probable multifactorial nature of the etiology of these conditions. In this presentation, a strategy to approach the multifactorial backgrounds of these defects with modern epidemiological techniques is described, and results are given from a follow-up study of 50,282 mother-child pairs, including 404 children with developmental defects of the cardiovascular system. A large number of maternal, fetal and other variables were explored, one at a time, to isolate factors related to the risk of congenital cardiovascular defects. Some putative risk factors were subsequently eliminated after linear discriminant function analysis, since their apparent effect disappeared in the presence of the concomitant influence of the covariates. Finally, quantitative estimates of the residual influence of each of the remaining risk factors, in the presence of other risk factors, were derived by application of a multiple logistic risk function model. Factors not previously suspected as being related to the risk of cardiovascular malformations have been identified.

AUTHOR'S NOTE

Since completion of this manuscript, an analysis of associations between drug use in early pregnancy and cardiovascular malformations has been completed. The results will be reported elsewhere. It is worth mentioning that incorporation of the associated drugs in the risk function model described here did not materially affect any of the adjusted relative risks presented in this report.

REFERENCES

1. C. Ferencz, J. Craft and H. Sultz, *Pediatrics 52,* 395, 1973.

2. M. Campbell, *Brit. Heart J., 35,* 189, 1973.

3. M. Lamy, J. de Grouchy and O. Schweisguth, *Am. J. Human Genet. 9,*

4. I. Emerit, J. de Grouchy, P. Vernant and P. Corone, *Circulation 36,* 886, 1967.

5. T.W. Rowland, J.P. Hubbel and A.S. Nadas, *J. Pediatr. 83,* 815, 1973.

6. W. Lenz, *in* Inter-American Conference on Congenital Malformations, compiled and edited for International Medical Congress, Lippincott, Philadelphia, p. 263, 1964.

7. T.P. Clemmer and I.R. Telford, *Proc. Soc. Exper. Biol. & Med. 121,* 800, 1966.

8. F. Beck and J.B. Lloyd, *in* Advances in Teratology, Vol. 1, D.H.M. Woollam, Logos Press, London, p. 131, 1966.

9. K.R Niswander and M. Gordon, The Collaborative Perinatal Study of The National Institute of Neurological Diseases and Stroke. Women and Their Pregnancies, W.B. Saunders, Philadelphia, 1972.

10. R. Van Praagh, P. Vlad and J.D. Keith, *in* Heart disease in Infancy and Childhood, J.D. Keith, R.D. Rowe and P. Vlad (Eds.), MacMillan, New York, 1967.

11. J. Cornfield, T. Gordon and W.W. Smith, *Bull. Inst. Int. Stat. 38, 3,* 97, 1971.

12. S.H. Walker and D.B. Duncan, *Biometrika 54,* 167, 1967.

13. M. Halperin, W. Blackwelder and J. Verter, *J. Chron. Dis. 24,* 125, 1971.

14. D.G. Siegel and S.W. Greenhouse, *Am. J. Epidemiol. 97,* 324, 1973.

15. S.C. Hartz and L. Rosenberg, *J. Chron. Dis. 28,* 379, 1975.

16. N.C. Myrianthopoulos and K.S. French, *Soc. Sci. Med. 2,* 283, 1968.

17. O.P. Heinonen, D. Slone and S. Shapiro (Eds.), Birth Defects and Drugs in Pregnancy, Publishing Sciences Group, Acton (in press).

MATERNAL DRUG EXPOSURE AND BIRTH DEFECTS*

Dennis Slone
Samuel Shapiro
Olli P. Heinonen
Richard R. Monson
Stuart C. Hartz
Victor Siskind
Lynn Rosenberg
Allen A. Mitchell

Introduction

During the years 1958 to 1965, some 55,000 pregnancies drawn from twelve institutions in different cities in the United States were entered into a cohort study. The offspring were followed to the eighth birthday. The study was designed and carried out by the Perinatal Research Branch of the National Institute of Neurological Diseases and Stroke. As originally envisaged, the principal aim of the study was to evaluate a variety of neurological defects in childhood as they may relate to intrapartum, peripartum and postpartum factors. However, as the design of the study was elaborated in greater detail, the objective was expanded to encompass a large variety of factors concerning pregnancy and their possible relationships to a large variety of outcomes in the offspring.

More specifically, as part of this expanded objective, information on drugs taken during pregnancy was recorded before the children were born. This information was obtained by interview of the pregnant mothers at each antenatal visit and by inspection of antenatal and hospital records. In most instances, the drug histories were confirmed by physicians participating in the project.

*Supported by contract NO1-NS-2-2322 with the National Institute of Neurological Diseases and Stroke, U.S. Public Health Service; contract NO1-GM-4-2148, with the National Institute of General Medical Sciences, U.S. Public Health Service; and by the Food and Drug Administration.

Information on a wide variety of factors was also recorded. This information included administrative data such as hospital and year of registration; descriptive data such as age; characteristics of the pregnancy such as duration and prior obstetrical history; complications of pregnancy such as hyperemesis, hydramnios or placenta previa; maternal diseases such as diabetes or epilepsy; and characteristics of the offspring such as weight, sex and survival.

An effort was made to achieve as complete a follow-up as possible and to determine and fully document the occurrence of congenital malformations. Over 90% of the offspring were successfully followed to the first birthday.

In 1970, our group undertook the task of analyzing relationships between antenatal drug exposure and malformations identified during the first year of life, or at autopsy, and thereafter up to the fourth birthday.

Before this analysis could commence, however, the material had to be extensively reorganized. This necessity arose because of a number of reasons. The chief reason was that the drug information, as originally coded, was unsatisfactory. It was necessary to devise a completely new drug dictionary and to recode the drug information. For certain drugs and drug classes, a substantial proportion of this task had to be accomplished by inspection of the original records to determine the actual drugs used.

There were over 600 distinct pharmacological entities taken by the mothers in numbers large enough to permit analysis and these had to be evaluated against a large variety of malformations identified in the children. In addition, in evaluating these relationships, it was essential to take a large group of potentially confounding variables into account. This, in turn, necessitated reorganization of a substantial amount of the remaining data in a manner suitable for the particular purposes of this study. Strategies adopted in this reorganization included verification of data items recorded in more than one place (for example, maternal age at different examinations), cross-tabulation of variables (for example, recorded duration of gestation against date of last menstrual period) and examination of tails of distributions (for example, birthweight against duration of pregnancy). Where discrepancies were noted (for example, a 4 kg baby born to a pregnancy lasting five lunar months; or a mismatch between last menstrual period and recorded length of gestation), the original records were inspected and the relevant data items were corrected. After three years of work, the files are now ready and analysis has commenced.

Pregnancies and Their Outcomes

The final material in this study consisted of 50,282 pregnancies (lasting at least five lunar months) occurring in White (22,811), Black (24,030) and Puerto Rican (3,441) mothers. There were 3,248 children with recorded malformations (6.5%).

The mean number of preparations taken by the mothers was approximately 3.8, and there was a steady increase in the number between the years 1958 and 1965, in spite of the wide publicity given to the thalidomide disaster in 1962; many of the preparations contained more than one drug and it is worth noting that almost one-third of the mothers took five or more products while pregnant. This does not include vitamins (other than B_{12}), iron (other than parenteral) and antacids: use of these agents was almost universal.

Analysis

Before proceeding to the analytical strategies we are employing in analyzing the data, it might be instructive to briefly review the thalidomide/malformation association since this relationship presents relatively few analytical or inferential difficulties. The drug was essentially given for one indication — insomnia — which is unlikely to be a risk factor for having a malformed child. In addition, prior to the epidemic, the most prominent malformation — phocomelia — was extremely rare. Correspondingly, the relative risk, given exposure to thalidomide during the first trimester or pregnancy, was high. In this situation, it is hard to imagine that any time of bias, or confounding by any factors in pregnancy, would eliminate or even weaken the association. The situation can be quite different if, for example, a diuretic is associated weakly, but significantly, with some common malformation, and if the drug is used for the treatment of some complication of pregnancy, such as toxemia, which is also independently associated with the malformation of interest.

In fact, even the foregoing example is a relatively simple one since it is common for certain drugs to be taken for more than one condition. Let us assume a diuretic is commonly taken for seven conditions (*e.g.*, toxemia, hypertension, edema, cardiac disease, hydramnios, twin pregnancies and excessive weight gain); we will make the further assumption that each of these conditions, independent of drug exposure, increases the risk of a specified class of malformations. These conditions, by definition, are confounding factors and due allowance must be made for their influence in the analysis by one or more of the usual strategies employed in epidemiology: *i.e.*, exclusion, and/or multiple stratification, and/or matching procedures, and/or multivariate analysis.

To complicate matters even further, there are many drugs, such as tranquilizers, for which the indication is not at all clear. If such drugs, hypothetically, tended to be given to mothers with, say, threatened abortion, a spurious relationship could be found when the suspect tranquilizer might not, in fact, be causal.

The problem with which we were confronted was the need to evaluate over 600 drugs against several hundred outcomes; data were recorded on some 200

TABLE 1

Distribution of Malformed Children by a History of Malformation in Siblings

Family History	Number of Children	Any Malformation		Relative Risk
		Number	Rate/1000	
Congenital malformation in one prior sibling	3,319	203	61	1.4
Congenital malformation in two prior siblings	347	32	92	2.1
Congenital malformation in three or more prior siblings	57	8	140	3.3
Firstborn child	15,166	676	45	1.0
No congenital malformation in prior siblings	30,613	1,321	43	1.0*

*reference category

pregnancy-related variables and, in theory, each of these variables had to be evaluated in relation to each putative drug/malformation combination to determine whether they required control. This would have required tens of thousands of analyses and was not feasible.

The strategy we have employed, instead, has been to use a combination of some of the options outlined above. For example, we have elected to exclude multiple pregnancies and those with documented rubella from consideration. Apart from exclusions, we have proceeded as follows:

1. The malformations were coalesced into large classes, *e.g.*, any malformed child, children with multiple malformations, gastrointestinal malformations, cardiovascular malformations and so on. The underlying principle was to go by degrees from more general to more specific malformation entities.

2. Each malformation class was screened by a large series of univariate analyses against all recorded pregnancy variables. Those variables related in any way to one or more of the malformation classes were selected for more detailed univariate analysis. This reduced the number of variables that had to be considered to 79, the remainder having shown no relationship to the outcomes.

3. Each of the 79 variables was broken down into categories and the categories were again evaluated against each class of malformations. Table 1 is an example of a variable, prior malformed siblings, that was strongly related to the outcome "malformed child" — which includes all children with identified malformations. Categories of the variable (one, two, or more than two, prior malformed siblings) showed a monotonic relationship to the risk of the outcome.

4. Remaining with the example of the "malformed child", all variables related to this outcome were subjected to linear discriminant function analysis. Such analysis eliminated some of the variables because they were accounted for by their covariates. For example, low placental weight was strongly related to the outcome but was eliminated by its covariate, low birthweight.

5. Factors that remained associated with the outcome after simultaneously controlling their influence by means of linear discriminant function analysis, were included in a multiple logistic risk function model. Applying a risk function for a given outcome (in this case "malformed child") to any mother-child pair, yielded a total risk score. Based on this univariate score, it was possible to calculate the probability of giving birth to a malformed child when the risk-score value was known. This probability was computed for each mother-child pair. Next, taking any group of mother-child pairs, one could derive an expected number of malformed children in the group and contrast this expected number with the number actually observed. The ratio of the observed number to the expected number was then the estimated relative risk

TABLE 2

Distribution of Observed and Expected Numbers of Malformed Children by Multiple Logistic Risk Function Scores

Percentile*	Observed Number of Malformed Children	Expected Number of Malformed Children
99–100	173	180.9
97–98	115	113.2
95–96	96	91.5
93–94	74	77.1
91–92	78	68.5
TOTAL (91–100)	536	531.2
81–90	284	286.6
71–80	223	235.4
61–70	222	209.9
51–60	188	191.1
41–50	166	191.0
31–40	209	185.2
21–30	157	155.1
11–20	145	145.6
1–10	147	145.9
TOTAL	2,277	2,277.0

*Each decile contains 5,025 pregnancies, except the lowest which contains 5,057 pregnancies.

adjusted for all variables in the model. (The lower portion of Table 3 shows the factors included as predicting the risk of giving birth to a malformed child.)

Table 2 classifies the pregnancies according to percentiles or risk score. It shows that there is good agreement between the predicted numbers of malformed children based on the multiple logistic risk function scores and the number of malformed children actually observed within each risk stratum. In addition, the ratio of the malformed children in the top decile of risk to the number in the lowest decile is over 3, indicating that the model is quite powerful in discriminating between degrees of risk. (The number of malformed children in this table excludes 971 children whose malformation rates showed gross hospital variability: these will be separately analyzed and considered elsewhere.

The overall malformation rate for the mother-child pairs displayed in Table 2 is 4.4% (2,277/50,282). For the purpose of understanding the utility of Table 2, assume that a group of 1,001 mothers in the top two percentiles of risk receive some drug and that 181 malformed children are born to them (18.1%). The crude relative risk would be 4.1 (18.1%/4.4%). However, the adjusted relative risk is 1.0 (ratio of observed to expected = 181/180.9). High risk, rather than the drug, accounts for the effect and there is no association. Similarly, it should be noted that if 5,057 mothers in the lowest decile of risk, after receiving some drug, were to give birth to 146 malformed children (2.9%), this would not imply that the drug is "protective". Once again, the adjusted relative risk is 1.0, as against a crude relative risk of 0.7. The apparent "protective" effect is accounted for by "low risk mothers" having received the drug. In fact, if 223 children were born to these mothers (4.4%), the crude relative risk would be 1.0, but the adjusted relative risk would be 1.5 (ratio of observed to expected = 223/145.9) implying that the effect of the drug is consistent with a 50% increased risk of having a malformed child. Comparison of crude unadjusted rates would fail to detect such an association.

It now becomes possible to proceed to drug evaluation and we will use, as an example, exposure to regular use of aspirin during the first four lunar months of pregnancy (Table 3). It will be observed that there were 5,128 exposed pregnancies; that the number of malformed children was 227 and that the expected number, after taking into account all recorded risk variables (a total of some 200), was 238.8. The ratio of the observed to the expected number is the adjusted point estimate of risk ratio for having a malformed child given exposure to aspirin: in this instance, 0.95. The narrowness of the 95% confidence limits around the estimated relative risk (0.84 to 1.08), indicates that the null hypothesis can be accepted. All risk variables (which, by definition, must include all confounding variables on which information was

TABLE 3

Regular Aspirin Use During Early Pregnancy in Relation to Malformations Among 50,282 Pregnancies

No. of Pregnancies Exposed in Lunar Months 1–4	No. of Malformed Children	Expected† No.	Standardized Risk Ratio	95% Confidence Limits
5,128	227	238.8	0.95	0.84 – 1.08

†Expected number adjusted for (multiple logistic risk function analysis)

1. Maternal age (<15 vs 15–34 vs 35+ years)
2. Sex of child
3. Duration of pregnancy
4. Single umbilical artery
5. Toxemia of pregnancy
6. Hydramnios
7. Maternal cardiac disorders (principally arrhythmias)
8. Maternal diabetes mellitus
9. Maternal hyperthyroidism
10. Maternal syphilis
11. Maternal convulsive disorder
12. Maternal abdominal/pelvic X-ray exposure
13. Family history of congenital defects
14. Birthweight

available) have been taken into account. One can, therefore, conclude that the regular use of aspirin in early pregnancy is not related to the risk of having a malformed child (although it must be stressed that specific malformations have not yet been considered).

One further point can also be made by returning to the example of a tranquilizer given for an unknown but "high risk" indication. Assume that the adjusted relative risk for ventricular septal defect, given exposure to the drug during the first trimester, is 3.0. This malformation can, presumably, only arise during early embryogenesis (and, indeed, this consideration applies with notable exceptions, to most malformations). If the adjusted relative risk for exposure in late pregnancy is also 3.0, it is possible that the indication for use is the underlying cause. On the other hand, if the latter relative risk is 1.0, then suspicion can more strongly be focused on the drug. In a more general sense, by comparing crude relative risks and adjusted relative risks, in early and late pregnancy, it is often possible to carry the inferential process further in evaluating potential drug teratogenicity. This topic requires more consideration than is possible within the scope of this paper.

The efficiency of the procedures outlined above is obvious. By controlling all risk variables, any confounding is automatically controlled. All that is required is the derivation of a small series of models, each tailored to the specific malformation class under consideration. One is then in a position to determine observed numbers and expected numbers for each drug exposure group, in turn. One can then identify associations that warrant further consideration, both by means of more detailed analysis within the existing data base and by using the hypotheses uncovered by this strategy as a springboard for further research in other bodies of data.

In this regard, we have already identified a number of interesting and important associations that are currently being further investigated.

Summary

A follow-up study of 50,282 pregnancies is described. Analytical strategies in use to evaluate potential drug teratogenicity are presented. These strategies have included exclusion, univariate analysis, linear discriminant function analysis and, finally, multiple logistic risk function analysis. Use of these procedures will enable screening of all drug exposures in pregnancy (in which there are sufficient numbers) against a variety of malformation classes. Associations identified in this way will serve as a resource for hypothesis generation and testing within the existing data. In addition, it will be possible to evaluate other bodies of data to confirm or reject hypotheses of interest.

AUTHOR'S NOTE

The following institutions participated in the Collaborative Perinatal Project of the National Institute of Neurological Diseases and Stroke: Boston Lying-in Hospital; Brown University; Charity Hospital, New Orleans; Children's Hospital of Buffalo; Children's Hospital of Philadelphia; Children's Hospital Medical Center, Boston; Columbia-Presbyterian Medical Center; Johns Hopkins Hospital; Medical College of Virginia; New York Medical College; Pennsylvania Hospital; University of Minnesota Hospitals; University of Oregon Medical School and University of Tennessee.

DISCUSSION

MERVYN SUSSER (Columbia University, New York City, New York): Dr. Heinonen, can you reduce the multivariant reduction of this complex body of data to quantitative terms and, once done, examine the logical structure of the variables that have been introduced into the multivariant analysis? Let's consider sequences which the variables introduced into the analyses might take. For instance, short gestation was set aside as a factor in congenital malformations of the heart because the whole of the relationship was explained by low birth weight. In reality, short gestation is a likely part of the causal sequence between whatever the precipitating or antecedent factor is, and low birth weight and the congenital malformation. There are two possibilities — either short gestation leads to low birth weight or, the improbable one, that low birth weight leads to the malformation. In fact, low birth weight is probably a consequence of the malformation. Furthermore, when you're controlling the low birth weight you may be actually controlling out risk because if low birth weight is a consequence and not an antecedent, by controlling it you are going to reduce a natural relative risk. Even though the quantitative approach which has been demonstrated gives us a tremendous tool, it still requires us to examine all the detailed relationships for early malformation and set up the quantities of relationship if they fit different logical sequences of the variables involved.

SAMUEL SHAPIRO (Boston University Medical Center, Boston, Massachusetts): Confounding is partially responsible for a difficult problem in epidemiology. What is confounding? When is a variable confounded? When is it antecedent? When does it follow? What is the causal chain? If we were to place the 15 factors related to the outcome into the model, death of the child would wipe out the 15 factors and leave only control data. Even though low birth weight may be a consequence, rather than a cause, a control is necessary because this, in turn, indicates that something else in the pregnancy put the pregnancy at high risk. Over-control is necessary because the degree of overlap between any drug exposure group and a particular factor are apt to be so small that variants that overlap are likely to be correspondingly "large". For example, where about 600 women suffered hydramnios in a total cohort of 50,000 pregnancies, it is not likely that we would eliminate an association between drug exposure and a particular outcome by over-controlling. The only examples of over-control we found in our data were in factors like maternal x-ray exposure when over half the cohort was exposed. Over-controlling for "small" factors has little effect. We always examine an interesting association more closely by this beautiful multivariant screening procedure. Also, if we find a 5-fold difference between crude and standardized relative risk we search for the cause and consider the possibility that we have over-controlled.

DR. HEINONEN: As to whether pelvic or abdominal x-rays have some influence on congenital heart disease, and if there is a temporal or dose relationship to the specific pregnancies in which these may occur, there are enormous amounts of information from the x-ray dates, doses of x-ray, number of x-rays, parts of the body x-rayed, etc., but we cannot pursue every detail when our goal is to evaluate drugs. We have limited it here to the pelvic and abdominal x-rays but we have not analyzed temporal or dose relationships.

DR. JANERICH: I think the importance of comparing the crude with the adjusted risk ratios has been overemphasized because interactions between conditions and drugs could be overlooked otherwise. Will you be examining the group that was excluded from analysis for the ratio?

DR. SHAPIRO: We are not planning to examine the exclusions.

HILDA KNOBLOCH (Albany Medical College, Albany, New York): Why didn't bleeding appear as a risk factor in pregnancy except for association of hemorrhagic shock?

DR. SHAPIRO: Bleeding did appear on univariate analysis, generally bleeding in the second trimester, which was most strongly related to malformation outcome. In relation to the malformed child, bleeding in pregnancy disappears when placed in the linear discrimination function model. The highest we found was about 1.1 for the first trimester, 1.3 for the second trimester and 1.1 again for the third trimester. Unfortunately, bleeding in pregnancy in this cohort was not clearly and well defined and did not appear because it was not a clear cut category. It varied from spurious menses, to threatened abortions, to vaginal polyps, to false onset of labor. We were unable to assess threatened abortion during the first trimester.

DR. KNOBLOCH: Dr. Stein, in order to evaluate your data adequately, one would have to assume that food was randomly distributed during the course of the famine. I suppose that the marked drop in birth weight was not randomly distributed even within the famine population, since the mean birth weight was 3,000 grams in a high socioeconomic area. You would not expect to find many survivors because the death rates were very high. I'm sure you did not mean to imply that a 400 calorie diet is recommended for pregnancy.

DR. STEIN: The food ration was available throughout the population. Black market and other methods were used more by those with influence, etc. More cohorts conceived in the heart of the famine were from the upper classes. Cohorts with reduction in birth weights do not show a relationship to social class nor a relationship between earlier low birth weight and lesser intelligence.

DR. KNOBLOCH: The cohort exposed to famine early in pregnancy represents those exposed when the central nervous system is undergoing its most active organization. You may have found no differences in later function because those children were born to the people who had the greatest access to food. One might assume that the fact that they became pregnant and were from the classes that had influence might have produced good later function. What are the social class differences between the famine area and the rest of Holland?

DR. STEIN: The numbers are large. Within social class there are differences but they were there through the three year period.

DR. KALTER: Dr. Stein, what central nervous system defects did 8 of the 3,600 young men have? Were you able to examine birth certificates to find the defects which occurred at birth in the population exposed to famine during early pregnancy?

DR. STEIN: The information noted at birth was not very specific. We examined chiefly the cohort which showed a reduced birth weight. Those exposed in the first trimester showed no defects as adults in the continuous distributions that were available. Nothing there shows any disadvantages from intrauterine exposure.

SECTION VI

GENETIC HETEROGENEITY: PROBLEMS OF ALLELIC DIVERSITY IN HETEROZYGOTE DETECTION AND IN THE DETERMINATION OF GENE FREQUENCY *

F. Gilbert
W.J. Mellman

"When I use a word", Humpty Dumpty said to Alice, "it means just what I choose it to mean — neither more nor less."[1] For the purpose of this discussion, genetic heterogeneity, which means different things to different people, will be used to refer to the effects that multiple alleles at one or more genetic loci may have on a specific gene product. Perhaps the most obvious, and certainly the most thoroughly explored, examples of allelic diversity are the mutations involving the β-chain locus of hemoglobin. These vary widely in phenotypic expression, from benign electrophoretic variants to those producing anemia with red cell sickling, cyanosis and polycythemia. This presentation will focus on several other genes responsible for human disease.

The demonstration of the biochemical basis of a large number of inherited disorders (a number which is over 100 at present and steadily increasing), while it has significantly advanced our understanding of the mechanisms of human disease, has also not been without its problems. The establishment of the individual enzyme deficiencies responsible for the production of specific metabolic disorders has made it possible, in some instances, to identify heterozygous carriers of these rare recessive genes and, thus, has made possible the counseling of individuals or couples who are at risk of transmitting such genes to their offspring. We are also now capable of determining the true frequencies of these rare genes in the population. The presence of variant enzymes of no pathological significance, a phenomenon which is now realized to be commonplace, however, may complicate both heterozygote detection and the calculation of gene frequencies.

That the exclusion of variants is not always simple is illustrated by the example of the galactosemia syndromes. There are at least two distinct disorders of galactose metabolism in man. A deficiency of the enzyme

---

*Supported in part by USPHS Grants GM-20138, HD-00599, HD-04861.

TABLE 1

Transferase (Gt) Activity Distribution

	n	Mean*	±	S.D.
Total Population	1700	6.03	±	.809
Obligate Heterozygotes for Gt Deficiency	32	3.15	±	.480

*μmoles/hr/ml packed RBC

galactose-1-phosphate uridyltransferase (recently renamed by the biochemists hexose-1-phosphate uridyltransferase) is involved in the conversion of galactose-1-phosphate to UDP galactose and glucose-1-phosphate and is associated with failure to thrive, liver disease, cataracts and mental retardation. A deficiency of the enzyme galactokinase (involved in the conversion of galactose to galactose-1-phosphate) is significantly milder in severity and usually results only in cataract formation.[2]

Estimates of the population frequency of the mutant genes for galactosemia, due to either galactokinase or transferase deficiency, are based either on determinations of carrier frequency or on disease incidence as detected in newborn screening surveys.[3,4]

There are several potential sources of error in determining gene frequency by analyzing newborn populations. Because a large sample is necessary to estimate homozygote frequency reliably, the surveys either must involve multiple clinical centers or be extended over many years. Among other potential sources of error which may be introduced into the calculations are the loss of transferase deficient homozygotes due to death in the neonatal period or, as has been speculated, due to intrauterine death.[5]

Carriers of the transferase deficiency gene can be identified by the presence of half-normal levels of enzyme activity in their erythrocytes.[2] There is no significant overlap evident between the distribution of enzyme activities of individuals who are carriers for this galactosemic gene and that for the general population (Table 1). Several estimates of the frequency of the transferase deficiency gene based on population surveys have been published.[6] The wide variation in these estimates reflects, at least in part, the existence of a third allele at the same locus. This is the so-called Duarte variant, first described by Beutler and co-workers, which results in reduced levels of red cell transferase activity when measured by standard assays.[7] Studies performed by several laboratories have demonstrated that the red cell transferase activities of individuals heterozygous and homozygous for the Duarte variant overlap with those of individuals heterozygous for the classical transferase deficiency gene.[8,9] Transferase from Duarte variant individuals can, however, be distinguished electrophoretically from that of carriers for galactosemia.[10]

The importance of distinguishing between the several transferase alleles was evident in a recent population survey of over 1700 obstetrical patients in Philadelphia.[6] Seventeen individuals were identified whose erythrocyte transferase activity was within the range of galactosemia heterozygotes. When red cell samples from these individuals were subjected to starch gel electrophoresis, nine of the seventeen were found to actually carry the Duarte variant gene and only eight were found to be true heterozygotes for the galactosemia gene. With the Duarte variants excluded from consideration, the observed frequency in the population of the gene for the transferase form of galactosemia is 1/212. By extrapolation, this would predict that the incidence of homozygous galactosemia in the population is 1/180,000, a figure which agrees remarkably well with the incidence previously reported in a screening of newborns in Massachusetts.[4]

Estimates of the frequency of the galactokinase gene have similarly been complicated by the presence of a common variant in the population.[11] This recently described variant, named the Philadelphia variant after its city of discovery, appears to be quite frequent among black individuals and produced a lowered red cell enzyme activity in the range observed with heterozygotes for galactokinase-deficient galactosemia. It can, however, be distinguished from true galactokinase deficiency by analyzing enzyme activity in leukocyte preparations. Carriers of the deficiency gene have approximately 50 percent of normal enzyme activity in their white cells as well as in their red cells, while carriers of the Philadelphia variant gene have normal levels of enzyme activity in their white cells. When individuals with the Philadelphia variant were excluded from the analysis, the frequency of the carrier state for galactokinase deficiency in the black population was estimated at 1/360, which is similar to the approximately 1/300 frequency we detected in the white population.

Families have also been described with variants that demonstrate high erythrocyte levels of galactokinase or transferase. This would indicate that there are at least four allelic classes at each of the genetic loci concerned with transferase and galactokinase activities — one specifying the normal enzyme, one coding for the classical deficiency state, one coding for apparently benign, low activity variants (the Duarte and Philadelphia variants respectively), and one coding for high red cell activity variants.

Awareness of the several variant alleles for these two loci makes it possible, albeit tedious, to determine the true population frequencies of the medically significant abnormal genes and to identify heterozygous carriers of these genes unequivocally. By analogy with these results, one would predict that as population screening for other recessive genes becomes more extensive, the number of described variants, both common and uncommon, will dramatically increase.

This prediction has already been realized with the gene for Tay-Sachs disease (TSD), a disorder that has attracted worldwide interest, because it is an example of a genetic disease that can be prevented by the identification of heterozygous individuals in the general population through community screening.[12,13] The enzyme disorder, a deficiency of the heat labile, so-called "A form" of hexosaminidase (Hex A), is recognizable by both serum and tissue assays.[14] In recent months there have been two individuals, and other members of one of the families, identified in widely divergent points of the globe (one in Tel Hashomer, Israel and the other in Portland, Oregon), who appear to have mutant genes that affect Hex A activity but which are different from the allele responsible for TSD.[15,16] Both individuals were studied because they had had a child with classical TSD and were therefore obligate heterozygous for the Tay-Sachs gene. Instead of demonstrating intermediate levels of enzyme activity as expected, however, each was found to have essentially no Hex A activity in their plasma or serum and an absence of the Hex A band on electrophoresis of tissue preparations. Both individuals were completely normal in all other respects and are presumed to represent "genetic compounds", heterozygotes for both the Tay-Sachs gene and for the mutant allele producing a deficiency of Hex A which is not clinically significant.

Additional studies of one of these individuals have demonstrated that the level of Hex A activity in skin fibroblasts and, presumably, other tissues as well, is similar to that found in carriers for TSD.[17] This situation is somewhat analogous to that described for the Philadelphia variant of galactokinase where there are different levels of enzyme activity in different tissues and would explain why some individuals with no apparent Hex A activity do not demonstrate classical TSD.

The serum determination of Hex A activity is the most common assay for this enzyme used in population surveys. Obviously, without additional testing, the presence of these variants would not only complicate, by falsely elevating, the measurement of the frequency of the Tay-Sachs gene, but might lead to the inappropriate labeling of individuals. Such individuals, who bear an apparently benign mutant allele, would be called carriers of the Tay-Sachs gene. Whether this variant for Hex A that mimics the Tay-Sachs gene is a common one, *i.e.,* is a polymorphism, or is a rare allele, has not yet been determined. Therefore, we do not yet know how often apparent carriers detected in a population survey are actually "pseudo-Tay-Sachs" carriers.

Conclusion

The remarkable number of electrophoretic variants of human genes detected over the past decade has resulted in an estimate of 6 percent for the average degree of heterozygosity at human gene loci.[18] This was considered by Harris to be most likely an underestimate. It is very possible that a similar degree of heterozygosity might exist due to alleles that are expressed as variations in the measured activity, both decreased and increased, of specific gene products. Some of these variants are expressed in the homozygotes as deficiency diseases. In general, such disease-producing alleles are of low frequency; they are lost by selection and maintained by mutation. On the other hand, variants at the same loci may have altered enzyme activity and, because they are not deleterious in the homozygous state, are not lost from the gene pool by selection. Such alleles, on the basis of their frequency, may be considered polymorphic and this appears to be the case for the Duarte variant of galactose-1-phosphate uridyltransferase and for the Philadelphia variant of galactokinase. These alleles can and have introduced errors in both the estimations of the population frequencies of their galactosemia-producing counterparts and in the identification of individuals as carriers for the two forms of galactosemia. A similar situation has recently been revealed with a Hexosaminidase A variant that mimics the Tay-Sachs gene. The degree of heterogeneity in the protein products, both structural and enzymatic, of specific genetic loci is, therefore, a significant problem which must be recognized if we are to deal effectively, in both individual and population terms, with the genes responsible for human disease.

REFERENCES

1. L. Carroll, The Annotated Alice Through the Looking Glass, Bramhall House, New York, p. 269, 1960.

2. H.M. Kalckar, J.H. Kinoshita and G.N. Donnell, *in* Biology of Brain Dysfunction, G.E. Gaull (Ed.), Plenum Press, p. 31, 1973.

3. S. Kelly, S. Katz, J. Burns and J. Boylan, *Publ. Health Rpts. 85,* 575, 1970.

4. V.E. Shih, L.H. Levy, V. Karolkewicz, S. Houghton, M.L. Efron, K.J. Isselbacher, E. Beutler and R.A. MacCready, *New Eng. J. Med. 284,* 753, 1971.

5. E. Beutler, M.C. Baluda, P. Sturgeon and R.W. Day, *J. Lab. Clin. Med. 68,* 646, 1966.

6. T.A. Tedesco, K. Miller, E. Rawnsley, M. Mennutti, R.S. Spielman and W.J. Mellman, Human erythrocyte galactokinase and hexose-1-phosphate uridyltransferase: a population survey (in preparation).

7. E. Beutler, M.C. Baluda, P. Sturgeon and R.W. Day, *J. Lab. Clin. Med. 68,* 646, 1966.

8. E. Beutler, *Israel, J. Med. Sci. 9,* 1323, 1973.

9. W.J. Mellman, T.A. Tedesco and P. Feigl, *Ann. Hum. Genet. (London) 32,* 1, 1968.

10. W.G. Ng, W.R. Bergren, M. Fields and G.N. Donnell, *Biochem. Biophys. Res. Comm. 37,* 354, 1969.

11. T.A. Tedesco, K.L. Miller, B.E. Rawnsley, M.D. Adams, H.J. Boedecker, K.G. Orkwiszewski and W.J. Mellman, Characterization of the Philadelphia variant of galactokinase (in preparation).

12. M.M. Kaback, R.S. Zeiger and H. Gershawitz, *Pediat. Res. 6,* 261, 1972.

13. J.S. O'Brien, S. Okada, D.L. Fillerup, M.L. Veath, B. Adornato, P.H. Boenner and J.G. Leroy, *Science 172,* 61, 1971.

14. S. Okada and J.S. O'Brien, *Science 165,* 698, 1969.

15. R. Navon, B. Padek and A. Adam, *Am. J. Hum. Genet. 25,* 287, 1973.

16. J. Vigdoff, N.R.M. Buist and J.S. O'Brien, *Am. J. Hum. Genet. 25,* 372, 1973.

17. J. Vigdoff, N.R.M. Buist, A. Miller, L. Tennant and J.S. O'Brien, Non-uniform Distribution of Hexosaminidase A (Abst.), presented at Am. Soc. of Hum. Genet., Oct. 16–19, 1974.

18. D.A. Hopkinson and H. Harris, *Ann. Rev. Genet. 5,* 5, 1971.

SCREENING: PERINATAL ASPECTS*

Harvey L. Levy

Perinatal screening for genetic diseases — that is, true general population screening in an essentially unselected manner — was planted, assiduously cultivated and brought to fruition by Dr. Robert Guthrie of Buffalo. Dr. Guthrie has received, at least in the United States, far too little recognition for his achievement, which may be one of the most significant medical discoveries of the modern era. For the simple Guthrie test[1] and the principles it illustrates have opened up an entire field for detection, study and treatment of human genetic disorders.

Dr. Guthrie, as all great scientists, has not labored in a vacuum, however. As indicated in Table 1, the development of the Guthrie test was significant because, many years before, Dr. A. Fölling, a Norwegian pediatrician and biochemist, had discovered phenylketonuria (PKU), a biochemical disorder that is associated with mental retardation[2] and because Dr. George Jervis, who is now in New York, discovered that PKU is an inborn error of amino acid (specifically phenylalanine) metabolism.[3-5] Finally, the concept that PKU is a truly important disease in regard to mental retardation and human genetics was sealed by the discovery of Bickel in 1953 that a special diet could not only control the biochemical abnormalities but could actually control certain of the manifestations of brain damage.[6] By the late 1950's it was known that a low-phenylalanine diet could probably prevent the brain damage in PKU, if only it were instituted in early infancy and before the brain damage became manifest.[7,8] The stage was set for the introduction of the Guthrie test which, far more than being a simple bacteriological assay for phenylalanine, established the concept that general population testing for biochemical disorders could be accomplished with a few drops of blood dried into filter paper and delivered by mail to a central laboratory. It is this concept which was truly revolutionary. From this have followed the brilliant paper chromat-

*Supported in part by MCHS-MR grant 01-H-000111-05-0 from the Health Services and Mental Health Administration of the U.S. Public Health Service and grant NS-05096 from the National Institutes of Health.

TABLE 1

Milestones in Perinatal Screening

1937	Fölling	Discovery of phenylketonuria
1939	Jervis	Familial nature of phenylketonuria
1940	Jervis	Accumulation of phenylalanine in phenylketonuria
1953	Jervis	Enzyme deficiency in phenylketonuria
1953	Bickel	Diet for phenylketonuria
1963	Guthrie	Screening test for phenylketonuria
1964	Efron	Screening for amino acids by paper chromatography
1966	Beutler	Enzyme spot screening test (galactosemia)

ographic technique for blood and urine developed by Efron and her colleagues[9] and the equally brilliant enzyme spot screening test for galactosemia, developed by Beutler and Baluda.[10]

The availability of such tests was not enough to insure perinatal screening for biochemical disorders. There was much opposition to such screening from both medical and lay individuals.[11,12] However, under the selfless and untiring direction of Dr. Robert MacCready, Massachusetts not only became the first state to routinely screen all newborns for PKU[13] but it also began screening these same newborns for many other disorders as the suitable tests became available. Table 2 lists these tests as they were added to the routine newborn blood specimen. As noted in Table 2, newborn urine testing for metabolic disorders was begun in 1968. This was instituted to enable the detection of those disorders that are not identifiable by blood testing, either because the metabolite accumulation in blood is below the sensitivity of the available tests or because there is no metabolite accumulation in blood. Disorders of renal transport, such as cystinuria or Hartnup "disease", are examples of the latter. Finally, the testing of umbilical cord blood was begun in late 1969, so that "classical"galactosemia could be detected in the neonate as early in life as possible.

Today, the Massachusetts program consists of multiple tests performed on these three filter paper specimens. Figure 1 lists the current program in Massachusetts, now known as the Massachusetts Metabolic Disorders Screening Program. In general, the tests have remained constant over the years. A comparison of Table 2 and Figure 1, however, reveals that testing for galactosemia has undergone several changes. Initially, the *E. coli* inhibition assay for galactose was applied to newborn blood. The technical difficulties with organism stability that were encountered prompted a change to the Beutler enzyme spot test, when the latter became available. When it was recognized that certain galactosemic infants die with sepsis within the first few days of life unless treated, a fact well documented by Dr. Sally Kelly,[14] umbilical cord blood collection was added to the program and the Beutler test was transferred to this specimen. Recently, the bacteriophage assay for galactose, developed by Paigen and Pacholec,[15] was added to the newborn specimen as insurance for "classical" galactosemia detection and for the detection of galactokinase deficiency.[16]

Table 3 lists the disorders that have been detected by such perinatal screening. PKU clearly represents the backbone of such a program at the present time, being the most frequent of the disorders that clearly result in clinical disease and for which early therapeutic intervention is both available and effective. Galactosemia, maple syrup urine disease, homocystinuria and argininosuccinic acidemia are placed in a second category of disorders with

TABLE 2

Screening Tests as Incorporated within the Massachusetts Program

Year	Specimen	Test	Disorder
1962	Newborn blood	Guthrie (Phe)	Phenylketonuria
1963		Guthrie (leu)	Maple syrup urine disease
1963		*"E. coli"*	Galactosemia
1965		Guthrie (Meth)	Homocystinuria
1967		Beutler	Galactosemia
1968		Guthrie (Tyr)	Tyrosinemia
1972		Paigen	Galactosemia
1968	Urine	Paper chromatography	Other amino acid disorders
1969	Umbilical cord blood	Beutler	Galactosemia
1970		Guthrie (Phe)	Maternal phenylketonuria

MASSACHUSETTS METABOLIC DISORDERS SCREENING PROGRAM

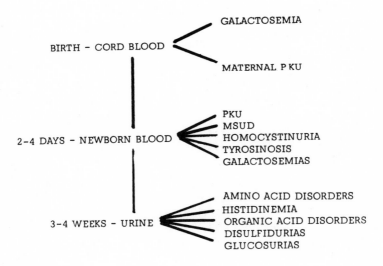

Fig. 1. Filter paper specimens obtained from infants routinely within the Massachusetts Metabolic Disorders Screening Program.

TABLE 3

Disorders Detected in the Massachusetts Metabolic Disorders Screening Program

Disorder	Newborns Screened	Number With Disorder	Frequency
* Phenylketonuria	1,095,519	78	1: 14,000
* "Atypical" PKU	1,095,519	64	1: 17,000
* Maternal PKU	232,227	8	1: 30,000
* Galactosemia	690,000	7	1:100,000
* Maple syrup urine disease	956,162	3	1:300,000
* MSUD (intermediate)	956,162	2	1:450,000
** MSUD (intermittent)	956,162	1	−
* Homocystinuria	563,773	3	1:190,000
* Tyrosinosis	498,313	0	−
* Argininosuccinic acidemia	414,329	6	1: 70,000
Histidinemia	414,329	22	1: 20,000
Histidinemia (atypical)	414,329	2	1:200,000
Hartnup "disease"	414,329	23	1: 18,000
* Cystinuria	414,329	27	1: 15,000
Iminoglycinuria	414,329	? 40	? 1: 10,000
* Hyperglycinemia (non-ketotic)	414,329	3	1:140,000
Cystathioninuria (B6-Response)	414,329	4	1:100,000
Cystathioninuria (B6-Resistant)	414,329	1	−
** Methylmalonic acidemia	414,329	2	1:200,000
Hyperprolinemia	414,329	2	1:200,000
* Propionic acidemia	414,329	1	−
* Rickets (Vit. D. Dependent)	414,329	1	−
Hyperlysinemia	414,329	1	−
* Fanconi Syndrome	414,329	1	−

*Clinically Significant Diseases: treatment is available for each one.

**"Missed" by routine neonatal screening but later identified on the basis of clinical disease.

clinical consequences and dietary efficacy but with a lower frequency than PKU. Methylmalonic acidemia and propionic acidemia would seem to be fit into a third category of disorders that are quite rare but which also are serious diseases and subject to therapy. Into a fourth category could be placed cystinuria, the Fanconi syndrome and vitamin-D resistant rickets, in which there may be no immediate neonatal need for therapy but in which identification early in life could be very important. A fifth category would include non-ketotic hyperglycinemia, which is associated with severe disease but for which no therapy is currently available.

The last category of disorders detectable by the current Massachusetts program includes those that are definitely benign or, on the basis of emerging evidence, may very likely be benign. Among the former, I would include iminoglycinuria and mild hyperphenylalaninemia and among the latter, histidinemia and Hartnup "disease" as well as hyperprolinemia. This is a very important category and one that certainly will be swollen by added disorders as we gain more information. The labeling of an infant as having a disease and especially the institution of treatment is a very serious matter, one that is likely to have a lifelong effect. Harm, both physical and emotional, as well as good, may result from such diagnosis and care. As physicians, it is most important that we bear in mind the dictum *"primum non nocere"* — first, do no harm. We have just as great a responsibility to learn of the benign biochemical findings as we do to diagnose and treat those disorders that are not benign.

The perinatal screening that I have described is hardly complete. There are many more genetic disorders not being sought routinely than there are those that are sought and discovered. Cystic fibrosis, the mucopolysaccharidoses and the hyperlipidemias are a few examples of disorders for which treatment may be available in the not-too-distant future and, in such circumstances, should certainly be detected in the perinatal period. The hemoglobinopathies, particularly sickle cell disease, may correctly be screened for in the neonates at some future time, though at present there would seem to be no clear justification for such screening. Screening for cretinism, as potentially valuable as is PKU screening, is already underway in Quebec[17] and probably should become a part of all perinatal screening programs.

Perinatal screening is just beginning. In the future a much wider array of genetic disorders than we can now imagine will be routinely sought in all newborns. It is of utmost importance that we now take as critical a look at such programs as possible, so that we retain and develop those programs that will lead to the prevention of disease.

REFERENCES

1. R. Guthrie and A. Susi, *Pediatrics 32,* 338, 1963.

2. A. Fölling, *Hoppe Seyler Z. Physiol. Chem. 227,* 169, 1934.

3. G.A. Jervis, *J. Ment. Sci. 85,* 719, 1939.

4. G.A. Jervis, R.J. Block, D. Bolling and E. Kanze, *J. Biol. Chem. 134,* 105, 1940.

5. G.A. Jervis, *Proc. Soc. Exp. Biol. Med. 82,* 514, 1963.

6. H. Bickel, J. Gerrard and E.M. Hickmans, *Lancet 2,* 812, 1953.

7. M.D. Armstrong, N.L. Low and J.F. Bosma, *Amer. J. Clin. Nutr. 5,* 543, 1957.

8. C.Y.-Y. Hsia, W.E. Know, K.V. Quinn and R.S. Paine, *Pediatrics 21,* 178, 1958.

9. M.L. Efron, D. Young, H.W. Moser and R.A. MacCready, *New Engl. J. Med. 270,* 1378, 1964.

10. E. Beutler and M.C. Baluda, *J. Lab. Clin. Med. 68,* 137, 1966.

11. S.P. Bessman, *J. Pediat. 69,* 334, 1966.

12. J.D. Cooper, *Medical Tribune,* Jan. 19, 1966.

13. R.A. MacCready and M.G. Hussey, *Amer. J. Publ. Health 54,* 2075, 1964.

14. S. Kelly, *J.A.M.A. 216,* 330, 1971.

15. K. Paigen and F. Pacholec (in preparation).

16. R. Gitzelmann, *Pediat. Res. 1,* 14, 1967.

17. J.H. Dussault and C. Laberge, *L'Union Med. Canada 102,* 2062, 1973.

ADVANCES IN THE DIAGNOSIS OF HUMAN GENETIC DISORDERS *

Betty Shannon Danes**

Since the term "advances" is more difficult to put into proper perspective than the word "diagnosis", I have arbitrarily limited my discussion to one clinic problem, the patient whose physical appearance is almost, but not quite, familiar — the patient without a diagnostic label, that is, an identifiable syndrome.

Webster's unabridged dictionary defines a syndrome as "a group of signs and symptoms that occur together and characterize a disease". Syndrome identification is one of the diagnostic cornerstones of clinical genetics. Occasionally, the clinical "picture" presented by the patient is suggestive of a known syndrome but does not meet all the recognized criteria for that syndrome.

The purpose of this communication is to discuss how the application of one methodology — the study of the cultured human cell — has added insight into understanding the genetic reasons for such disparate clinical phenotypes. A mutant genotype not recognizable and/or understandable *in vivo* can often be recognized *in vitro* by studying the metabolism and morphological characteristics of the cultured cell.

Two syndromes will be used as illustrations of this principle — the genetic mucopolysaccharidoses and cystic fibrosis.

GENETIC MUCOPOLYSACCHARIDOSES

Diagnosis of a human disorder in mucopolysaccharide metabolism starts with the clinician's recognition of the signs and symptoms which fit one of the syndromes in the McKusick classification of genetic mucopolysaccharide

---

*This research was made possible through a grant from the National Foundation-March of Dimes and partially supported by the Cystic Fibrosis Children's Fund and the National Cystic Fibrosis Research Foundation.

**Career Scientist of the Health Research Council of New York City (I-797).

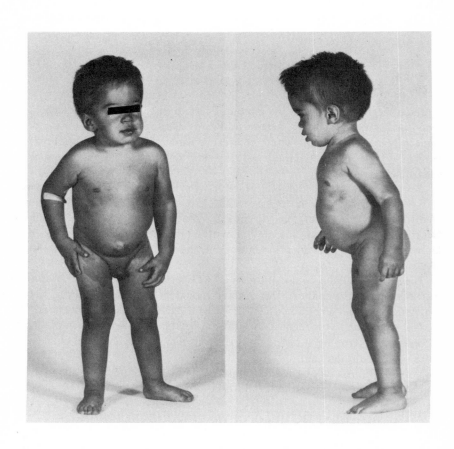

Fig. 1. Hurler/Scheie compound heterozygote at age 17 mos.

disorders.[1] The clinic phenotypes for each of these known syndromes are so constant that the diagnosis is usually made on seeing the patient and the subsequent laboratory tests confirm the initial impression.

This constancy of clinical phenotype is so well recognized that when a patient is seen whose clinical signs are suggestive but not diagnostic of one of the recognized mucopolysaccharidoses, the clinician recounts the atypical features to his colleagues.

The following clinical summary is an example: a caucasian male was first seen at the New York Hospital at the age of 17 months for recurrence of a left inguinal hernia. His previous clinical history was non-informative except for bilateral inguinal hernias at age 3 months. At 16 months the diagnosis of a mucopolysaccharide disorder was made (Fig. 1), on the basis of physical findings (mild coarsening of facies, limitation of joint mobility, faint corneal clouding, hepatosplenomegaly) and laboratory tests (mucopolysacchaduria composed of 50% dermatan sulfate and 48% heparan sulfate, leukocyte inclusions and metachromatic cultured fibroblasts). On the basis of cloudy corneas and evidence of mucopolysaccharide storage in other tissues by x-ray (Fig. 2), the diagnosis of the Hurler syndrome was made, although the clinical expression of the Hurler syndrome was milder than expected for the chronological age of the patient.

At 28 months of age the patient was seen in the Moore Clinic, the Johns Hopkins Hospital, with signs of progression of mucopolysaccharide storage, particularly involving the skeletal system (Fig. 3). At approximately the same time the enzyme deficient in both the Hurler and Scheie syndromes was determined to be a-L-iduronidase.[2] This patient's cultured fibroblasts were shown to lack the same enzyme. McKusick[3] thought that the clinical phenotype of this patient was difficult to categorize as Hurler, primarily due to the mild expression at two years of age. On the basis of this intermediate phenotype in combination with a deficiency of a-L-iduronidase, McKusick suggested that this patient was a mixed heterozygote — having inherited a Hurler gene from one parent and a Scheie gene from the other parent, resulting in an intermediate phenotype. However, on the basis of enzyme deficiency it was not possible to determine which of the two mutated genes had been transmitted from each parent.

At 5 years of age the patient has normal intelligence but he had delayed speech development and a hearing deficit.

Cell culture offered an opportunity to answer this question and to understand the genetic reason for this patient's disparate clinical phenotype. If the presence of the gene for the Hurler and Scheie syndromes could be distinguished in culture by differences in cell culture phenotype, then assignment of each gene to one of the two parents would be possible.

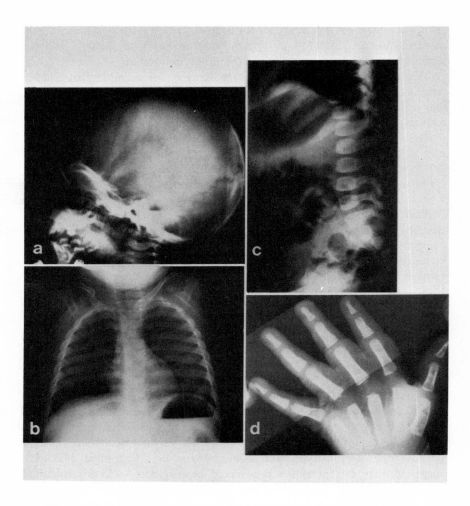

Fig. 2. Roentgenograms of Hurler/Scheie compound heterozygote at age 17 months.

(a) Skull, (b) chest, (c) spine and (d) hand.

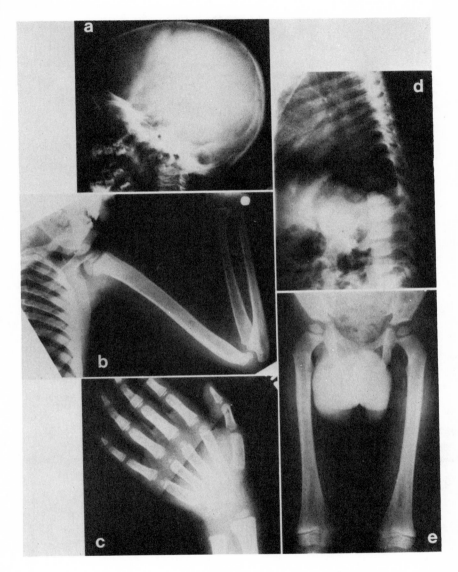

Fig. 3. Roentgenograms of Hurler/Scheie compound heterozygote at age 3 years.

(a) Skull, (b) chest and upper limb, (c) hand and wrist, (d) spine and (e) pelvis and lower limbs.

METHODOLOGY FOR STUDIES ON THE MUCOPOLYSACCHARIDES OF CULTURED FIBROBLASTS

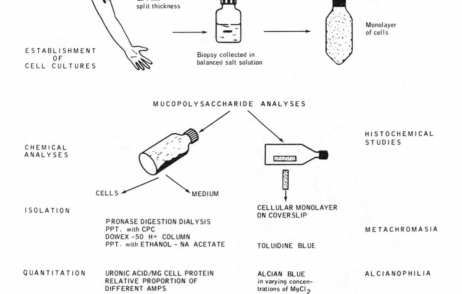

Skin biopsy
1x4 mm
split thickness

ESTABLISHMENT
OF
CELL CULTURES

Biopsy collected in
balanced salt solution

Monolayer
of cells

MUCOPOLYSACCHARIDE ANALYSES

CHEMICAL
ANALYSES

HISTOCHEMICAL
STUDIES

CELLS   MEDIUM

ISOLATION

CELLULAR MONOLAYER
ON COVERSLIP

PRONASE DIGESTION DIALYSIS
PPT. with CPC
DOWEX -50 H+ COLUMN
PPT. with ETHANOL - NA ACETATE

METACHROMASIA

TOLUIDINE BLUE

QUANTITATION   URONIC ACID/MG CELL PROTEIN
RELATIVE PROPORTION OF
DIFFERENT AMPS

Sensitive to hylauronidase
Nitrous acid reaction for N-sulfated
hexosamines
Electrophoresis

ALCIAN BLUE
in varying concen-
trations of MgCl$_2$

alcianophilia
in 0.3 M MgCl$_2$

ALCIANOPHILIA

Fig. 4

302

The cellular mucopolysaccharides of the cultured skin fibroblasts from two normals, an individual each with the Hurler and Scheie syndromes, their parents and the patient and his parents were studied (Fig. 4).

Methodology

Split thickness biopsies were taken without anesthesia from the extensor surface of the arm (Fig. 4). The establishment of the cell lines from skin biopsies by standard culture methods[4] requires about 6 weeks so that the cells studied have been grown as monolayer cultures from 1 to 2 months (two to six subcultures by trypsinization) prior to studies. Culture medium used in all cultures was reinforced Eagle's medium containing 10% by volume of new-born calf serum. Prior to each experiment, cell lines were grown in large round bottles on a roller apparatus, so that cell samples for both morphological and chemical studies came from one parent culture.

Histochemical Studies. Approximately 20,000 cells were inoculated into each 2-ounce glass flask which contained a coverslip. One week later the coverslip was removed, washed in warm balanced salt solution for 1 minute and cut into three parts. The first part was immediately immersed in methanol for 5 minutes and stained with the metachromatic dye, toluidine blue O[5]. The other two parts were stained for the presence of specific mucopolysaccharides in a simple one-step procedure, using Alcian blue 8 GX solutions containing 0.1 or 0.3 M $MgCl_2$.[6]

Chemical Studies. Roller bottle cultures of a cell line were established with approximately 10^8 cells and grown for about 2 weeks (with one medium change) prior to harvesting for chemical analyses.

Isolation of Mucopolysaccharides. After decanting the medium, the monolayer was trypsinized (0.25%) for 10 minutes and the sheet of cells shaken into suspension. The mucopolysaccharides of the cell suspension and used medium were then isolated by digestion with Pronase dialysis and precipitated with cetylpyridinium chloride (CPC).[7] Total polysaccharide was estimated as uronic acid by the carbazole method.[8]

The CPC-precipitate was then washed repeatedly with 95% ethanol containing 10% potassium acetate and dissolved in water.[9] This aqueous solution of CPC-precipitate was then passed through a column (5 X 1 cm) of Dowex 50 (X4, 50-100 mesh, H^+ form) and the effluent applied to a column (7 X 1 cm) of AG 1 (X2, 200-400 mesh, Cl^-), washed with saline and the mucopolysaccharides eluted with 2.0 M NaCl.[10,11] The eluate was precipitated with ethanol at 4° C, and redissolved in 1 ml distilled water. Total polysaccharide was estimated as uronic acid by the carbazole method.[8] Dermatan sulfate was measured by a modification of the periodate Schiff reaction.[11] Heparan sulfate was detected by the nitrous acid reaction for

TABLE 1

Mucopolysaccharides of the Human Skin Fibroblast Cultures

| | | Skin Fibroblast Cultures | | | | | | |
| | | Hurler | | Scheie | | Family | | |
Characteristics	NORMAL	Hom.	Het.	Hom.	Het.	Mother	Father	Compound
Histochemical								
Metachromasia[5]	−	++++	++++	+	+	++++	+	++++
Alcianophilia in 0.3 M MgCl2[6]	−	++++	++++	+	+	++++	+	++++
Chemical analyses								
Total cellular content[7] (μg uronic acid/mg cell protein)	1.8	16.8	12.9	7.0	3.4	11.9	4.1	19.0
Relative proportion of mucopolysaccharides								
Hyaluronic acid	68	28	36	48	46	30	59	25
Chondroitin sulfates	14	6	4	10	10	10	9	20
Dermatan sulfate	16	54	50	40	40	50	40	36
Heparan sulfate	2	12	10	2	4	10	2	19
α-L-iduronidase activity (Hurler factor[2,13])		dec.	dec.	dec.	dec.			dec.

Cytoplasmic staining with toulidine blue 0 is referred to as metachromasia (pink) (+) or orthochromasia (blue) (−); cytoplasmic staining with alcian blue solution containing 0.3 M MgCl2 is alcianophilia (+) and no staining is (−).

N-sulfate hexosamines.[12]   A portion was subjected to testicular hyaluronidase digestion and the undigested material was reprecipitated with ethanol-sodium acetate.   Hyaluronic acid and chondroitin sulfates were determined as the material susceptible to testicular hyaluronidase.

The phenotype for the cultured fibroblasts from the families with the Hurler and Scheie syndromes could be readily distinguished (Table 1).[14] (1) The cultured cells from both the homozygotes and heterozygotes for the Hurler syndrome showed intensive staining (both metachromasia and alcianophilia), whereas those for the Scheie syndrome showed much less staining. (2) Total mucopolysaccharide content was 2-3 times greater in the Hurler than in the Scheie cell.   The relative distribution of the different mucopolysaccharides was distinct for each.   In the Hurler cell both dermatan sulfate and heparan sulfate were increased, whereas only dermatan sulfate was increased in the Scheie cell.

The cultured skin fibroblasts from the mother had the culture phenotype of the Hurler cell (intense staining, increased total mucopolysaccharide content and a marked relative increase in both dermatan sulfate and heparan sulfate).   The cells from the father had the culture phenotype of the Scheie cell (slight staining, modest increase in total mucopolysaccharides and a relative increase in dermatan sulfate).   The cells from the patient had the Hurler phenotype.

On the basis of the culture phenotype, it was possible to determine that the mother was a carrier of the Hurler gene and the father the Scheie gene, resulting in their offsprings being a mixed heterozygote, that is, a genetic compound.   A genetic compound is defined as the condition when two different rare alleles are present at a given locus.[3]

By studying the cultured cell not only from the affected individual but also both his parents, (1) his clinical phenotype was shown to reflect a lack of a-L-iduronidase,[2,13] (2) the difficulty in syndrome categorization was attributed to his being a genetic compound, having received a Hurler gene from his mother and a Scheie gene from his father.

The genetic cause for his clinical phenotype which almost, but not quite, fit the Hurler syndrome was solved through the application of chemical and histochemical assays to the cultured skin fibroblast. Without this research approach, the diagnosis of "atypical Hurler syndrome" would have been used in genetic counselling with the family members which would have been far from satisfactory in the ensuing genetic discussions.

CYSTIC FIBROSIS (CF)

The second case I would like to describe as an illustration of the basic

TABLE 2

Clinical History of Cystic Fibrosis Patient P.C.

P.C.   ♀   age 20 years

Clinical Evidence of Cystic Fibrosis	Presence + = positive − = negative
LUNGS	
Chronic bronchiolar obstruction	+
Lung infections	+
Staph. aureus	+
Hemophilis influenza	+
Antibiotic therapy	intermittent
Chest x-ray	+ (6/6 fields)
Pulmonary function studies	
FEV_1	2150
Fvc	2900
Nasal polyps	−
Pulmonary osteopathy	+
GASTROINTESTINAL	
Malabsorption	+ (without RX)
steatorrhea	+
azotorrhea	+
Malnutrition	−
Meconium ileus	−
Rectal prolapse	−
Intestinal obstruction	−
Pancreatic supplements	+
Cirrhosis	−
Hepatosplenomegaly	−
Liver function tests	NL
Diabetes mellitus	−
Hirsuitism	−
GROWTH	
Height	5 feet, 4 inches
Weight	110 pounds (nl 108−116)

concept of this paper — that a mutant genotype not recognizable *in vivo* can often be recognized by studying the cultured cell — is patient P.C. (Table 2).

P.C. is a 20 year old female typist who was first seen at Queen Elizabeth Hospital for Children, London, at the age of 6 months for "large bulky stools and a cough". The diagnosis of cystic fibrosis was made on the basis of the clinical picture and the presence of a positive quantitative sweat test (Na 107 meq/1, upper limit of normal 60 meq/1 for the laboratory). The patient was placed on pancreatic supplement which improved both intestinal absorption and bowel function. For the next 17 years she continued to take pancreatic supplements but no antibiotic treatment was required for pulmonary infections. At the age of 17 years clinical treatment for chest symptoms was required. As staphylococcus aureus and hemophilus influenza were cultured from her sputum, intermittent antibiotic therapy was started. At present (age 20 years), her pulmonary and liver function studies are within normal limits but changes associated with cystic fibrosis are seen in all lung fields by x-ray. The only clinical complication associated with cystic fibrosis is pulmonary osteopathy (clubbing of the fingers).

A wide variation in the clinical course of CF has been recognized for many years. In Shwachman's series of 2200 patients with CF,[15] approximately 12% (260 patients) reached the age of 17 years. P.C. fits into this category. At the age of 20 years, P.C. is a patient with an atypical clinical course. At age 6 months she had the clinical triad for CF — evidence of malabsorption, cough and elevated sweat electrolytes. Thus, she had the clinical picture and laboratory evidence indicating CF. There are few tests in pediatrics that carry the same degree of reliability as the sweat test. No other commonly encountered condition in pediatrics yields a consistently positive sweat test.[15]

Shwachman[15] had no explanation for the mild course of this group of CF patients nor does he think that one can identify CF patients who will have a mild expression with a good prognosis at the time of the initial diagnosis.

Such variation in clinical expression in a genetic disorder raises at least three possible explanations: (1) variable expressivity of the same gene (*i.e.*, CF is the result of the mutation of one gene), (2) more than one gene mutation may be expressed as the clinical phenotype known as CF (*i.e.*, genetic heterogeneity) and (3) two different alleles at a given locus produce a mixed heterozygote, a genetic compound.[3,16]

Cell culture has offered an opportunity to study the isolated human cell with the CF genotype to answer this question — is CF one or more genetic disorders?

Some of the characteristics of the cultured CF fibroblast have been established (Table 3). Although all the abnormalities noted so far, which

TABLE 3

Abnormalities of Cultured Cells Derived from Homozygotes for
Cystic Fibrosis

CULTURE ABNORMALITY	REFERENCES*
Metachromasia	17, 4, 18
Heterogeneity in staining metachromasia and ametachromasia	17, 18
Variable mucopolysaccharide content intra- and extracellular	4, 8
Increased glycogen storage	19
Decreased collagen synthesis and collagenolysis	20
Longer generation time	20
Increase in lysosomes number and size	21
Alteration in total hexosaminidase and ratio of isoenzymes A to B	22
Cystic fibrosis factor activity (CFFA) in culture medium of metachromatic CF cultures	17, 23, 24, 25, 26
Abnormality in complement	27
Metabolic cooperation between fibroblasts of normal (non-CF) genotype and CF (metachromatic, CFFA positive) but not between the latter and CF (ametachromatic, CFFA negative)	28
Increased sulfate and heparan incorporation	29, 30, 31
Relative increase in dermatan sulfate with a normal total mucopolysaccharide content in CF lymphoid lines derived from families whose cultured fibroblasts have either culture phenotype	32
Undermethylation of RNA in cultured lymphocytes and fibroblasts	33

*Numbers refer to papers identified in References.

distinguish the cultured CF cell from the normal cultured cell, are not specific for CF, they suggest that a cell with a CF gene adapts differently to an artificial-culture environment, as displayed by abnormalities in both morphology and metabolic activity.

Three of these characteristics have been used together as a cell culture phenotype in studying the genetic expression of the CF gene in culture: metachromasia, cystic fibrosis factor activity (CFFA) and metabolic cooperation. An evaluation of the present status of each of these three characteristics will be presented to establish the criteria for the CF culture phenotype.

Metachromasia

Metachromasia is a non-specific staining reaction given by any macromolecule containing electronegative radicals and exhibiting a periodic negative surface charge.[34] Substances such as metaphosphates, nucleic acids, polypeptides, mucopolysaccharides and lipids show tissue metachromasia.[35] If cells are grown under controlled conditions with the pH of the medium maintained in the acid range (6.8–7.4),[36] approximately 5 to 10% of a normal population will yield cultured fibroblasts which show metachromasia.[37–39] When studied for mucopolysaccharide content (qualitative and quantitative — see Methodology — and by specific histochemical staining, using alcian blue in varying concentrations of $MgCl_2$), these fibroblasts show no abnormality in cellular mucopolysaccharides.[6] Thus, the specific substance causing the metachromasia has not been determined for fibroblasts from 5 to 10% of normal, unrelated individuals in the general population.

When technical precautions of controlled cultured conditions are used in culturing,[36] fibroblasts from 80% of CF patients and their parents show cellular metachromasia.[17] The mucopolysaccharide content of the CF cell has been found to be normal[40] and variable[18,41] in chemical content but not to be mucopolysaccharides, by specific histochemical staining. The significance of the metachromasia to the as yet unknown basic defect in cystic fibrosis has not been established.

Cystic Fibrosis Factor (CFF)

A factor named the cystic fibrosis factor (CFF) has been recognized in the serum and media from skin fibroblast cultures established from the majority of patients with CF. Two biological assays have been used for the detection of CFF. Ciliary dyskinesis is evidence of activity in the rabbit tracheal bioassay,[26] whereas ciliary stoppage is, in the oyster cilia test.[43] These two assays have been used in studies on the characterization of the factor but each study has utilized only one assay.[43,25,44] It has been assumed that the same factor is being assayed, irrespective of the cilia source or the culture and assay

TABLE 4
Culture and Assay Conditions which Differed in the Oyster Cilia Test and the
Rabbit Tracheal Bioassay to Detect Cystic Fibrosis Factor Activity (CFFA)[26,43]

	Assays for Cystic Fibrosis Activity	
CONDITIONS	Oyster Cilia Test	Rabbit Tracheal Bioassay
pH of medium during culture and assay	7.5 – 7.8	6.8 – 7.4
Assay preparation sealed	Yes	No
Assay temperature	25° C	37° C
Ciliary actions monitored	stoppage within 60 min.	dyskinesis within 6 min.

conditions being used. Recent experimental evidence suggests that the two assays are detecting different biological substances. The data in Tables 4 and 5 indicate that culture and assay conditions which influence CFF detection in one system appear to have no effect in the other assay system. This disparity was shown clearly in the fibroblast cultures tested in the two assays.

The chemical nature of the CFF is not known. Conover, Conod and Hirschhorn[27] have suggested that the CFF identified in the rabbit tracheal bioassay is a complex of a complement component, C3a (known as ana-phylatoxin) with IgG. If C3a is the substance responsible for CFF activity in the rabbit tracheal bioassay and a different, as yet unknown, substance is being detected in the oyster test, the inactivation of C3a by specific antiserum would be expected to influence activity in the rabbit and not in the oyster test. CFF assayed in the oyster cilia test was found to be associated with a low molecular weight, negatively charged molecule that contained no uronic acid.[44]

Awareness that the two assay systems are probably detecting different substances should help in the characterization of the specific factor and its role in the pathology of CF.

CFF in the family PC was detected by a modification of the oyster cilia test, in which CFF activity was measured as the ability of culture media to stop oyster cilia.

Metabolic Cooperation

Correction of a mutant phenotype which requires cell-to-cell contact has been named metabolic cooperation.[45] This process has been extensively studied in the Lesch-Nyhan syndrome where metabolic cooperation between normal cells and mutant cells deficient in hypoxanthine-guanine or adenine phosphoribosyltransferase may have been the result of transfer of the enzyme product, nucleotide or nucleotide derivative from normal to mutant cells. Separation of Lesch-Nyhan cells from normal cells resulted in prompt reversion to the mutant phenotype. The molecular basis of metabolic cooperation in this defect, however, is not known.

Several reports[22,37,46,47] have established the existence in culture of metachromatic and ametachromatic classes of CF fibroblasts, which show intrafamilial agreement. Although the metachromatic class was distinguished in cell culture by the staining reaction and CFF activity, the ametachromatic class was indistinguishable from cultures derived from non-carriers. The mixing experiments[28] revealed a distinct difference. When positive CF cells were mixed with normal cells, correction (*i.e.*, metabolic cooperation) occurred, whereas positive CF cells mixed with negative cells were not corrected.

The mutant phenotype was not corrected by growing CF cells in used

TABLE 5

Cystic Fibrosis Factor Activity (CFFA) in Culture Medium from Three Different Cell Types from Cystic Fibrosis and Normal Families Assayed Using the Oyster Cilia Test and the Rabbit Tracheal Bioassays[26,43]

	SUBJECTS					
	NORMAL		CYSTIC FIBROSIS			
			Metachromatic		Ametachromatic	
CULTURED CELL TYPES			CILIA ASSAYS			
	Rabbit**	Oyster	Rabbit*	Oyster	Rabbit	Oyster
Skin fibroblasts						
non-confluent						
without addition of IgG	−	−	−	+	−	−
with addition of IgG	−	−	+	+	+	−
confluent	+	−	+	+	+	−
Short-term white blood cells	−	−	+	+	+	+
Long-term lymphoid lines	−	−	+	−	+	−

*References 8 and 9.
**The experiments involved the addition of 50 µl of monoclonal human immunoglobulin IgG subclass 1/ml used culture medium.

Results are shown as presence (+) or absence (−) of CFFA.

medium from normal cultures or with normal cells in the same vessel but separated to avoid cell-to-cell contact.[2]

Cells from patients, such as P.C. and her obligatory heterozygote parents, were examined for CF culture phenotypes in an attempt to answer the question — does phenotypic diversity reflect more than one genetic defect?

Before proceeding, I should point out that the two classes of CF fibroblasts (Class I — metachromatic, CFF positive, metabolic cooperation positive; Class II — ametachromatic, CFF negative) have been found to relate to the degree of clinical expression. In Danish families with CF, for example,[48] the propositus in each family was discovered earlier in Class II than in Class I, suggesting a poorer prognosis for Class II patients. A relationship of class to clinical expression and/or prognosis was suggested also by the frequency of Class I fibroblasts in adults with CF in a London group, with the diagnosis made before puberty. Of the 42 adult CF patients studied in collaboration with Drs. Batten, Herrick and Hodson at The Brompton Hospital, 39 were Class I, as expected, and 3 were Class II. As predicted. two of these three Class II patients had extensive clinical involvement and succumbed in the past year. The clinical course of our patient, P.C., was relatively mild, in fact uneventful on pancreatic supplement, even though diagnosis was made at an early age. If she were Class II CF, she should have succumbed by the age of 20 years, or at least shown extensive clinical involvement. At 20 years of age, her physical condition was good with the exception of evidence of lung involvement by x-ray.

Study of cultured fibroblasts from her parents added new insight into the clinical expression of her disorder. Her mother's cell culture phenotype was Class I (Table 6) and her father's was Class II. The mating between the Class I and Class II CF heterozygotes resulted in a child with cystic fibrosis which followed an atypical clinical course.

In summary, the patients described were selected to demonstrate how the use of cell culture adds insight into the diagnosis of human genetic disorders.

The first patient's atypical expression of the Hurler syndrome was clarified by cell culture studies. The patient was presumed to be a genetic compound for the Hurler/Scheie syndromes because: (1) his clinical phenotype was intermediate between those of the Hurler and Scheie homozygotes, (2) his cells were deficient in α-L-iduronidase, the same enzyme as is deficient in the Hurler and Scheie syndromes,[2] (3) complementation did not occur between cultured cells from the patient, his parents and the Hurler or Scheie syndromes,[3] and (4) cell culture phenotype of the mother was that of the Hurler gene (Table 1) and of the father, the Scheie gene.[14] Although these observations are evidence. for allelism, proof will be provided only when the structure of the enzyme α-L-iduronidase is determined in the Hurler and

TABLE 6

Characteristics of the Cultured Skin Fibroblasts from Cystic Fibrosis Families and Family P.C.

SUBJECTS	CYSTIC FIBROSIS CULTURE PHENOTYPES[17]		
	Metachromasia	Cystic Fibrosis Factor Activity	Metabolic Cooperation
CF Class I	+	+	+
CF Class II	–	–	–
Family P.C.			
Proband	–	–	–
Mother	+	+	+
Father	–	–	–

314

Scheie syndromes as well as in our patient.

The second patient, P.C., illustrated how cell culture studies added information but not necessarily understanding. Evidence (Table 6) that P.C. might represent a genetic compound was: (1) The clinical course for CF was milder than expected. (2) If the assumption is made that the different culture phenotypes of the heterozygous CF parents reflected different CF mutations, the fact that these two different genes combined in the offspring to produce disease, (3) complementation (metabolic cooperation) did not occur between the cultured cells from the mother, father and offspring. Until the basic defect in CF is known, it is not possible to prove that the CF cell culture Classes I and II reflect different alleles at the same locus, capable of producing a genetic compound. Thus, the answer to whether the clinical phenotype of P.C. reflected a genetic compound (mixed heterozygote) or variable expressivity of one or more genes will have to await future research.

In conclusion, the study of the cultured human cell has and will aid in advancing our ability to diagnose human genetic disorders.

REFERENCES

1. V.A. McKusick, Heritable Disorders of Connective Tissue, 4th Ed., St. Louis, 1972.

2. U. Wiesmann and E.F. Neufeld, *Science 169,* 72, 1970.

3. V.A. McKusick, I.E. Hussels, R.R. Howell, E.F. Neufeld and R.E. Stevenson, *Lancet 1,* 993, 1972.

4. B.S. Danes and A.G. Bearn, *J. Exp. Med. 129,* 775, 1969.

5. B.S. Danes and A.G. Bearn, *J. Exp. Med. 123,* 1, 1966.

6. B.S. Danes, J.E. Scott and A.G. Bearn, *J. Exp. Med. 132,* 765, 1970.

7. B.S. Danes and A.G. Bearn, *J. Exp. Med. 124,* 1181, 1966.

8. T. Bitter and H.M. Muir, *Anal. Biochem. 4,* 330, 1962.

9. N. Di Ferrante, G. Neri, M.E. Neri and W.E. Hogsett, *Connect. Tissue Res. 1,* 93, 1973.

10. S.S. Schiller, G.A. Slover and A. Dorfman, *J. Biol. Chem. 236,* 982, 1961.

11. N. Di Ferrante, P.V. Donnelly and R.K. Berglund, *Biochem. J. 124,* 549, 1971.

12. D. Lagunoff and G. Warren, *Arch. Biochem. Biophys. 99*, 396, 1962.

13. R. Matalon, J.A. Cifonelli and A. Dorfman, *Biochem. Biophys. Res. Commun. 42*, 340, 1971.

14. B.S. Danes, *Lancet 1*, 680, 1974.

15. H. Shwachman, *Birth Defects: Orig. Art. Ser. 8*, 102, 1972.

16. V.A. McKusick, *Am. J. Hum. Genet. 24*, 446, 1973.

17. B.S. Danes, *Birth Defects: Orig. Art. Ser. 8*, 114, 1972.

18. R. Matalon and A. Dorfman, *Biochem. Biophys. Res. Commun. 33*, 954, 1968.

19. J.C. Pallavicini, U. Wiesmann, W.B. Uhlendorf and P.A. di Sant'Agnese, *J. Pediatr. 77*, 280, 1970.

20. J.C. Houck and V.K. Sharma, *Proc. Soc. Exp. Biol. & Med. 135*, 369, 1970.

21. J. Bartman, U. Wiesmann and W. A. Blanc, *J. Pediatr. 76*, 430, 1970.

22. J.H. Conover, E.J. Conod and K. Hirschhorn, *Lancet 1*, 1122, 1973.

23. B.S. Danes and A.G. Bearn, *J. Exp. Med. 136*, 1313, 1972.

24. B.H. Bowman, D.R. Barnett, R. Matalon, B.S. Danes and A.G. Bearn, *Proc. Nat. Acad. Sci. USA 70*, 548, 1973.

25. J.H. Conover, N.G. Beratis, E.J. Conod, E. Ainbender and K. Hirschhorn, *Pediat. Res. 7*, 224, 1973.

26. J.H. Conover, R.J. Bonforte, P. Hathaway, S. Paciuc, E.J. Conod, K. Hirschhorn and F.B. Kopel, *Pediat. Res. 7*, 220, 1973.

27. J.H. Conover, E.J. Conod and K. Hirschhorn, *Lancet 2*, 1501, 1973.

28. B.S. Danes, *Lancet 2*, 765, 1973.

29. B.S. Danes and A.G. Bearn, *Lancet 2*, 437, 1969.

30. M. Caudill, I. Schafer and R. Stjernholm, *Lancet 1*, 32, 1974.

31. J.A. Robertson, B. Chernik, D.J. Segal and E.E. McCoy, *Lancet 1*, 1256, 1974.

32. B.S. Danes, J.E. Backofen and B.K. Rottell, *Biochem. Genet. 12* (in press), 1974.

33. O. Rennert, J. Frias and D. LaPointe, *in* Fundamental Problems of Cystic Fibrosis and Related Diseases, J.A. Mangos and R.C. Talamo (Eds.), Intercont. Med. Book Corp., New York, p. 41, 1973.

34. B. Sylvén, *Acta Histochem. suppl. 1,* 79, 1958.

35. T. Barka and P.J. Anderson, Histochemistry, Theory, Practice and Bibliography, Harper and Row, New York, p. 84, 1963.

36. O.S. Lie, V.A. McKusick and E.F. Neufeld, *Proc. Nat. Acad. Sci., USA 69,* 2361, 1972.

37. B.S. Danes, *Birth Defects: Orig. Art. Ser. 7,* 139, 1971.

38. A. Dorfman, Personal Communication, 1969.

39. H. Nadler, *Birth Defects: Orig. Art. Ser. 6,* 26, 1970.

40. U. Wiesmann and E.F. Neufeld, *J. Pediatr. 77,* 685, 1970.

41. B.S. Danes and A.G. Bearn, *Biochem. Biophys. Res. Commun. 36,* 919, 1969.

42. A. Spock, H.M.C. Heick, H. Cress and W.S. Logan, *Pediat. Res. 1,* 173, 1967.

43. B.H. Bowman, M.L. McCombs and L.H. Lockhart, *Science 167,* 871, 1970.

44. B.S. Danes, S.D. Litwin, T.H. Hutteroth, H. Cleve and A.G. Bearn, *J. Exp. Med. 137,* 1538, 1973.

45. R.P. Cox, M.R. Krauss, M.E. Balis and J. Dancis, *Exp. Cell Res. 74,* 251, 1972.

46. J. Bartman, U. Wiesmann and W.A. Blanc, *J. Pediatr. 76,* 430, 1970.

47. H.L. Nadler, J.M. Wodnicki, M.A. Swae and M.E. O'Flynn, *Lancet 2,* 84, 1969.

48. B.S. Danes and E.W. Flensborg, *Am. J. Hum. Genet. 23,* 297, 1971.

EXPERIENCES DEVELOPING A HUMAN GENETIC MUTANT CELL REPOSITORY *

Arthur E. Greene

INTRODUCTION

We have needed contaminant-free and well characterized reference cell lines for more than a decade,[1,2] a need stimulated by the widespread application of cell cultures to problems in cancer research, cytologic and biochemical genetics, immunology, virology, toxicology, nutrition and many other areas of biology and medicine.

The revelation of widespread contamination and admixture of cell cultures at three *ad hoc* conferences in 1959 cast serious doubts on the validity of much research utilizing cultured animal cells. Many or most cell lines were contaminated with bacteria or mycoplasma or with another cell species. Cell characteristics were unstable on serial passage yet there were no established techniques for rapid characterization of cells or detection of contaminants. Cell lines often transformed spontaneously and were thought to have been contaminated by another cell line by faulty techniques. Our objective was to determine whether these problems could be solved by improved or new culture techniques and thus eliminate waste of time and money. The method of approach involved basic research on many aspects of the above general problems.

We, and our collaborating laboratories, have since been able to develop and perfect new and improved techniques for species identification,[3,4] elimination and prevention of contamination of cell cultures,[5,6] characterization by chromosome morphology, growth requirements for numerous cell lines, techniques of mass production of cell cultures without antibiotics, preservation and long term storage of cells in liquid nitrogen[7] and the recovery of cells from the frozen state without damage to or deterioration of their original

---

*Supported by Contract N01-GM-3-2112 from the National Institute of Medical Sciences; and Grant-in-Aid Contract M-43 from the State of New Jersey.

properties. Each phase was conducted to solve the technical problems and to train a highly competent team to carry out the meticulous details. Individualized treatment is especially necessary with cell lines with genetic, biochemical and functional abnormalities.

BACKGROUND AND HISTORY OF THE HUMAN GENETIC MUTANT CELL REPOSITORY

Of 1,800 human genetic diseases, many can now be successfully predicted, prevented, controlled or treated. The techniques are at hand for improving our understanding of still others. With this in mind, the National Institute of General Medical Sciences (NIGMS) in 1972 coordinated research efforts involving several clinical centers, a central repository and others interested in genetic mutant diseases. A contract was awarded to the Institute for Medical Research, Camden, New Jersey, to establish and operate the repository, or bank, of genetic mutant cell cultures and normal control cultures stored in liquid nitrogen to facilitate and support expanded clinical and basic research programs in the field.[8]

The bank's supply of mutant and control cell cultures should promote genetic research because (1) the diseases may be rare and material not readily available to all interested physicians, (2) some cell types are cultured only with difficulty, (3) many examples of a given genetic defect are needed to explore its permutations and (4) time and money can be saved if new investigators can obtain standard cell cultures and procedures without having to develop cell lines and techniques.

The NIGMS also organized a scientific advisory committee to guide the development and research aspects of the Repository. It presently consists of Drs. Frank H. Ruddle, Chairman; Arthur Bloom; Elizabeth Neufeld; Stanley Gartler and Kurt Hirschhorn, assisted by the Projects Officers from NIGMS, Fred Bergmann and William Gartland, Jr., and formerly included Drs. William Mellman, Robert Krooth and Gordon Sato. The committee meets twice a year to establish general and recommend specific policies, such as the inclusion of particular cell lines or classes of cells.

The Repository stores viable cells in low passage with single and multiple gene defects, both defined and undefined at the molecular level; chromosome abnormalities (translocations, deletions and others); polymorphisms (isozymes, antigens); carrier and normal control cultures. Although most lines will be of human origin, a few non-human mammalian lines with unique or valuable genetic characteristics may be accepted.

Types of Cells Stored in the Repository

Additions to the collection can be made in the form of low passage cell cultures or, preferably, skin biopsies from patients with confirmed genetic variant diseases. The cell culture from excised tissue assures preservation of the *in vivo* karyotype, metabolic and enzyme characteristics in low passage, maximum cultural life span and minimum chance of contamination. All cultures are grown in laminar flow rooms or hoods without antibiotics after primary culture and stored in liquid nitrogen.

1. Fibroblast cultures

The collection of fibroblast cultures has been emphasized during the first two years of operation. The advice of other investigators is sought to ensure the responsiveness of the collection to the needs of the scientific community. Experts in specific biochemical diseases are acting as curators for the selection of additional cells. Our initial efforts are directed toward collecting mutant conditions for which known enzyme or protein defects have been established. although mutations of unknown molecular etiology, such as cystic fibrosis, will be included. The curator structures the collection from the significant family groups he or other investigators have thoroughly studied. Collections which include variant forms of the disease and appropriate controls are desirable. If necessary the curator may confirm the biochemical deficiency.

The Repository now contains cell cultures from patients with disorders expressed in cell culture including (1) amino acid metabolism, (2) carbohydrate metabolism, (3) lipid metabolism and (4) nucleic acid metabolism as well as several in which the defect is not presently expressed in culture.

The collection of cell cultures with chromosome abnormalities has also been given high priority. The important recent advance in somatic cell genetics, the demonstration of somatic cell fusion in man-mouse or man-hamster cell hybrids, makes possible the assigning of human genes to specific chromosomes and specific areas on the chromosomes.[9] Thus, somatic cell genetics is beginning to fulfill its promise as a powerful tool in mapping human chromosomes. Regional mapping will be made easier if cell lines representing well characterized translocation, inversions and deletions are available.

2. Lymphoid cultures

The lymphoid cell cultures now widely used in hybridization and in study of the inborn errors, can be grown more rapidly than fibroblast cell lines and thus provide relatively large numbers of cells quickly. Other advantages over fibroblast cell lines are their ready cloning, giving definable cell populations, and free growth in suspension, making them more suitable for metabolic investigation.[10] Their contamination with a possible oncogenic virus (the

Epstein-Barr virus[11]), however, has been a major concern. A subcommittee of the Advisory Committee to the Repository, consisting of Drs. Arthur Bloom, Kurt Hirschhorn and Lewis Coriell, met with Dr. Alfred Hellman, Office of Biohazards of the National Cancer Institute and Dr. Earl Chamberlayne of the National Institute of Allergy and Infectious Diseases, to formulate minimum safety guidelines and assurances necessary and desirable for the handling of lymphoid and virus transformed cell lines. Two documents were drafted as a result of the meeting, entitled "Agreement on Lymphoid and Virus Transformed Cells" and "Minimum Safety Guidelines Recommended for Working with Lymphoid and Virus Transformed Human Cell Lines". The former document requests that the recipient of lymphoid cells be aware of (1) the potential biohazard of these cells and not to distribute cells to other laboratories; (2) not to use the cells in human experimentation without the written approval of the Project Officer of the Contract. This agreement, when appropriately executed and signed, will be kept on file at the Institute for Medical Research and allow the signatories to receive lymphoid cells from the Repository. The second document, "Minimum Safety Guidelines Recommended for Working with Lymphoid and Virus Transformed Human Cell Lines", suggests to the recipient of the cultures a number of recommended procedures to reduce to a minimum the opportunities for accidental infection of laboratory personnel by any known or unknown viruses that might be in a cell culture. The acquisition and distribution of lymphoid cell cultures will be actively pursued now that the question of biohazards has been resolved.

3. Amniotic cells

Amniocentesis is now a widely established procedure for the prenatal diagnosis of a number of chromosomal and biochemical defects of the fetus.[12] Standardization of cultures of amniotic cells is difficult, however, because the sources of the cells are so variable and long-term culture is beset with technical problems. We are adding them to the Repository collection only at a pilot study level.

We recently established 46 cell cultures from amniocentesis fluids, preserved them in liquid nitrogen between the 2nd and 5th passage and later recovered them from the frozen state with little loss of viability. Five to ten percent glycerol was an optimal preservative for storage in liquid nitrogen and growth was initiated from as few as 5×10^5 viable cells per frozen ampule. Storage in liquid nitrogen did not affect the G6PD, LDH, MDH, leucine aminopeptidase, acid phosphatase or 6-phosphogluconic acid dehydrogenase isozymes, and the cells survived subculturing for approximately 25-30 passages before senesence.

322

PUBLICATION OF A CATALOG OF CELL CULTURES STORED IN THE HUMAN GENETIC MUTANT CELL REPOSITORY

The Repository has periodically published catalogs or lists of cell cultures available for distribution to interested investigators. The first official edition of the catalog was published in April 1973 by NIGMS and contained a list of 92 biochemical, chromosomal aberrant and 18 normal cultures. The second edition of the catalog was available for distribution late in 1974.[13] It contains 331 cultures, including 195 cultures classified under biochemical diseases, 64 cultures with chromosomal aberrations, 16 human lymphoid cultures, including controls, 2 SV_{40} transformed cell lines, 9 animal cell lines used in gene mapping, 5 human amnion cultures and 40 apparently normal fibroblast cell lines. The age of the individual from whom the culture was established, passage level of the cells stored in liquid nitrogen and contributor of the biopsy or culture are included. More detailed documentation about the cell culture is forwarded when a culture is shipped to a requesting investigator. Permission to include a brief description of diseases and key references from the third edition of "Mendelian Inheritance in Man" has been obtained from V.A. McKusick, M.D. and the Johns Hopkins Press. Chromosome cultures stored in the Repository are also listed in a computerized catalog of variations and anomalies compiled by D.S. Borgaonkar, Ph.D., which will also be published by the Johns Hopkins Press.

The Repository, with the concurrence of the Advisory Committee, allows contributors to store their cultures at the Repository without distribution until the appearance of their first publication or for a period of 12 months after submitting the culture to the Repository.

Publication of Data on Chromosome Abnormalities

Arrangements were made by the Repository and Advisory Committee and Dr. Harold Klinger, Editor of *Cytogenetics and Cell Genetics,* to publish short descriptions of cell cultures with chromosome abnormalities available from the Repository. The report consists of a brief history of the individual donating the cells, clinical data when appropriate, family pedigree when available, description of the chromosome abnormality using the Paris nomenclature and references listing previously published data. A photograph of the trypsin-giemsa banded karyotype prepared on cells recovered from liquid nitrogen to verify the abnormality after frozen storage is also included in the short description. The contributor or originator of the biopsy or culture and co-workers are listed as senior authors on the paper.

PROCEDURES FOR PLACING CULTURES IN THE REPOSITORY

1. Quarantine. Fresh biopsies or cell cultures sent to the Repository are placed in a quarantine laboratory and are cultured in his laboratory until proven free of contamination.

2. Sterility. Samples from cultures or biopsies are removed aseptically for sterility testing the first time the flask or container is opened. Bacterial contamination is determined by inoculation of the test samples in a variety of culture media and on an agar blood plate. Sabouraud dextrose broth and agar are used for the isolation of mold and fungi. Mycoplasma contamination of culture and biopsies is assayed for by growth in mycoplasma broth and on mycoplasma agar, using aerobic and anaerobic culturing techniques developed in our laboratory[14] as well as recently developed radioisotope methods. Mycoplasma growth is confirmed by microscope observation, staining techniques and serological identification. Cell cultures are kept in quarantine for 3 weeks or until they are known to be free of microbial contamination. Contaminated cell cultures or biopsies are immediately discarded to prevent cross contamination of clean cell cultures.

3. Expansion of Cell Cultures for Storage in Liquid Nitrogen. Cell cultures free of microbial contamination are expanded in culture medium similar to that used by the originator but without antibiotics. Antibiotics have a place in establishing primary cultures from contaminated tissues but should be removed at the time of the first subculture. Experience with amnion and skin biopsy cultures demonstrated that it is possible to prepare approximately 100 frozen ampules containing 5×10^5 viable cells per ampule within 3 or 4 cell passages from a fresh biopsy. All cell culture studies are carried out in laminar air flow rooms or hoods.[6]

4. Characterization of Cell Lines from the Frozen State. After storage in liquid nitrogen one or two ampules from each frozen cell line are removed and the cells studied for viability, morphology and sterility. Viability is determined by trypan blue dye exclusion test and by cell growth in antibiotic-free medium in culture. Species of origin of the cell line when required is determined by a combination of the immunodiffusion,[15] immunofluorescence[3] or cytotoxic-antibody dye exclusion tests.[4]

A brief surveillance karyotype is determined on all frozen cell lines to verify species and previously observed genetic abnormalities. A detailed karyotype by trypsin-giemsa banding technique is undertaken when the information is considered vital for the further characterization of the cell lines, *i.e.,* publication.

Isozyme analysis on cell lines is often undertaken when this is an important genetic character of the culture.

5. Procedures for Shipping Cell Lines to Users. The cells are distributed only to qualified professional persons who are associated with recognized research, medical educational or industrial organizations engaged in health-related research or health delivery.

Cultures are shipped as vegetative cells in plastic 30 cm^2 tissue culture flasks by air mail special delivery. The flasks are filled with culture medium and packed in styrofoam containers. Upon arrival the flasks should be placed in a 37° C incubator overnight before the flask is opened to allow recovery from the trauma of shipping.

Cell lines shipped from the Repository are accompanied by a data sheet which includes: (1) the original diagnosis of the patient, (2) the originating laboratory and original references or publications, (3) number of cell passages since the original isolate was made, (4) karyotype, if the data are available, (5) any other pertinent data of value to the investigator receiving the cells, (6) conditions for growing the cells, culture media, culture conditions, etc., and special characteristics or peculiarities of the specific cell line, as well as a brief description of the disease and key references from the third edition of "Mendelian Inheritance in Man", by V.A. McKusick, M.D., published by the Johns Hopkins Press.

RESEARCH PROGRAMS APPLIED TO IMPROVING THE PERFORMANCE OF THE REPOSITORY

The Institute has demonstrated that the development of a successful cell repository requires the skills of many different specialists and strong basic research programs aimed at improving the quality, adaptability, availability and reliability of the techniques used in cell culture. Our past experience indicates that success of the Human Genetic Mutant Cell Repository program will also depend on research programs using cell culture techniques to resolve the problems that develop. Some of our more recent investigations are: (1) development of techniques to establish and freeze cells from human amniotic fluid; (2) optimal methods for establishing lymphoblasts in long-term culture for genetic studies; (3) aging studies in genetically abnormal cells; (4) transformation of biochemical deficiency fibroblast cell cultures with SV$_{40}$ virus; (5) evaluation of the toxicity of the serum and culture medium by plating efficiency methods; (6) development of more sensitive methods for the isolation of mycoplasma from cell cultures. These programs are in addition to numerous smaller projects that arise in connection with cultivation, characterization and storage of mutant cells, many of which require special conditions that cannot be predicted from experience with normal cells.

SUMMARY

A Human Genetic Mutant Cell Repository has been established at the Institute for Medical Research, Camden, New Jersey by the National Institute of General Medical Sciences. The function of the Repository is to store valuable mutant and normal cultures in liquid nitrogen for the purpose of stimulating and facilitating research, diagnosis, teaching and prevention of human genetic diseases. Included are the historical development and descriptions of the need for a genetic cell repository, its organization, types of cells accepted, methods for informing the scientific community of the cultures available, procedures for characterizing cells and research programs applied to improving the performance of the Repository. The aid of interested investigators in anticipating and meeting these needs is earnestly solicited.

REFERENCES

1. Cell Cultures Collection Committee, *Science 146,* 241, 1964.

2. W.F. Scherer, *Nat. Canc. Inst. Mono. 7,* 3, 1962.

3. W.F. Simpson and C.S. Stulberg, *Nature 199,* 616, 1963.

4. A.E. Greene, L.L. Coriell and J. Charney, *J. Nat. Canc. Inst. 32,* 779, 1964.

5. L.L. Coriell, *Nat. Canc. Inst. Mono. 7,* 33, 1962.

6. G. McGarrity and L. Coriell, *In Vitro 6,* 257, 1971.

7. A.E. Greene, R. Silver, M. Krug and L. Coriell, *Proc. Soc. Exp. Biol. & Med. 116,* 462, 1964.

8. L.L. Coriell, *Science 180,* 427, 1973.

9. F.H. Ruddle, V.M. Chapman, F. Ricciuti, M. Murane, R. Klebe and P. Meere Khan, *Nature New Biol. 232,* 69, 1971.

10. W.J. Mellman, *Hosp. Pract.,* June, p. 103, 1973.

11. P. Gerber, *Birth Defects: Orig. Art. Series,* Vol. IX, No. 1, p. 20, 1973.

12. H.L. Nadler and A.B. Gerbie, *New Eng. J. Med. 282*, 596, 1970.

13. The Human Genetic Mutant Repository. List of Genetic Variant, Chromosomal Aberrations and Normal Cultures. 2nd Edition, October, 1974. Institute for Medical Research, Camden, N. J.

14. G.J. McGarrity and L.L. Coriell, *In Vitro 9*, 1973.

15. A.E. Greene, J. Charney, W.W. Nichols and L.L. Coriell, *In Vitro 7*, 313, 1972.

ADVANCES IN THE TREATMENT OF GENETIC DISEASES:
AN OVERVIEW*

R.J. Desnick**
M.B. Fiddler

INTRODUCTION

Major advances have been made in the elucidation of the molecular pathologies of inherited metabolic diseases during the past two decades. The clinical and pathophysiologic manifestations have been delineated and the metabolic derangements have been characterized in an ever increasing number of these myriad disorders.[1-4] Sophisticated chemical and enzymatic techniques, as well as *in vitro* tissue culture systems, have been developed to identify the specific enzymatic defects in more than 120 of the over 400 catalogued, recessively inherited inborn errors of metabolism.[2,4] Implementation of these techniques in major centers has made the diagnosis of these disorders a reality. Indeed, the demonstration of the specific enzymatic deficiency, at the level of the biochemical defect, has provided for the accurate diagnosis of affected homozygotes or hemizygotes, detection of heterozygous carriers, and the capability to prenatally diagnose and prevent the birth of affected fetuses. In spite of these major diagnostic achievements, however, patients and their families have become increasingly disappointed by the absence of specific therapies for most of these debilitating disorders.

During the past decade, considerable attention has been focused on the development of strategies to treat patients with inherited metabolic diseases

*Supported in part by Grant No. CBRS-273, National Foundation-March of of Dimes; Grant No. 74-915, American Heart Association; Grants. No. AM 15174 and AM 14470, National Institutes of Health; Grant No. RR-400, Clinical Research Centers Program of the Division of Research Resources, National Institutes of Health and a predoctoral fellowship (to M.B.F.) from the National Science Foundation.

**Recipient of a National Institutes of Health Career Development Award, No. 1-K04-AM0042.

TABLE 1

Approaches for the Treatment of Inherited Metabolic Diseases

METABOLIC MANIPULATION

Dietary Restriction
Surgical Bypass Procedures
Chelation
Metabolic Inhibitors
Product Replacement

GENE PRODUCT THERAPY

Cofactor Supplementation
Enzyme Induction
Allotransplantation
Enzyme Replacement Therapy

GENE THERAPY

PREVENTIVE THERAPY

Heterozygote Screening
Genetic Counseling
Prenatal Diagnosis

(Table 1). Theoretically, the ideal cure for these inherited disorders would be the insertion of the normal segment of DNA coding for the synthesis of the normal gene product. Therapeutic intervention at the level of the primary genetic defect or gene therapy, however, is presently precluded by our limited biochemical and cellular technology. Early therapeutic endeavors primarily involved attempts to alter the disease course by manipulations at the level of the metabolic or biochemical defects (Table 1). In selected diseases, investigators have attempted to reduce the levels of the accumulated substrate or precursors to the metabolic block by dietary restriction, chelation or administration of appropriate metabolic inhibitors. Alternatively, the deficient metabolic product has been supplied with documented examples of chemical and clinical success. Therapeutic trials at the level of the biochemical defect have involved direct administration of the appropriate gene product, the specific active enzyme or deficient cofactor or by the transplantation of allografts capable of producing the normal gene product. The limitations, as well as the encouraging experiences, of various strategies for the treatment of genetic disease have been the subject of recent symposia and reviews.[5-9]

A major thrust of current research is directed at the lysosomal storage diseases which have become a focus of exploratory therapeutic endeavors. Perhaps the experience and information gained from the study of these disorders, as prototypes, may provide the basis for future therapeutic endeavors specifically modified for other inherited metabolic diseases. The development of these strategies has been and will continue to be dependent on the further elucidation and understanding of the basic molecular pathology of specific inherited enzymatic deficiencies. Thus, my discussion will provide an overview of the various strategies for the treatment of genetic diseases.

METABOLIC MANIPULATION

As illustrated in Figure 1, therapeutic manipulation of the metabolic alterations resulting from an enzymatic defect has been designed either (1) to limit the intake or deplete the accumulation of the toxic substrate and/or its precursors or (2) to supply adequate concentrations of crucial metabolic products. In each amenable disorder, the metabolic manipulation is based on an understanding of the specific pathogenic compound, the accumulated substrate or deficient product. Table 2 lists the genetic diseases that have been treated by various metabolic manipulations.

Dietary Restriction

Dietary restriction was the first therapeutically successful manipulation for an inborn error of metabolism. In 1953, Bickel *et al.*[10] demonstrated the

331

TREATMENT OF INHERITED METABOLIC DISEASES

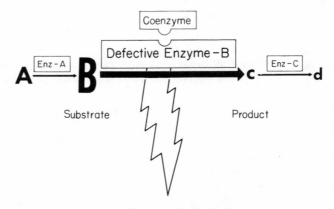

Therapeutic Strategies

SUBSTRATE:
1. Limit toxic metabolites – dietary therapy
2. Deplete stored metabolites – chelators
3. Metabolic inhibitors
PRODUCT:
4. Supply deficient metabolic product
ENZYME:
5. Supply coenzyme – cofactor, vitamin
6. Enzyme induction – ↑residual activity/alternate pathway
7. DIRECT GENE PRODUCT REPLACEMENT – ENZYME THERAPY

Fig. 1

TABLE 2

Genetic Diseases Treated by Metabolic Manipulation

DIETARY RESTRICTION
Argininosuccinicaciduria
Branched-Chain Ketoacidosis
Citrullinuria
Cystinuria
Galactosemia
Hereditary Fructose Intolerance
Histidinemia
Hyperammonemia
Hyperargininemia
Lactose Intolerance
Phenylketonuria
Tyrosinemia

CHELATION
Cystinuria
Primary Gout
Wilson's Disease

METABOLIC INHIBITORS
Hyperlipoproteinemia, Type III
Lesch-Nyhan Syndrome

PRODUCT REPLACEMENT
Adrenogenital Syndromes
Congenital Hypothyroidism
Orotic Aciduria
Pituitary Dwarfism

value of a low phenylalanine diet to limit the accumulation of the toxic substrate in patients with phenylketonuria (phenylalanine hydroxylase deficiency). Subsequent experience with this rationale has proven effective not only for patients with phenylketonuria but in other inborn errors whose pathogenesis is characterized by toxic substrate accumulation, including galactosemia,[11,12] hereditary fructose tolerance,[13] lactose intolerance[14] and tyrosinemia.[15] However, experimental attempts to treat cystinuria,[16,17] histidinemia[18, 19] and other aminoacidurias by appropriate dietary restriction have met with limited success.

Surgical Bypass Procedures

Intriguing surgical strategies have been accomplished for the treatment of patients with glucogenoses, types I[20] and III,[21] and hyperlipoproteinemia, type IIa.[22] In the glycogenoses, the progressive incorporation of absorbed glucose into hepatic glycogen is reversed by a surgical anastamosis between the portal vein and inferior vena cava. This portacaval shunt permits some of the circulating glucose, absorbed from the intestine, to bypass the hepatocyte where glucose is pathologically and irreversibly deposited as glycogen; the glucose-rich blood is shunted to nourish the tissues. In addition to re-establishing normoglycemia, these patients have documented clinical improvement. Similarly, ileal-jejunal bypass procedures have been successful in reducing the hypercholesterolemia in patients with hyperlipoproteinemia, type IIa, by decreasing the absorption of cholesterol from the gut.

Chelation

Another approach to decrease the concentrations of the noxious substrate and/or precursors and metabolic derivatives is the administration of chelators or other drugs to mobilize the excretion of these compounds. In Wilson's disease,[23,24] the copper accumulation may be depleted by the administration of penicillamine, a chelating agent which binds to, mobilizes and promotes the excretion of the intracellularly accumulated copper ions. Penicillamine has also been used for the treatment of cystinuria,[25] although for this disorder the drug participates in a mixed disulfide reaction to promote urinary clearance. Analogous therapy in primary gout has utilized various uricosuric drugs to decrease the systemic uric acid accumulation by increasing its renal excretion and mobilizing the intracellular deposits of uric acid salts.[26]

Metabolic Inhibitors

Metabolic inhibitors have been used to inhibit the synthesis of accumulated substrates or precursors. In patients with Lesch-Nyhan syndrome (hypoxanthine-guanine phosphoribosyl transferase deficiency) and primary gout

334

allopurinol has been used therapeutically to inhibit the precursor enzyme, xanthine oxidase, in order to reduce the uric acid concentrations.[27] Clofibrate, which inhibits the synthesis or release of glyceride from the liver, has been found effective in reducing blood lipids to normal levels in patients with hyperlipoproteinemia, type III.

Product Replacement

The clinically most effective metabolic manipulations involve direct product replacement in disorders whose pathogenesis results from the defective enzyme's failure to produce a metabolically crucial product. The administration of appropriate steroids to patients with the congenital adrenal hyperplasia syndromes,[29] thyroid hormone for hypothyroidism,[29] growth hormone for pituitary dwarfism,[30] and RNA or uridine for orotic aciduria[31] have provided therapeutically effective approaches to override the inherited metabolic block.

GENE PRODUCT THERAPY

Therapy at the level of the biochemical defect, the defective enzyme, is the focus of recent efforts to treat inherited metabolic diseases. Characterization of the molecular nature of a specific enzymatic defect provides the biochemical rationale for the development of effective therapeutic strategies at the level of the gene product as indicated in Table 3.

Cofactor Supplementation

Many enzymatic reactions require specific cofactors, often a vitamin or its derivative, for normal catalytic activity. In certain inborn errors, the enzymatic defect may involve the binding site for a specific cofactor or vitamin. Experience with the vitamin-dependent enzymatic deficiency diseases has indicated that, for certain mutations, cofactor supplementation may increase the residual activity of the mutant enzyme. This strategy has been applied to the treatment of a number of cofactor or vitamin responsive disorders (Table 3).

In several of these disorders, vitamin-responsive and non-responsive subtypes involving the same deficient enzymatic activity have been identified. Based on *in vivo* and *in vitro* studies, it has been hypothesized that responsive and unresponsive forms of a particular disease represent different structural mutants of the enzyme; in the responsive mutation, the cofactor binding site may be altered, but is still capable of binding when large concentrations of the cofactor are provided; the unresponsive mutation presumably has irreversibly altered the enzyme's conformation so that the residual enzymatic activity is not increased with the administration of large doses of the appropriate cofactor.

TABLE 3

Gene Product Therapy in Genetic Diseases

COFACTOR SUPPLEMENTATION

Branched-chain Ketoaciduria

Cystathioninuria

Dihydrofolate Reductase
    Deficiency

Familial Hypophosphatemia

Formiminotransferase Deficiency

Glutamic Acid Decarboxylase
    Deficiency

Hartnup Disease

Homocystinuria

Hyperoxaluria

Lactic Acidosis

Leigh's Disease

Methylmalonic Aciduria

Propionic Acidemia

Thiamin Responsive Anemia

Xanthurenic Aciduria

ENZYME INDUCTION

Crigler-Najjar Syndrome

Gilbert's Syndrome

ENZYME OR CORRECTIVE
FACTOR REPLACEMENT

Agammaglobulinemia

Diabetes Mellitus

Fabry's Disease

Gaucher's Disease

Glycogenosis Types II and IV

Hemophilia A and B

Metachromatic Leukodystrophy

Mucopolysaccharidoses
    Types I, II, III

Sandhoff's Disease

Von Willebrand's Disease

Overall, the clinical effectiveness of cofactor supplementation therapy. which is often accompanied by other dietary manipulations, has been variable; it is not anticipated, however, that even slight elevations in enzyme activity may prove beneficial, and follow-up studies are still required in these disorders. The therapeutic value of cofactor supplementation, as well as a theoretical discussion of the nature of the molecular pathologies in this group of diseases, has recently been reviewed.[3,9]

Enzyme Induction

Another approach at the level of the enzymatic defect involves the use of drugs which are capable of increasing a residual enzymatic activity. Phenobarbital and related drugs apparently stimulate the production of smooth endoplasmic reticulum as well as the synthesis of specific enzymes of the endoplasmic reticulum, including hepatic glucuronyl transferase. These findings have provided the basis for administering phenobarbital to patients with Gilbert's syndrome and Group 2 Crigler-Najjar syndrome.[32] Although enzyme modification or stabilization has not been ruled out, the drug presumably induces the glucuronyl transferase activity, resulting in increased conjugation of unconjugated bilirubin and a decrease in the plasma bilirubin levels. This approach may be of value in selected enzymatic defects resulting from a decreased rate or failure of synthesis of a specific enzyme.

Allotransplantation

An intriguing means for transferring normal genetic information into patients with selected structural and metabolic gene defects is allotransplantation. This approach exploits the grafting of cells, tissues or organs containing the normal DNA for the production of active enzymes or other gene products in the recipient. For structural gene defects limited to specific organs· or tissues, successful transplantation of the appropriate allograft may provide effective treatment. The selection of the allograft in a particular inherited disorder must be based on the specific nature of the defective gene product, the pathophysiology of the disease, as well as the probable mechanism by which the allograft might provide the normal gene product.

Figure 2 summarizes the various genetic diseases in which allotransplantation has been accomplished. Several of these endeavors were specifically designed to be therapeutic — to continuously replace defective enzymes hormones or immunologic factors or effectively restore the functional alterations resulting from structural gene defects.

Bone marrow, thymus and fetal liver have been transplanted in immunodeficiency diseases.[33] Bone marrow has been effective in reconstituting normal immunocompetence in over 20 patients with severe combined immuno-

ALLOTRANSPLANTATION IN GENETIC DISEASES

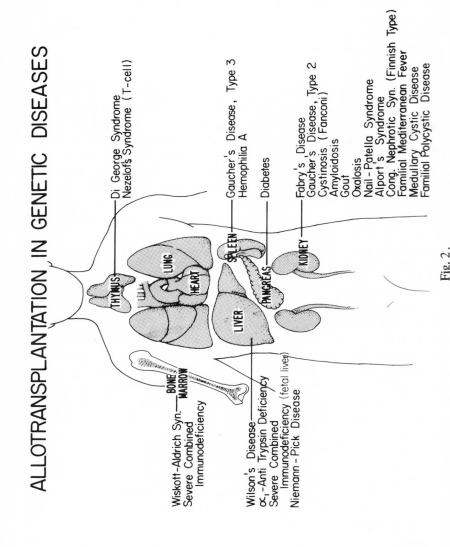

Fig. 2.

deficiency[34] and in several patients with the Wiskott-Aldrich syndrome,[35] an X-linked disorder characterized by thrombocytopenia, eczema and recurrent infections. Fetal thymus allografts have reconstituted the immunologic and thymic deficiencies in the Di George syndrome[36] and corrected the immunologic defect in Nezelof's syndrome, a rare T-cell immunodeficiency.[37]

Total liver allografts have been attempted in 2 patients with Wilson's disease[38] and 2 patients with a_1-antitrypsin deficiency.[39] Although the specific defect has not been identified in Wilson's disease, the levels of serum ceruloplasmin and copper increased from low to normal levels 2 weeks after transplantation. Urinary copper excretion also increased after transplantation and homograft biopsies have shown no copper accumulation. Hepatic transplantation in a_1-antitrypsin deficiency resulted in normal levels of plasma a_1-antitrypsin during the short period before the recipient expired from graft rejection. Transplantation of the pancreas has been accomplished in more than 20 patients with juvenile diabetes mellitus.[40] Almost immediately after transplantation, the insulin levels became homeostatic and the patients became normoglycemic. Several patients have had normal glucose and hormone levels and survived for more than one year after transplantation. Splenic transplantation has been accomplished in patients with hemophilia A[41] and juvenile or Type 3 Gaucher's disease.[42] The levels of Factor VIII were essentially unchanged; however, the level of plasma glucocerebroside, the Gaucher substrate, was decreased after transplantation. Unfortunately, the spleen is an extremely immunogenic organ and these grafts were rejected because of host reaction.

Extensive experience with renal transplantation has demonstrated that the kidney is the most successfully transplanted organ. Renal transplantation has been accomplished in over a dozen genetic diseases. The majority of these disorders involve primary renal pathology and the allograft corrects the abnormal renal function. Renal transplantation in familial polycystic disease, medullary cystic disease, familial Mediterranean fever with amyloidosis, congenital nephrotic syndrome, Alport's syndrome, nail-patella syndrome and amyloidosis results in excellent renal function and no apparent recurrence of renal disease. The protein and lipid levels in patients with the congenital nephrotic syndrome became normal after transplantation.[43] Recipients with primary gout have normal renal function but the hyperuricemia and gouty symptoms persist.[44] Kidney transplantation in several patients with primary oxalosis has been unsuccessful due to the rapid reaccumulation of calcium oxalate crystals in the allograft.[45]

Renal transplantation has been accomplished in more than 20 children with cystinosis.[46] Most recipients have received allografts from their parents who were obligate heterozygotes for the cystinotic gene. The cystine levels in

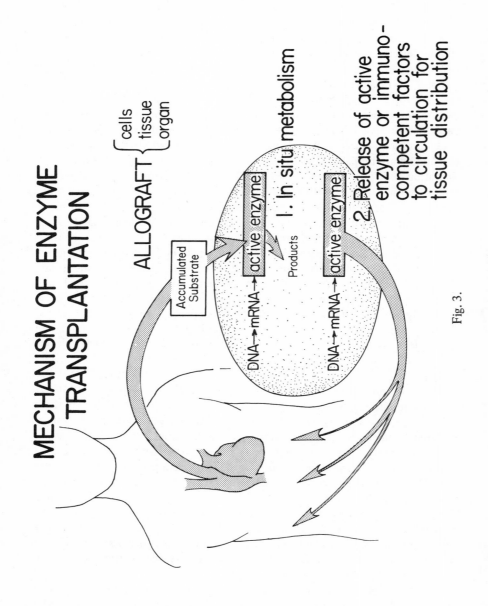

MECHANISM OF ENZYME
TRANSPLANTATION

ALLOGRAFT { cells, tissue, organ

Accumulated Substrate

DNA→mRNA→ active enzyme

Products

1. In situ metabolism

DNA→mRNA→ active enzyme

2. Release of active enzyme or immuno-competent factors to circulation for tissue distribution

Fig. 3.

cornea, bone marrow and peripheral leukocytes have not decreased after transplantation. Cystine has not reaccumulated in the proximal renal epithelium of the allografts, but reaccumulation has occurred in the renal interstitial cells, presumably due to infiltration by the recipient's macrophages. However, no cystine reaccumulation was demonstrated two years after transplantation in a patient who received a cadaver allograft; this finding suggests that the unrelated, normal allograft is more capable of handling cystine than heterozygous kidneys.[46]

For inherited metabolic defects, allotransplantation may provide a strategy for the grafting of appropriate tissues for the continuous synthesis of active gene products. Figure 3 illustrates the concept of "enzyme transplantation" and indicates two potential mechanisms by which the allograft might therapeutically metabolize the accumulated substrate in recipients with selected inherited enzymatic deficiencies. In disorders characterized by substrate accumulation in the plasma, the active enzyme in the allograft may metabolize or clear the accumulated substrate which is delivered to the transplanted tissue by the circulation. As the accumulated substrate is cleared from the plasma, a concentration gradient would be established between the plasma and the tissue sites of substrate deposition, allowing for the continuous resaturation of the plasma and continual clearance of the systemic substrate load. *In situ* metabolism would probably be the major mechanism of substrate metabolism by transplanted organs such as liver, spleen and kidney.

Alternatively, the normal allograft may synthesize active enzyme, an essential cofactor, hormone or immunocompetent factor, which is either released by the turnover of allograft cells or by direct secretion into the circulation. The active enzyme or gene product is then distributed to the tissues where it may gain access to cells for substrate metabolism. The release and distribution of normal gene products conceivably would be a therapeutic mechanism of transplanted pancreas, bone marrow, thymus and, to a lesser degree, liver and kidney.

Renal transplantation in patients with Fabry's disease was undertaken to monitor the biochemical and clinical effectiveness of enzyme transplantation. Fabry's disease is an X-linked, inborn error of glycosphingolipid metabolism. In 1963, Sweeley and Klionsky[47] identified the accumulating Fabry substrate as trihexosyl ceramide; the primary defect was subsequently identified by Brady and associates[48] in 1967 as the deficient activity of the lysosomal enzyme, ceramide trihexosidase or a-galactosidase A.

Since patients with Fabry's disease present with renal failure and since renal tissue contains active a-galactosidase A, it was hypothesized that a renal allograft might provide active enzyme to correct the metabolic defect of Fabry's disease. The biochemical results of successful renal transplantation in five recipients with Fabry's disease have been similar.[49,50] Following transplantation, the levels of a-galactosidase A activity in the recipients' urines were within normal range and could not be distinguished from normal control urine, based on thermolability and myoinositol inhibition studies. Initially, increased levels of total a-galactosidase activity were observed in the recipients' plasmas; however, this reflected a non-specific increase of the thermostable a-galactosidase B activity, presumably due to immunosuppression therapy.[51] Evidence of a-galactosidase A activity in the plasma will require the development of more sensitive techniques, such as radioimmunoassay. Significantly, the levels of trihexosyl ceramide, the accumulated substrate, in plasma and urinary sediment decreased to levels in, or slightly above, the normal range. Concomitant with these biochemical results, there has been a marked amelioration of the painful crises of Fabry's disease and improvement in the general well-being of the recipients.

The mechanism by which the renal allograft is responsible for the chemical and clinical observations in recipients with Fabry's disease is the focus of current investigations. At present, the data support the mechanism of renal filtration and *in situ* metabolism; the allograft may filter the accumulated lipid substrate from the plasma and catabolize the lipid within the kidney. Then, as the accumulated lipid is cleared from the plasma, a concentration gradient would be established between the plasma and tissue sites of lipid deposition, allowing for the continuous resaturation of the plasma and eventual clearance of the lipid accumulation. Further studies are in progress, however, to determine if active enzyme is released into the circulation by the allograft and taken up by the recipient's tissues.

Several recent reports have described the successful transplantation of heterotopic allografts and cell implants for the correction of metabolic deficiencies in animal model systems. Heterotopic liver allografts have corrected the glucuronyl transferase deficiency in recipient Gunn rats,[52] and pancreatic islet cell implants have re-established normal insulin and glucose levels in alloxan-induced diabetic rates.[53] An intriguing, but preliminary, report describes the successful orthotopic liver graft in a recipient with Niemann-Pick Type A disease.[54] After transplantation, the sphingomyelinase activity in plasma, urine, and most notably, cerebrospinal fluid, appears to be markedly increased, suggesting that normal hepatic tissue is capable of secreting active enzyme which can be distributed to various tissues and fluids of the recipient's body.

Thus, the grafting of enzyme-producing tissues for the continuous production of the normal gene products may provide another strategy for the treatment of appropriate recessively-inherited, metabolic diseases. It must be emphasized, however, that this approach is exploratory and further study of the results in patients with transplanted organs must be evaluated before enzyme transplants are undertaken in other inherited metabolic diseases.

Enzyme Replacement Therapy

The thrust of current research is directed at the treatment of inherited metabolic diseases at the level of the primary defect — the specific enzymatic lesion. Since these disorders are caused by a critical mutation in a segment of DNA whose resultant gene product is a defective enzyme, the rationale of enzyme replacement therapy is obvious. The major requisites for effective enzyme therapy are summarized in Table 4.

With the identification of the specific enzymatic defects in several lysosomal storage diseases, investigators were immediately intrigued with the therapeutic possibilities of enzyme replacement. The initial experiments, performed in the mid-1960's, involved the administration of crude preparations of heterologous enzymes into severely debilitated patients. In 1964, Baudhuin and associates[55] were the first to intravenously administer an enzyme-rich extract from *Aspergillus niger* as a source of a-glucosidase to a patient with glycogenosis type II (Pompe's disease). Further trials using fungal enzymes were attempted in patients with glycogenosis types II[56–60] and IV[61] and indicated that the active exogenous enzyme could gain access to visceral tissues for the catabolism of the accumulated glycogen substrates. These studies were complicated, however, by pyrogenic contaminants and immunologic reactions to the fungal proteins.

In 1966, enzyme replacement in patients with metachromatic leukodystrophy was accomplished by intravenous and intrathecal administration of arylsulfatase A partially purified from beef brain.[62] Following intravenous administration, levels of enzymatic activity increased significantly in serum and excised hepatic tissue. After intrathecal administration, enzymatic activity increased in cerebrospinal fluid for 20 hours but could not be demonstrated in excised brain tissue. The studies indicated that future trials of enzyme therapy would clearly require the use of non-immunogenic enzymes, presumably from human sources.

Austin,[63] recognizing the need for homologous enzyme, intrathecally administered human urinary arylsulfatase A to a patient with metachromatic leukodystrophy. Seven and one-half hours after injection, the arylsulfatase A activity in the cerebrospinal fluid had increased approximately fifty-fold. Concomitantly, the patient developed an immunologic hypersensitivity reaction, a febrile episode (105° F), and a polymorphonuclear leukocytosis in the cerebrospinal fluid.

Stymied by the previous clinically unsuccessful attempts to administer partially purified exogenous enzymes, investigators turned to the use of normal plasma and leukocyte preparations for therapy. In 1970, Mapes and co-workers[54,65] administered fresh heparinized plasma containing active ceramide trihexosidase (a-galactosidase A) to patients with Fabry's disease. Not

TABLE 4

Requisites for Effective Enzyme Therapy

ENZYME

Sufficient quantities of highly active, stable non-immunogenic, sterile enzyme.

ADMINISTRATION

DELIVERY of sufficient enzymatic activity to target tissue and subcellular sites for effective substrate metabolism at reasonable intervals.

PROTECTION of enzyme from inactivation, degradation and immunologic surveillance.

IN VIVO TEST SYSTEM

Mammalian model systems to evaluate and maximize enzyme stability, protection, tissue distribution and uptake, subcellular localization and substrate metabolism prior to human trials.

THERAPEUTIC EVALUATION

Demonstration of biochemical and clinical improvement.

only did enzymatic activity increase in the plasma of the recipients, but the level of the specific plasma substrate, trihexosyl ceramide, significantly decreased, providing evidence of the catabolic activity of the exogenously supplied enzyme. Similar results were observed when plasma concentrates were administered to a patient with Sandhoff's disease.[66] Hexosaminidase levels were increased in the plasma and the concentration of plasma globoside, a substrate of the enzyme, was significantly reduced after injection.

Shortly thereafter, several investigators reported enzyme replacement studies in mucopolysaccharidoses I, II and III by infusion of normal plasma[67-70] and leukocytes.[71] The chemical results of these studies were highly variable; some authors reported evidence for mucopolysaccharide catabolism,[72] while others found none.[69,70] The current concensus is that this approach is unlikely to have significant therapeutic effect.

Recent trials of enzyme replacement therapy have utilized highly purified enzymes isolated from human tissues. Pilot intravenous administrations of the appropriate enzymatic activity have been accomplished in patients with Sandhoff's disease (urinary hexosaminidase A),[73] glycogenosis type II (placental a-glucosidase),[74] Fabry's disease (placental a-galactosidase)[75] and most recently, Gaucher's disease type 1 (placental β-glucosidase.[76] In each case, the highly purified human enzyme was shown to hydrolyze its natural substrate *in vitro* prior to *in vivo* trials. The plasma clearances of the injected enzymes were rapid, and exogenous enzymatic activity was recovered in excised liver samples from each of the patients. The approximate plasma activity half-lives were 10 minutes in Sandhoff's disease, 20 minutes in Pompe's disease, 10–12 minutes in Fabry's disease and 18 minutes in Gaucher's disease. Evidence for concomitant substrate catabolism was demonstrated; decreased concentrations of plasma globoside (Sandhoff's disease), hepatic glycogen (Pompe's disease), plasma trihexosyl ceramide (Fabry's disease), and plasma, erythrocytic and hepatic glucocerebroside (Gaucher's disease) were found following enzyme administration. These preliminary, but encouraging, results support the feasibility of enzyme therapy with highly purified human enzymes. The major limitations of these endeavors, however, were the short half-lives of the circulating exogenous enzymatic activities (instability ? bioinactivation ?) and the lack of evidence for substrate catabolism in the target tissue and subcellular sites of pathologic deposition.

Furthermore, these studies have identified the need for enzyme and cellular engineering techniques to (1) establish the enzyme for optimal activity under physiologic conditions; (2) protect the administered enzyme from degradation, bioinactivation and immunologic surveillance; and (3) deliver the enzyme to the sites of pathology.

Various strategies for enzyme protection and delivery are shown in Figure 4.

ADMINISTRATION OF ENZYME PREPARATION

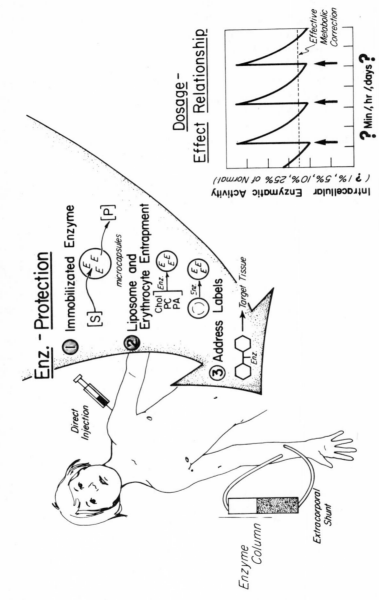

Fig. 4.

Enzyme entrapment techniques including the use of enzymes immobilized in microcapsules,[77] liposomes[78] or erythrocytes,[79,80] may prove useful for protection from bioinactivation and immunologic processes and delivery to specific tissue and subcellular sites. Furthermore, the entrapped enzyme may be delivered to specific tissue and subcellular sites by the chemical addition of an "address label", a specific oligosaccharide or glycopeptide, *a la* Morrell *et al.*;[81] these workers have identified the specific carbohydrate code for the uptake of circulating glycoproteins by hepatocytes. Extension of these findings to the identification of the specific "address codes" for uptake by other cells and tissues would be a major breakthrough for the delivery of various therapeutic agents, particularly the glycoprotein enzymes, to target sites.

In summary, the recent advances in the enzyme technology, including the development of affinity chromatographic methods for enzyme purification[82-84] and chemical methods for the modification of enzymes for optimal *in vivo* activity and stability,[85] should enhance the feasibility and potential practicality of enzyme replacement. In addition, the rapid and anticipated progress in cellular engineering should provide the technology to deliver these highly-purified and chemically modified enzymes to the target tissue and subcellular sites required for maximal therapeutic effectiveness. Thus, future prospects for enzyme therapy in selected inborn errors of metabolism are promising.

GENE THERAPY

The search for the ideal treatment for inherited genetic diseases has stimulated investigations which could lead to the permanent introduction of new genetic information into a patient's genome. The rapid developments in biochemistry, immunology and somatic cell genetics may make the insertion and integration of specific DNA segments a reality in the future. Achievements in isolating and purifying specific messenger RNA's[86] capable of *in vitro* synthesis of macromolecules[87] and the *in vitro* synthesis of DNA, complementary to mRNA templates,[88] have laid the groundwork for strategies to accomplish the synthesis and transplantation of a normal gene into recipient patients.

Figure 5 illustrates one potential approach for the treatment of inherited enzymatic defects by "gene transplantation". Using normal human tissues as the source of a selected normal enzyme and crude polysomes, specific human genes may be produced *in vitro*. Antibodies made to the purified human enzyme will bind nascent polypeptide chains of the specific enzyme-synthesizing polysomes. The addition of excess purified enzyme, which binds

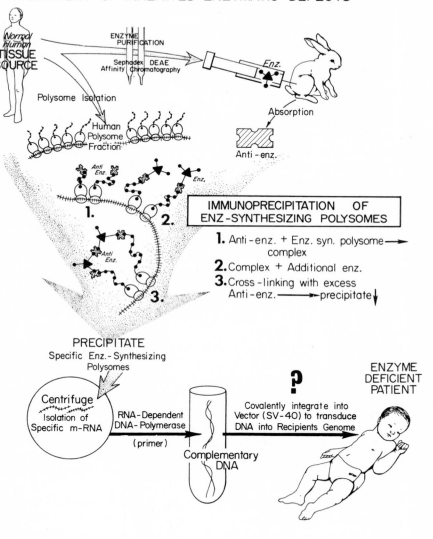

"GENE TRANSPLANTATION"
TREATMENT OF INHERITED ENZYMATIC DEFECTS

Fig. 5.

to the anti-enzyme portion of the complex and finally, the addition of excess antibody, which cross-links adjacent enzyme antigen determinants, will immunoprecipitate specific enzyme-synthesizing polysomes. With special care to exclude ribonuclease activity, the specific messenger-RNA for the selected enzyme can be isolated from the precipitated polysome complexes. Utilizing RNA-dependent DNA polymerase (reverse transcriptase) and the isolated mRNA as template, the complementary DNA can be synthesized *in vitro*. This DNA segment has the specific genetic information to code for the synthesis of the active enzyme. The feasibility of this strategy for isolating DNA has already been proven by Schimke and his colleagues.[86,87]

The major hurdle for gene therapy is the actual insertion and integration of the specific DNA segment into the recipient's genome. The exogenous DNA must be covalently integrated in a genetically stabilized manner for normal replication, transcription and regulation processes. One possible solution to this problem may be the use of a vector, such as SV_{40} or polyoma viruses. DNA may be covalently integrated into the viral genome using the methods of Berg and colleagues.[89] Transduction of the new DNA segment into the recipient's chromosomes may then be accomplished by infecting the patient with the virus. Alternatively, a pseudo-virion, or virus-like particle, containing the human DNA instead of viral DNA may be employed for transduction of the new genetic material.

Many of these developments must await new information and insights into the structure, regulation and accessibility of the human genome; however, this approach need not be considered a mere geneticist's fantasy. The task, however, is not without serious pitfalls and potential dangers, both ethical and biological, the latter strongly emphasized by a recently proposed ban on specific genetic engineering experiments by leading investigators in the field.[90]

PREVENTIVE THERAPY

The delivery of medical care is best when it can be preventive; for many genetic diseases, preventive therapy is, in fact, the only treatment currently available. With the increasing capabilities of *in utero* diagnosis, prenatal recognition of many genetic defects can be achieved.[91] Over 60 inborn errors of metabolism, all the known chromosomal aberrations and an increasing number of congenital malformations, can be identified early in pregnancy. Thus, the combination of amniocentesis, ultrasonic techniques and amniotic fluid and cell analyses have made many fatal or severely debilitating disorders preventable through optional termination.

The future success of preventive therapy will come from the dissemination of pertinent information by genetic and family counseling and community prevention programs which focus on groups of individuals at high-risk for genetic disorders.   Indeed, the recent initiation of Tay-Sachs prevention programs in over a dozen cities in the United States is exemplary. These proto-type programs for the control of genetic disease[92] are designed to educate and identify heterozygotes for the Tay-Sachs gene in the at-risk community. Identified carrier couples are then counseled with respect to their various reproductive options, including prenatal diagnosis.   These programs have already confirmed the feasibility and practicality of preventive therapy for genetic disease.

REFERENCES

1.   J.G. Stanbury, J.B. Wyngaarden and D.S. Frederickson (Eds.), The Metabolic Basis of Inherited Disease, 3rd ed., McGraw-Hill, New York, 1972.

2.   V.A. McKusick, Mendelian Inheritance in Man, 3rd ed., Johns Hopkins Press, Baltimore, 1971.

3.   C.R. Scriver and L.E. Rosenberg, Amino Acid Metabolism and Its Disorders, W.B. Saunders Co., Philadelphia, 1973.

4.   K.O. Raivio and J.E. Seegmiller, *Ann. Rev. Biochem. 41,* 543, 1972.

5.   R. Howell, *in* Medical Genetics, V.A. McKusick and R. Claiborne (Eds.), Hospital Practice Publishing Co., New York, p. 271, 1972.

6.   H.N. Kirkman, *Progr. Med. Genet. 8,* 125, 1972.

7.   R.J. Desnick, R.W. Bernlohr and W. Krivit (Eds.), Enzyme Therapy in Genetic Diseases, Birth Defects: Orig. Art. Series, Vol. IX, Williams and Wilkins, New York, 1973.

8.   P.J.G.M. Rietra, F.A.J.T.M. vander Bergh and J.M. Tager, *in* Enzyme Therapy in Lysosomal Storage Diseases, J.M. Tager, G.J.M Hooghwinkel and W.T. Daems (Eds.), North-Holland, Amsterdam, 1974.

9.   J.W.T. Seakins, R.A. Saunders and C. Toothill (Eds.), Treatment of Inborn Errors of Metabolism, Churchill Livingstone, Edinburgh, 1973.

10.   H. Bickel, J. Gerrard and E.M. Hickmans, *Acta Pediatr. 43,* 64, 1954.

11.   H.L. Nadler, T. Inouye and D.Y.Y. Hsia, *in* Galactosemia, D.Y.Y. Hsia (Ed.), C.C. Thomas, Springfield, 127, 1969.

12. G.N. Donnell, R. Koch and W.R. Bergren, *in* Galactosemia, D.Y.Y. Hsia (Ed.), C.C. Thomas, Springfield, p. 247, 1969.

13. E.R. Froesch, *in* The Metabolic Basis of Inherited Disease, J.G. Stanbury, J.B. Wyngaarden and D.S. Frederickson (Eds.), 3rd ed., (McGraw-Hill, New York, p. 128, 1972.

14. G.M. Gray, *in* The Metabolic Basis of Inherited Disease, J.G. Stanbury, J.B. Wyngaarden and D.S. Frederickson (Eds.), 3rd ed., McGraw-Hill, New York, p. 1457, 1972.

15. S. Halvorsen, *Amer. J. Dis. Child. 38,* 113, 1967.

16. F.O. Kolb, J.M. Earll and H.A. Harris, *Metabolism 16,* 378, 1967.

17. H.H. Zinneman and J.E. Jones, *Metabolism 15,* 915, 1966.

18. B.D. Corner, J.B. Holton, R.M. Norman and P.M. Williams, *Pediatrics 41,* 1074, 1968.

19. P.D. Gatfield, R.M. Knights, M. Deveraux and J.P. Pozsonye, *Can. Med. Ass. J. 101,* 71, 1969.

20. A.G. Riddell, R.P. Davies and A.D. Clark, *Lancet 2,* 1146, 1966.

21. T.E. Starzl, B.I. Brown, H. Blanchard and L. Brettschneider, *Surgery 65,* 504, 1969.

22. R.B. Moore, R.L. Varco and H. Buchwald, *Amer. J. Cardiol. 31,* 148, 1973.

23. Y.E. Hsia, J.T. Coombs, L. Hook and I.K. Brandt, *J. Pediatr. 68,* 921, 1966.

24. J. Richard, Y.M. Rosenoer, S.L. Tomsett, I. Draper and J.A. Simpson, *Brain 87,* 619, 1964.

25. J.C. Crawhill, E.F. Scowen and R.W.E. Watts, *Br. J. Med. 1,* 1411, 1964.

26. J.B. Wyngaarden and W.N. Kelley, *in* The Metabolic Basis of Inherited Disease, J.B. Stanbury, J.B. Wyngaarden and D.S. Frederickson (Eds.), 3rd ed., McGraw-Hill, New York, p. 930, 1972.

27. *Ibid.,* p. 986.

28. C.G.D. Brook, M. Zachmann, A. Prader and G. Mürset, *J. Pediatr. 85,* 12, 1974.

29. A.H. Klein, S. Meltzer and F. Kenny, *J. Pediatr. 81,* 912, 1972.

30. J.M. Tanner, R.H. Whitehouse, P.C.R. Hughes and F.P. Vince, *Arch. Dis. Child. 46,* 745, 1971.

31. L.H. Smith, C.M. Huguley and J.A. Bain, *in* The Metabolic Basis of Inherited Disease, J.G. Stanbury, J.B. Wyngaarden and D.S. Frederickson (Eds.), 3rd ed., McGraw-Hill, New York, p. 1022, 1972.

32. R.P.H. Thompson, *in* Treatment of Inborn Errors of Metabolism, J.W.T. Seakins, R.A. Saunders and C. Foothill (Eds.), Churchill Livingstone, Edinburgh, p. 215, 1973.

33. C.C. Congdon, *Science 171,* 1116, 1971.

34. E.R. Stiehm, G.J. Lawlor, Jr., M.S. Kaplan, H.L. Greenwald, R.C. Neerhout, D.P.S. Sengar and P.I. Terasaki, *New Engl. J. Med. 286,* 797, 1972.

35. F.H. Bach, R.J. Albertini and P. Joo, *Lancet 2,* 1364, 1968.

36. C.S. August, F.S. Rosen, R.M. Filler, C.A. Janeway, B. Markowski and H.E.M. Kay, *Lancet 2,* 1210, 1968.

37. D.G. Tubergen, *J. Pediatr. 84,* 915, 1974.

38. R.S. Dubois, G. Giles, D.O. Rodgerson, J. Lilly, G. Martineau, C.G. Halgrimson, G. Shroter, T.E. Starzl, I. Sternlieb and I.H. Scheinberg, *Lancet 1,* 505, 1971.

39. H.L. Sharp and J.S. Najarian, unpublished results.

40. E.P. DiMagno, J. Hermon-Taylor, V.L.W. Go, R.C. Lillehei and W.H.J. Summerskill, *Gastroenterology 61,* 363, 1971.

41. T.L. Marchioro and T.E. Starzl, *Transplant 7,* 73, 1969.

42. C.G. Groth, L. Hagenfeldt, S. Dreborg, B. Lofstrom, P.A. Ockerman, K. Samuelson, L. Svennerholm, B. Werner and G. Westberg, *Lancet 1,* 1260, 1971.

43. J.R. Hoyer, C.M. Kjellstrand, R.L. Simmons, J.S. Najarian, S.M. Mauer, T.J. Buselmeier, A.F. Michael and R.L. Vernier, *Lancet 1,* 1410, 1973.

44. L.B. Sorensen, *Proc. Nat. Acad. Sci., USA, 55,* 571, 1966.

45. S.D. Deodhar, K.S.K. Tung, V. Zühlke and S. Nakamoto, *Arch. Path. 87,* 118, 1969.

46. C.P. Mahoney, G.E. Striker, G.H. Fetterman, R.O. Hickman, J.A. Schneider and T.L. Marchioro, *in* Enzyme Therapy in Genetic Diseases, R.J. Desnick, R.W. Bernlohr and W. Krivit (Eds.), Birth Defects: Original Article Series, Vol. IX, Williams and Wilkins, Baltimore, p. 141, 1973.

47. C.C. Sweeley and B. Klionsky, *J. Biol. Chem. 238,* 3148, 1963.

48. R.O. Brady, A.E. Gal, R.M. Bradley, E. Martensson, A.L. Warshaw and L. Laster, *New Engl. J. Med. 276,* 1163, 1967.

49. R.J. Desnick, R.L. Simmons, K.Y. Allen, J.S. Najarian and W. Krivit, *Surgery 72,* 203, 1972.

50. M. Philippart, S.S. Franklin and A. Gordon, *Ann. Int. Med. 77,* 195, 1972.

51. R.J. Desnick, K.Y. Allen, R.L. Simmons, J.E. Woods, C.F. Anderson, J.S. Najarian and W. Krivit, *in* Enzyme Therapy in Genetic Diseases, R.J. Desnick, R.W. Bernlohr and W. Krivit (Eds.), Birth Defects: Original Article Series, Vol. IX, Williams and Wilkins, Baltimore, p. 88, 1973.

52. A.B. Mukherjee and J. Krasner, *Science 182,* 68, 1973.

53. R.J. Leonard, A. Lazarow and O.D. Hegre, *Diabetes 22,* 413, 1973.

54. E. Delvin, F. Glorieux, P. Daloze, J. Gorman and P. Bloch, *Abstracts, Amer. Soc. Human Genetics,* Portland, Oregon, p. 25A, 1974.

55. P. Baudhuin, H.G. Hers and H. Loeb, *Lab. Invest. 13,* 1139, 1964.

56. H.G. Hers, *Biochem. J. 86,* 11, 1963.

57. R.M. Lauer, T. Mascarinas, A.S. Racela, A.M. Diehl and B.I. Brown, *Pediatrics 42,* 672, 1968.

58. G. Hug and W.K. Schubert, *J. Cell Biol. 35,* C1, 1967.

59. G. Hug and W.K. Schubert, *J. Clin. Invest. 46,* 1073, 1967.

60. G. Hug, W.K. Schubert and G. Chuck, *Clin. Res. 14,* 345, 1968.

61. J. Fernandes and F. Huijing, *Arch. Dis. Child. 43,* 347, 1968.

62. H.L. Greene, G. Hug and W.K. Schubert, *Arch. Neurol. 20,* 147, 1969.

63. J.H. Austin, *in* Inborn Disorders of Sphingolipid Metabolism, S.M. Aronson and B.W. Volk (Eds.), Pergamon Press, Oxford, p. 359, 1967.

64. C.A. Mapes, R.L. Anderson, C.C. Sweeley, R.J. Desnick and W. Krivit, *Science 169,* 987, 1970.

65. C.C. Sweeley, C.A. Mapes, W. Krivit and R.J. Desnick, *in* Sphingolipids, Sphingolipidoses and Allied Disorders, B.W. Volk and S.M. Aronson (Eds.), Plenum Press, New York, p. 287, 1972.

66. R.J. Desnick, W. Krivit, P.D. Snyder, S.J. Desnick and H.L. Sharp, *in* Sphingolipids, Sphingolipidoses and Allied Disorders, S.M. Aronson and B.W. Volk (Eds.), Plenum Press, New York, p. 351, 1972.

67. N. Di Ferrante, B.L. Nichols, P.V. Donnelly, G. Neri, R. Hrgovcic and R.K. Berglund, *Proc. Natl. Acad. Sci., USA, 68,* 303, 1971.

68. M.F. Dean, H. Muir and P.F. Benson, *Nature New Biol. 243,* 143, 1973.

69. A.S. Dekaban, K.R. Holden and G. Constantopoulos, *Pediatrics 50,* 688, 1972.

70. R.P. Erickson, R. Sandman, W. van B. Robertson and C.J. Epstein, *Pediatrics 50,* 693, 1972.

71. A.G. Knudson, Jr., N. Di Ferrante and J.E. Curtis, *Proc. Natl. Acad. Sci., USA, 68,* 1738, 1971.

72. N. Di Ferrante, B.L. Nichols, A.G. Knudson, K.B. McCredie, J. Singh and P.V. Donnelly, *in* Enzyme Therapy in Genetic Diseases, R.J. Desnick, R.W. Bernlohr and W. Krivit (Eds.), Birth Defects: Original Article Series, Vol. IX, Williams and Wilkins, Baltimore, p. 120, 1973.

73. W.G. Johnson, R.J. Desnick, D.M. Long, H.L. Sharp, W. Krivit, B. Brady and R.O. Brady, *in* Enzyme Therapy in Genetic Diseases, R.J. Desnick, R.W. Bernlohr and W. Krivit (Eds.), Birth Defects: Original Article Series, Vol. IX, Williams and Wilkins, Baltimore, p. 120, 1973.

74. Th. De Barsy, P. Jacquemin, F. van Hoof and H.G. Gers, *in* Enzyme Therapy in Genetic Diseases, R.J. Desnick, R.W. Bernlohr and W. Krivit (Eds.), Birth Defects: Original Articles Series, Vol. IX, Williams and Wilkins, Baltimore, p. 184, 291, 989, 1974.

75. R.O. Brady, J.F. Tallman, W.G. Johnson, A.E. Gal, W.R. Leahy, J.M. Quirk and A.S. Dekaban, *N. Engl. J. Med. 289,* 9, 1973.

76. R.O. Brady, P.G. Penchev, A.E. Gal, S.R. Hibbert and A.S. Dekaban, *N. Engl. J. Med. 291,* 989, 1974.

77. T.M.S. Chang, Artificial Cells, Charles C. Thomas, Springfield, 1972.

78. G. Gregoriadis and R.D. Leathwood, *FEBS, Letters 14,* 95, 1971.

79. G.M. Ihler, R.H. Glew and F.W. Schnure, *Proc. Natl. Acad. Sci. 70,* 2663, 1973.

80. M.B. Fiddler, S.R. Thorpe, W. Krivit and R.J. Desnick, *in* Enzyme Therapy in Lysosomal Diseases, W. Th. Daems, G.J.M. Hooghwinkel and J.M. Tager (Eds.), North Holland Publishing Co., Amsterdam, 1974.

81. A.G. Morell, G. Gregoriadis, I.H. Scheinberg, J. Hickman and G. Ashwell, *J. Biol. Chem. 246,* 1461, 1971.

82. N.S. Radin, J.C. Hyun and R.S. Misra, *Fed. Proc. 33,* 1226. 1974.

83. C.A. Mapes and C.C. Sweeley, *J. Biol. Chem. 248,* 2461, 1973.

84. A.G.W. Norden and J.S. O'Brien, *Biochem. Biophys. Res. Comm. 56,* 193, 1974.

85. P.D. Snyder, Jr., F. Wold, R.W. Bernlohr, C. Dullum, R.J. Desnick, W. Krivit and R.M. Condie, *Biochim, Biophys. Acta 350,* 432, 1974.

86. R. Palacios, R.D. Palmiter and R.T. Schimke, *J. Biol. Chem. 247,* 2316, 1972.

87. R. Palacios and R.T. Schimke, *J. Biol. Chem. 248,* 1424, 1973.

88. J. Ross, H. Aviv, E. Scolnick and P. Ledu, *Proc. Nat. Acad. Sci. 69,* 264, 1972.

89. D.A. Jackson, R.H. Symons and P. Berg, *Proc. Nat. Acad. Sci. 69,* 2904, 1972.

90. P. Berg, D. Baltimore, H.W. Boyer, S.N. Cohen, R.W. Davis, D.S. Hogness, D. Nathans, R. Roblin, J.D. Watson, S. Weissman and N. D. Zinder, *Science 185,* 303, 1974.

91. A. Mulinsky, The Prenatal Diagnosis of Hereditary Disorders, L.C.

92.   M.M. Kaback and J.S. O'Brien, *in* Medical Genetics, V.A. McKusick and R. Claiborne (Eds.), Hospital Practice Publishing Co., p. 253, 1973.

PRENATAL TREATMENT OF METHYLMALONIC ACIDEMIA WITH VITAMIN B$_{12}$

Mary G. Ampola
Maurice J. Mahoney
Eiichi Nakamura
Kay Tanaka

Until recently, amniocentesis was primarily limited to situations in which therapeutic abortion was anticipated if a positive result was obtained; *e.g.,* Down's syndrome and Tay-Sachs disease. For many workers in the field, the hope has been that at least some genetic diseases detectable by amniocentesis would prove to be treatable *in utero* and that thereby some of these babies might be salvaged.

I shall be reporting such a case of successful prenatal treatment of a fetus.

Methylmalonic acidemia is characterized by vomiting, ketoacidosis, hepatomegaly, bone marrow depression, failure to thrive and mental retardation. Biochemically, there is hyperglycinemia and accumulation of methylmalonic acid.

This acid is derived primarily from protein via four amino acids: isoleucine, methioine, threonine and valine. Most patients with methylmalonic acidemia have a defect of conversion of L-methylmalonyl Co A to succinyl Co A, either in the enzyme itself or in the ability to produce the necessary coenzyme, 5´deoxyadenosylcobalamin.

Two coenzymes, 5´ deoxyadenosylcobalamin and methylcobalamin, are normally formed from vitamin B$_{12}$ and the postulated defect here is beyond the branch point. Usually this block is not complete and is partially bypassed by massive amounts of B$_{12}$. This form is referred to as the B$_{12}$ responsive type, while the apoenzyme defect is designated B$_{12}$-nonresponsive.

The only sibling of the present patient entered the Boston Floating Hospital at three months of age in a moribund condition, following two weeks of vomiting and ketoacidosis. Hepatomegaly and pancytopenia were present but, despite heroic measures, the child died shortly thereafter. Autopsy revealed only a terminal pseudomonas sepsis.

A urine sample later revealed marked elevation of lysine on amino acid

357

screening and a large spot suggestive of methylmalonic acid on organic acid screening. The acid's identity was confirmed by gas-liquid chromatography and mass-spectroscopy. Urine methylmalonic acid measured 4.3 mg/ml or approximately 1.7 gm/day (normal = $<$ 5 mg/day). Serum analysis revealed a 3-fold increase in glycine and lysine. No frozen tissue was available for enzyme assay.

The parents were given genetic counseling as to the probable autosomal recessive nature of the disease and the possibility of prenatal diagnosis, although this had not yet been achieved. The couple decided to have another baby. Even without the question of pregnancy termination, amniocentesis was planned for the following reasons: (1) to establish the reliability of enzyme assay from amniotic fluid cells, (2) if the fetus was shown to have the disease, to try to establish its precise form and (3) if the cells suggested B_{12} responsiveness, vitamin therapy later in pregnancy would be considered.

In early 1973, the mother again became pregnant and amniocentesis was carried out at 19 weeks. Enzyme assays kindly performed by Dr. Maurice Mahoney, of Yale-New Haven Medical Center, yielded the following results: propionate and succinate oxidation were measured. Propionate is *proximal* to the block and succinate *beyond*. Propionate oxidation was only about 8% that of the controls while succinate oxidation was excellent.

Spontaneous B_{12} coenzyme accumulation was measured. There was no detectable 5′deoxyadenosyl derivative while the methyl form was adequate.

With this coenzyme *added* to the culture, succinate formation was 76% of controls as compared with an apoenzyme-defective patient who did not respond significantly.

Cell growth was not adequate to test the question of responsiveness to B_{12}; however, it is known that the majority of patients with a B_{12} error respond to the vitamin clinically.

Because of previous evidence gathered by Dr. Grant Morrow[1] that methylmalonic acid accumulation is progressive during pregnancy, particularly in the last two months, we carefully considered giving the mother large doses of B_{12}. A literature search revealed that the vitamin crosses the placenta readily and has no known adverse effects on the fetus. After the entire situation was discussed with the couple and they were eager to prevent any accumulation of acid which might harm the fetus, the decision was made to give B_{12} during the last two months of pregnancy.

Urines were collected at intervals and it became obvious to Dr. Tanaka at Yale, who performed analyses on the specimens, that the standard Giorgio and Plaut technique,[2] which involved a colorimetric reaction with paranitroanaline, was not sufficiently sensitive for minute amounts of methylmalonic acid. He and Dr. Nakamura therefore proceeded to develop a microanalytical method involving combined ion-exchange and gas-liquid chromatography, which will soon be published in detail.

The first urine collected at 23 weeks contained about 6 micrograms of methylmalonic acid per milligram of creatinine. The level rose sharply over the next few weeks so that by 31 weeks she was excreting 4 times as much.

At 32 weeks, the mother was begun on oral cyanocobalamin, 10 mg/day, in divided doses. On this regimen, however, serum B_{12} rose only slightly above the normal range. Since we were using this parameter to determine therapy, we elected to change to intramuscular therapy, 5 mg daily for the last six weeks of pregnancy. It was here that the mother truly showed her determination, since this involved 5 mg in 5 cc's of solution daily. Subsequently, the serum B_{12} level climbed to about 6500 during pregnancy. The final figure is not comparable to the others, since it was taken shortly after that morning's injection. Maternal and cord B_{12} were very similar at delivery. On oral therapy, even though the serum level of B_{12} had not risen well, urine methylmalonic acid declined. Intramuscular therapy lowered it further. Indeed, the methylmalonic acid in the sample just before delivery was lower than that at 23 weeks. Following delivery, the mother's urine level dropped promptly to within the normal range by day three.

Of special interest are the data collected by Dr. Mahoney[3] on a presumed heterozygote who was carrying a normal fetus. Here the methylmalonic acid never rose above normal, strongly suggesting that it is not the heterozygous state of the mother but rather the homozygous fetus which causes the accumulation.

Amniotic fluid was analyzed at 19 weeks and at delivery. The methylmalonic acid was three times the mean of controls on each of these specimens. The content for the patient doubled in this interval, as did that of the controls.

At 41 weeks gestation, labor was induced and the baby was born in excellent condition. A skin biopsy for fibroblast studies was forwarded to Dr. Mahoney's laboratory and confirmed the amniotic fluid cell studies.

In addition, the cells were studied for propionate oxidation after growing in culture, with and without added B_{12}. Although the oxidation of the control cells improved somewhat with B_{12} (2.7 times), the patient's cells improved by a greater factor (6 times). On another occasion, when the same assay was performed under slightly different conditions, no increase over the controls was seen. Dr. Mahoney has observed similar *in vitro* variability of B_{12} response with cell lines from other patients known to be B_{12} responsive *in vivo*.

The child was placed on a formula calculated to provide 1.5 grams of protein and 150 calories per kilogram per day. This was achieved by using an Enfamil base and adding appropriate amounts of Lipomul, Karo syrup, Pedialyte and calcium lactate pentahydrate.

Since there was presumably adequate B_{12} from maternal sources, it was elected to give no vitamin initially but to follow the response to low protein diet alone.

The baby's urine methylmalonic acid was measured both by the new method and the standard technique. The methylmalonic acid scale is 100 times that for maternal urine. The baby's first voided urine contained about 10 times the methylmalonic acid of the maternal urine just before delivery. To put this in perspective, although this urine contained about 30 times the amount of methylmalonic acid excreted by normal newborns, this was only about 1/1000th the levels in the urine of clinically ill patients with this disease.

From birth to about 6 weeks, excretion plateaued at 100 to 200 micrograms/milligram of creatinine. Serum B_{12} dropped as the baby cleared maternal B_{12}. By 9 weeks, it was normal. Between 6 and 16 weeks, a new plateau for methylmalonic acid excretion was reached at about 800. We then raised her protein intake over a 2 week period to 2.5 grams per kilo per day. After one week, methylmalonic acid was 5 times greater than the previous urine. She then appeared to adjust somewhat and the next 3 levels were in the range of 2 to 3000. B_{12} was then given on a trial basis and she received 1 mg intramuscularly daily for 11 days. This raised the serum B_{12} well and the methylmalonic acid dropped from 2600 to 400; that is, to less than 1/6 as much.

Serum methylmalonic acid rose gradually from about 2 micrograms/ml to 5.4 at 15 weeks, which is the latest result available. For comparison, clinically ill patients generally average about 200 μgm/ml.

At age 5½ months, the protein intake was again raised, this time to 3.5 gm/kg/day. Twenty-four hours later, she developed severe vomiting and irritability. Urine methylmalonic acid rose to almost 10,000 μgm/mg creatinine, twice as high as during the previous stress period. We then lowered the protein intake to 3.0 gm/kg/day. Vomiting ceased but she continued to be irritable, with some somnolence. Five days after the initial increase to 3.5 gm protein/kg/day, B_{12}, 1 mg intramuscularly daily, was begun. Within 24 hours after beginning the vitamin, she lost her irritability and became progressively more alert and energetic. Two weeks after the vitamin was begun, the urine methylmalonic acid level had dropped to 1800 μgm/mg creatinine – virtually the same as before increasing protein intake and again demonstrating *in vivo* B_{12} responsiveness.

Currently, the child is receiving 2 gm protein/kg/day, without added B_{12}. This is achieved with a formula containing Enfamil, Lipomul, Karo syrup and low protein foods such as cereals, fruits and vegetables.

Arterial gasses, electrolytes and amino acids have been carefully followed and have remained consistently normal.

Physically, she is now growing along the 75th percentile in terms of height, weight and head circumference. At the present age of 11 months, she is beginning to take steps independently and has a vocabulary of ten words and one three-word phrase. Incidentally, this little girl seems to have established her priorities, right or wrong: her first word beyond "Mama" and "Dada" was "diamond".

A number of comments may be made concerning these data.

First, in terms of the *first affected* sibling: A urine was collected at one month of age (before the child became symptomatic) for the Massachusetts Metabolic Screening Program and was run by paper chromatography for methylmalonic acid. On staining with aniline-xylose, no accumulation was detectable. Recently, however, a new staining method using Fast Blue B has been used for screening.[4] The original filter paper on the affected baby who died was run again and this time a *large spot* was demonstrable. Hopefully, this will prove to be a much more reliable screening stain but to save some of these babies, it may well be necessary to collect the urines in the newborn period.

In the *second* sibling, the vitamin B_{12}-responsiveness form of methylmalonic acid was established on amniocentesis and later this led to the *in utero* treatment of the affected fetus with the vitamin. By following the maternal urine, the status of the fetus' production of the acid could be accurately followed using the sensitive new micromethod.

Urinary methylmalonic acid declined after treatment to a level *even below* that in the first urine tested at 23 weeks. Comparison can be made of the excretion of methylmalonic acid by this mother, with Dr. Grant Morrow's patient who was carrying an affected fetus with the non-B_{12}-responsive form of the disease. While the acid content was similar at about 25 and 31 weeks gestation, our mother was excreting at term only about one-third as much as the other.

The question of whether prenatal treatment was absolutely necessary for the survival and/or normal mentality of this child may logically be raised, particularly in view of the fact that her sibling did not become symptomatic until after one month of age. However, the onset of symptoms of many if not most patients with this disorder is within the first few days. This makes it very likely that significant amounts of the acid accumulate prenatally, perhaps related to variables such as maternal protein intake. It is not yet known whether any permanent injury to the fetus is done by this *in utero* exposure to excesses of methylmalonic acid.

In summary, a fetus with the vitamin B_{12}-responsive form of methylmalonic acidemia was detected using amniocentesis. We have demonstrated that administration of large doses of vitamin B_{12} to the mother during pregnancy can lower excretion of the acid in her urine and, by inference, its accumulation in fetal tissues. To our knowledge, this is the first instance of *in utero* treatment of an inborn error using large doses of a vitamin.

REFERENCES

1.   G. Morrow, R.H. Schwarz, J.A. Hallock and L.A. Barness, *J. Pediat. 77*, 120, 1964.

2.   A. Giorgio and G.W.E. Plant, *J. Lab. Clin. Med. 66*, 667, 1965.

3.   Personal communication, Dr. M. Mahoney.

4.   Personal communication, Dr. H. Levy.

THE MOLECULAR BASIS OF THE THALASSEMIAS

Corrado Baglioni

The thalassemias are inherited diseases caused by an inborn defect in hemoglobin synthesis, as shown by the characteristic microcythemia and hypochromia of the erythrocytes of affected individuals.[1] The etiology of thalassemia has been traced to "ineffective erythropoiesis", with massive bone marrow proliferation which results in an inadequate output of erythrocytes with a shortened life span. The first clear theory on the molecular basis of thalassemia was put forward by Ingram and Stretton in 1959.[2] These authors have taken into proper consideration the molecular structure of human adult hemoglobin, made up of two a and two β chains, and postulated that the thalassemias can be explained by a quantitative defect in the synthesis of either peptide chain. When a thalassemic gene is present together with an allele for an abnormal hemoglobin, two possible situations are observed: in the "non-interacting" case, the ratio of Hb A to abnormal hemoglobin remains unchanged, whereas in the "interacting" case, the abnormal hemoglobin becomes the predominant hemoglobin species.[3] The thalassemic gene can thus be considered an allele of the abnormal hemoglobin gene with which it interacts.

Fifteen years of active research have elapsed between the initial postulate of the two basic types of thalassemia; i.e., a-thalassemia and β-thalassemia. During this period of time, several important discoveries have been made and we are very close today to a full understanding of the molecular basis of thalassemia. Mainly, it has been recognized that the thalassemias are an heterogenous group of inherited hemoglobinopathies, both from the clinical and the molecular point of view. In the following discussion, a brief historical description of the different types of thalassemias and a critical review of those forms of thalassemia for which there is not yet a clear cut molecular explanation will be presented.

A classification of the thalassemias based on the genetic and molecular defect is shown in Table 1. I have included among the thalassemias those hemoglobinopathies which are characterized by the synthesis of an abnormal hemoglobin; i.e., Hb Lepore and Hb Constant Spring, and result in hemato-

TABLE 1

Genetic and Molecular Classification of Thalassemias

	β and δ Locus	α^1 and α^2 Locus
Synthesis of an abnormal peptide chain	Lepore (gene deletion from unequal X-over)	Constant Spring (mutation of chain termination codon)
Reduced synthesis of a normal peptide chain	βThal$^+$ (reduced amount of mRNA)	αThal$^+$ (reduced amount of mRNA)
Absence of the synthesis of one peptide chain	βThal^0 (gene deletion?)	αThal^0 (gene deletion?)
Absence of the synthesis of two peptide chains	β–δThal^0 (gene deletion?)	α_1–α_2Thal^0 (gene deletion)

logical diseases similar to the other forms of thalassemias. The heterozygote for a thalassemic gene is clinically asymptomatic. The presence of two β-type thalassemic genes causes severe anemia. The genetics of a-thalassemia is somewhat complicated by the likely duplication of the a-locus.[12] When three out of four a-genes are affected, an a-thalassemia, characterized by over-production of β chains, is observed (Hb H disease); when all a genes are non-functional, a severe a-thalassemia is observed, which is incompatible with life and results in stillbirth and hydrops fetalis.

Thalassemias Characterized by the Synthesis of an Abnormal Peptide Chain

The first thalassemia type for which a molecular explanation has been provided is the Lepore hemoglobinopathy. In 1962, I described the chemical composition of the Lepore chain (Fig. 1) as an hybrid peptide chain, with the N-terminal sequence characteristic of the δ chain and the C-terminal sequence characteristic of the β chain.[4] The δ chain is present in hemoglobin A$_2$, a minor hemoglobin species present at about 2.5% the concentration of Hb A in normal adults. The structure of the Lepore peptide chain results from a non-homologous unequal crossing-over, leading to one chromosome with a deletion of part of the β and δ genes and to another chromosome with a duplication.[4] The peptide chain synthesized by the latter abnormal gene has been called anti-Lepore, since it has a sequence opposite in a complementary way to that of the Lepore chain.[5]

Hb Lepore represents 15% or less of the total hemoglobin in heterozygotes. Thus, the decreased synthesis of this hemoglobin accounts for the hemato-logical manifestations of the carriers. The reasons for the decreased synthesis are not fully understood but may be related to the control of the synthesis of the δ chain, of which the Lepore chain shares the same 5' nucleotide sequence. Synthesis of Hb A$_2$ occurs in bone marrow cells and to much less extent in more mature erythroid cells;[6] the mRNA for the δ chain is thought to be less stable and to be degraded more rapidly than the mRNA for the β chain. A similar situation exists for the Lepore chain[7,8] and for the anti-Lepore chain.[9] The stability of mRNA and the level of synthesis of the corresponding peptide chain cannot thus be related in a simple way to the nucleotide sequence presumably present. One possible explanation for this rather puzzling observation is that untranslated regions of mRNA play an important role in mRNA stability and translational efficiency.[10]

The other thalassemia in which the synthesis of an abnormal peptide chain is observed is the a-thalassemia characterized by the presence of Hb Constant Spring (Hb CS). This hemoglobin is present as 1–3% of the total hemo-globin and has a chains 31 amino acid residues longer than the a^A chain.[11] These residues are presumably translated from a normally untranslated portion

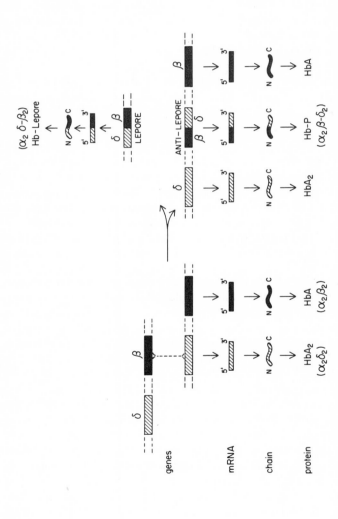

Fig. 1. Schematic representation of the non-homologous unequal crossing over leading to the formation of the Lepore gene. The two products of the crossing over are shown on the right. The mRNA molecules transcribed from each gene and the peptide chains translated from each mRNA represented diagrammatically to show that there are untranscribed portions of each gene and untranslated regions of each mRNA. The role that these nucleotide regions might play in the regulation of transcription, translation and mRNA stability is discussed in the text.

TABLE 2

Molecular Basis of the Thalassemias

Structural Genes Mutations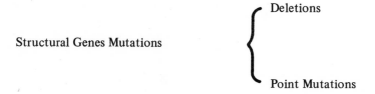
Deletions

Point Mutations

Mutations in Non-Coding Regions — unstable mRNA

Regulatory Genes Mutations — reduced amount of mRNA

(Translational Defects) — ruled out by lack of trans effect

TABLE 3

Studies on Molecular Mechanisms of the β^+ and α^+ Thalassemia

Year	Experimental Approach	Results	References
1960–63	Search for amino acid substitution	negative	Baglioni, Guidotti[3,2]
1964–66	Synthesis of globin chains in intact cells (determination of α/β ratios)	descriptive	Heywood et al.[25] Weatherall et al.[26]
1970	Synthesis of globin chains in marrow	mRNA instability?	Schwartz[28]
1963	Synthesis of globin in cell-free system (normal ribosomes)	uninformative	Marks et al.[29,30]
1968	Rate of chain assembly — Dintziz plot	normal assembly time faster translation	Clegg et al.[31] Rieder[32]
1971	Rate of assembly — Polysome profile	normal polysome size	Nathan et al.[33]
1970–73	Initiation of globin synthesis	normal ribosomes	Anderson et al.[34,35,36]
1972	Chain termination (β^{Thal0})	normal	Dreyfus et al.[37]
1971	Translation from mRNA^{Thal} (from homozygotes) in cell free systems	poor translation β chain	Nienhuis and Anderson[38] Benz and Forget[39]
1973–74	Quantitation of mRNA by hybridization	reduced amounts of mRNA	Housman et al.[21] Forget et al.[24] Kacian et al.[22]

be similar and less than 1.[16,17] In the intact cells of some patients a balanced α/β chain synthesis is observed in marrow cells but not in reticulocytes.[16,17] A detailed discussion of this problem has been presented by Forget.[10]

Thalassemias with Absence of the Synthesis of One or Two Peptide Chains

The incubation of reticulocytes or marrow cells of patients with homozygous β^0-thalassemia shows that β chain synthesis is not detectable.[17—19] The possibility exists, however, that some inactive mRNA for β globin is present in erythroid cells. Direct assay of mRNA not based on translation is necessary to rule out such an hypothesis. Hybridization experiments utilizing cDNA as a probe have thus been devised to test this hypothesis. The cDNA complementary to α mRNA has initially been synthesized, using mRNA isolated from postribosomal supernatant fluid of rabbit reticulocytes;[19] cDNA complementary to β mRNA can also be synthesized with mRNA obtained from large polysomes of rabbit reticulocytes treated with the isoleucine analog 0-methyl-threonine.[20] These cDNA's hybridize with human globin mRNA's and can thus be used as probes to determine the relative amount of mRNA present in erythroid cells of thalassemic patients.[21—23]

Two procedures have been used for the hybridization reaction: (1) saturation hybridization[21] and (2) kinetics of hybrid formation.[22] The first procedure gives results which are somewhat easier to quantitate.[10] Comparable results have been obtained with both procedures. In the case of Hb H disease, the ratio of α mRNA/β mRNA found is $1/6$. The deficiency of α mRNA is thus much greater than that expected from the α/β synthetic ratio. In the case of β-thalassemia mRNA assay, a complication arises from the presence in erythroid cells of a substantial amount of α chain mRNA, since this mRNA hybridizes with the cDNA$^\beta$rabbit probe.[21] A different strategy has been thus used to synthesize a better probe by using human mRNA from a patient with Hb H anemia. Moreover, by selecting more stringent hybridization conditions it is possible to eliminate the hybridization to α chain mRNA.[21] The α mRNA/β mRNA ratio observed is $10/1$, similar to that of the synthetic α/β ratio in erythroid cells of the same patient.[21] It is important to point out that the mRNA used in this assay has been extracted from total lysates rather than from polysomes; this rules out the possibility that some inactive mRNA not associated with polysomes is present in thalassemia erythroid cells.[21]

Similar experiments have been carried out with mRNA obtained from patients with homozygous β^0-thalassemia or with homozygous β-δ-thalassemia.[24] These experiments have shown that β chain mRNA is definitely absent in β-δ-thalassemia and quite likely also absent in β^0-thalassemia. In the latter case, some hybridization to the cDNA probe is observed at high RNA input but this can be .attributed to the small amount of δ chain mRNA present.[24] This explanation is somewhat contradictory with the finding that δ chain synthesis does not occur in circulating reticulocytes discussed above. Two possible explanations are that δ chain synthesis does not decay in thalassemic reticulocytes in comparison to reticulocytes of normal individuals or that translation of δ chain mRNA decays but untranslated mRNA remains present and is detected by the hybridization assay.

A direct assay for a chain genes by hybridization to specific cDNA probes has recently been reported by two groups of investigators.[40,41] DNA has been obtained from liver and spleen of stillborn infants with homozygous a-thalassemia. A cDNA highly enriched for a chain sequences has been prepared either by using as template mRNA from patients with homozygous β-thalassemia,[40] or by reannealing cDNA complementary to a and β chain mRNA with mRNA from the stillborn infants[40] or with mRNA obtained from patients with Hb H anemia.[41] These mRNA preparations do not contain a chain mRNA, in the case of the stillborn infants, or contain a very small amount of a chain mRNA, in the case of Hb H anemia. The cDNA-mRNA hybrids are then removed by chromatography on hydroxyapatite; the non-reannealed cDNA should contain only sequences complementary to the a chain genes. This cDNA probe has then been annealed with DNA from the stillborn infants and, as a control, with DNA from normal individuals. In the first case, hybridization occurs to a final level of 40%, whereas with normal DNA, hybridization to a 70% level is observed.[40] This demonstrates the deletion of all or a substantial part of the a chain genes in a^0-thalassemia.[40,41]

Therapeutic Prospectives

The only therapy presently available for homozygous thalassemia is blood transfusions. These are administered at 3 to 6 week intervals and provide a symptomatic relief of the severe anemia. Deposition of iron in the tissues of the affected individuals is a severe problem and the prospects for survival beyond early adulthood are indeed slim.

Various potential approaches to the therapy of thalassemia have been proposed. A brief outline of potential research lines is described here, without any attempt to cover this important aspect of the research on thalassemia in a comprehensive way. These different approaches can be considered: (1) amelioration of present management; (2) attempt to change the pattern of hemoglobin synthesis; (3) substitution of bone marrow by transplantation and (4) gene substitution.

The first approach is directed at finding an effective way of preventing iron accumulation, by administering chelating compounds. Although an effective agent has not yet been found, some way of preventing iron accumulation appears feasible. Attempts to change the pattern of hemoglobin synthesis may be directed at either prolonging the synthesis of fetal hemoglobin beyond fetal life or at depressing the synthesis of the globin chain made in excess, thus reducing the formation of inclusion bodies and prolonging the life span of erythrocytes. There is no known way of affecting either of these processes.

The relevant switch from synthesis of Hb F to Hb A occurs during the first few weeks of neonatal life. Synthesis of Hb A is already active during fetal hematopoiesis but after birth there is a period of inactive erythropoiesis (newborns are relatively polycythemic and reach a lower hematocrit level within a few weeks), followed by a rapid substitution of Hb F by Hb A.* It is during this period of time that erythrocytes containing predominantly Hb A replace the erythrocytes of the newborn containing predominantly Hb F. If some way were found to prevent this developmental switch, β-thalassemia might be cured. Persistence of the synthesis of Hb F throughout adult life seems to have little pathological consequence, as shown by the occurrence of this condition in homozygotes for a mutation affecting this developmental switch.[42]

Bone marrow transplantation is a definite possibility but involves high risk of graft vs host reaction for the recipient. The risk is somewhat reduced if a donor with good matching of histocompatibility antigens can be found. It seems unlikely, however, that bone marrow transplantation can be effective at a time of extreme hyperplasia of the recipient bone marrow. Since the transplanted erythroid cells have no known selective advantage, they will be diluted into a vastly proliferated erythroid cell population. In order to be potentially effective, bone marrow transplantation should take place shortly after birth, at the time of relatively inactive erythropoiesis. However, techniques for the diagnosis of β-thalassemia at birth should be developed and tested.

Gene substitution involves the administration of DNA containing the relevant nucleotide sequence of the globin gene affected, either carried by a virus known to integrate in the genome or as free DNA. DNA complementary to mRNA is not likely to contain the entire nucleotide sequence deleted in the case of globin gene deletion, or the nucleotide sequence affected by the thalassemia mutation, if this involves an untranscribed part of the globin gene or a regulatory gene. Selection of the relevant nucleotide sequence to be transferred into potential recipients has to follow a completely different strategy, possibly starting from the complete genome from a fraction of DNA enriched in globin genes through hybridization. In any event, this seems to be a quite remote approach which will only be developed after several years and after an animal model for genetic engineering has been tested.

---

*B. Colombo, personal communication.

Conclusions

The molecular basis of many types of thalassemia are fully understood today. A major gap in our knowledge exists with respect to the α^+- and β^+-thalassemia. We do not know whether these diseases are caused by mutations of regulatory genes, which control the rate of globin mRNA production during erythropoiesis, or by mutations of nucleotide sequences which are either not transcribed or transcribed in the nuclear precursor to globin mRNA. The presence of such an altered nucleotide sequence or of a deletion may slow down transcription, for example, by decreasing the affinity of RNA polymerase for a binding site, or may slow down nuclear processing, thus decreasing the output of mRNA. Some of the techniques necessary to test these hypotheses are already available; the difficulty of obtaining human cells active in globin mRNA synthesis and of keeping these cells under tissue culture condition is the principal obstacle to these experiments. We can reasonably expect, however, that the cause of the molecular defect of all types of thalassemia will be detected within a few years.

REFERENCES

1. D.J. Weatherall and J.B. Clegg, *in* The Thalassemia Syndromes, 2nd ed., Blackwell Scientific Publications, Oxford, 1972.

2. V.M. Ingram and A.O.W. Stretton, *Nature 184,* 1903, 1959.

3. C. Baglioni, Mol. Gen., Part 1, J.H. Taylor (Ed.) Academic Press, New York, p. 405, 1963.

4. C. Baglioni, *Proc. Natl. Acad. Sci. USA 48,* 1880, 1962.

5. Y. Ohta, K. Yamaoka, I Sumida and T. Yanase, *Nat. New Biol. 234,* 218, 1971.

6. A.V. Roberts, D.J. Weatherall and J.B. Clegg, *Biochem. Biophys. Res. Commun. 47,* 81, 1972.

7. J.M. White, A. Lang, P.A. Lorkin, H. Lehmann and J. Reeve, *Nat. New Biol. 235,* 208, 1972.

8. F. Gill, J. Atwater and E. Schwartz, *Science 178,* 623, 1972.

9. A.V. Roberts, J.B. Clegg, D.J. Weatherall and Y Ohta, *Nat. New Biol. 245,* 23, 1973.

10. B.G. Forget, *Critical Rev. in Biochem.* (in press), 1974.

11. J.B. Clegg, D.J. Weatherall and P.F. Milner, *Nature 234,* 337, 1971.

12. P. Wasi, *Br. J. Haematol. 24,* 267, 1973.

13. P.F. Milner, J.B. Clegg and D.J. Weatherall, *Lancet 1,* 729, 1971.

14. Y.W. Kan, D. Todd and A.M. Dozy, *Clin. Res. 20,* 471, 1972.

15. J.B. Clegg and D.J. Weatherall, *Nat. New Biol. 240,* 190, 1972.

16. A.W. Nienhuis, P.H. Canfield and W.F. Anderson, *J. Clin. Invest. 52,* 1735, 1973.

17. C. Natta, J. Banks, G. Niazi, P.A. Marks and A. Bank, *Nat. New Biol. 244,* 280, 1973.

18. L.W. Dow, M. Terada, C. Natta, S. Metafora, E. Grossbard, P.A. Marks and A. Bank, *Nat. New Biol. 243,* 114, 1973.

19. M. Jacobs-Lorena and C. Baglioni, *Proc. Natl. Acad. Sci. USA 69,* 1425, 1972.

20. G. Temple and D. Housman, *Proc. Natl. Acad. Sci. USA 69,* 1574, 1972.

21. D. Housman, B.G. Forget, A. Skoultchi and E.J. Benz, Jr., *Proc. Natl. Acad. Sci. USA 70,* 1809, 1973.

22. D.L. Kacian, R. Gambino, L.W. Dow, E. Grossbard, C. Natta, F. Ramirez, S. Spiegelman, P.A. Marks and A. Bank, *Proc. Natl. Acad. Sci. USA 70,* 1886, 1970.

23. D. Housman, A. Skoultchi, B.G. Forget and E.J. Benz, Jr., *Ann. N.Y. Acad. Sci.* (in press), 1974.

24. B.G. Forget, E.J. Benz, Jr., *Nature 247,* 379, 1974.

25. J.D. Heywood, M. Karon and S. Weissman, *Science 146,* 530, 1964.

26. D.J. Weatherall, J.B. Clegg and M.A. Naughton, *Nature 208,* 1061, 1965.

27. A. Bank and P.A. Marks, *Nature 212,* 1198, 1966.

28. E. Schwartz, *Science 167,* 1513, 1970.

29. E.R. Burka and P.A. Marks, *Nature 199,* 706, 1973.

30. P.A. Marks and E.R. Burka, *Science 144,* 552, 1964.

31. J.B. Clegg, D.J. Weatherall, S. Na-Nakorn and P. Wasi, *Nature 220,* 664, 1968.

32. R.F. Rieder, *J. Clin. Invest. 51,* 364, 1972.

33. D.G. Nathan, H. Lodish, Y.W. Kan and D. Housman, *Proc. Natl. Acad. Sci. USA 68,* 2514, 1971.

34. J.M. Gilbert, A.G. Thornton, A. Nienhuis and W.F. Anderson, *Proc. Natl. Acad. Sci. USA 67,* 1854, 1970.

35. A.W. Nienhuis, D.G. Laycock and W.F. Anderson, *Nat. New Biol. 231,* 205, 1971.

36. R.G. Crystal, N.A. Elson, A. Nienhuis, A.C. Thornton and W.F. Anderson, *N. Engl. J. Med. 288,* 1091, 1973.

37. J.C. Dreyfus, D. Labie, M. Vibert and F. Conconi, *Eur. J. Biochem. 27,* 291, 1972.

38. A.W. Nienhuis and W.F. Anderson, *J. Clin. Invest. 50,* 2458, 1971.

39. E.J. Benz, Jr. and B.G. Forget, *J. Clin. Invest. 50,* 2755, 1971.

40. S. Ottolenghi, W.G. Lanyon, J. Paul, R. Williamson, D.J. Weatherall, J.B. Clegg, J. Pritchard, S. Pootrakul and H.B. Wong, *Nature 251,* 389, 1974.

41. J.M. Taylor, A. Dozy, Y.W. Kan, H.E. Varmus, L.E. Lie-Tngo, J. Ganeson and D. Todd, *Nature 251,* 392, 1974.

42. C. Baglioni, *Nature 198,* 1177, 1963.

DISCUSSION

DR. PORTER: Dr. Baglioni, have you now concluded that you are dealing with a gene deletion in thalassemia?

DR. BAGLIONI: In the a-thalassemias, yes.

DR. PORTER: Can the sequencing be worked out now that you know you are dealing with a deletion?

DR. BAGLIONI: Nobody has been able to establish the sequencing in DNA. We can detect the deletion by hybridization, which is in progress in β-δ-thalassemia. We need a source of DNA sperm, which is difficult to obtain because the boys usually die before they are old enough to produce sperm. Another possibility is to grow fibroblasts from the skin, as has now been done for β-δ-thalassemia. My contribution was to provide access to homozygous patients whom we knew in Sicily. Their fibroblasts are now growing at the Boston Children's Hospital and may indicate whether there is a deletion in β-δ-thalassemia.

DR. LAMM: You related the problem of thalassemia to the problem of malaria. Is there a relationship of thalassemia and malaria in the sub-Sahara and African or the Indian sub-continent as here in populations with sickle hemoglobin?

DR. BAGLIONI: Malaria has been an important selective factor in survival of human populations. Different populations use different genetic strategies to cope with malaria. The African population used hemoglobin S, sickle cell anemia or hemoglobin C. The Mediterranean area developed thalassemia and G6PD deficiency. I'm not familiar with the Indian situation but there is clear evidence from Sardinia that thalassemia provides a similar type of protection against malaria as the sickle cell gene.

DR. PORTER: Dr. Meuwissen, did you imply that people with G6PD deficiency are more susceptible to infection?

DR. MEUWISSEN: Yes, that seems to be the case.

DR. LAMM: Is the oxygen tension in thalassemic cells reduced?

DR. BAGLIONI: If you are thinking of sickle cells, I should like to point

377

out that the oxygen tension is not reduced in sickle cell anemia. The protection afforded the heterozygotes is related to the development of the malarial organism within the normal red cell and its ability to complete a growth cycle. In thalassemia, the increased fragility — with shorter life span of the red cell — may interrupt the plasmodium life cycle, as has been proven quite clearly in sickle cell anemia.

DR. VALLET: Dr. Ampola, some patients with methylmalonic acidemia slip in and out of acidosis, in association with loading of the specific branch chain amino acids rather than an increase in total proteins. Were you able to identify the source of intolerance in your patient?

DR. AMPOLA: No. The pathway is well enough delineated to incriminate 4 amino acids. We know from other patients that we can't lower the four without using synthetic diets. Protein diet is preferable and the growth rate on it substantiates its success.

DR. VALLET: We found Ketostix useful in monitoring and correcting ketosis in a patient who was not receiving vitamin B_{12}. Did your patient slip into ketosis before deteriorating?

DR. AMPOLA: She has never been ketoacidotic, not even with infection. We shall, however, give the mother Ketostix to test for it occasionally, particularly if there's an infection. So far, we've regulated her amino acids well enough so that stress, infection and a certain amount of catabolism have not unbalanced her.

SUBJECT INDEX

M

Male abortion rate, 11
Maple syrup urine disease, 291
Mastoiditis, 120
Malformations
  of head and spine in siblings,
    259, 260
Malignant melanoma, 121
Marijuana, 199, 201
Maternal
  age, 30, 45, 122, 124, 139, 141,
    145, 157, 240
    by birth order, 52, 145
    by parity, 14
    -dependent risk, 103
    -specific pattern, 92
  anxiety, 82
  birth cohort, 14
  cardiac disorders, 271
  continent of birth, 51
  convulsive disorder, 271
  diabetes, 129, 252, 259, 260, 271
  diet, 173
  drug exposure and birth defects,
    265-273
  education, 125, 141, 143,
    145-148, 157, 169
  -fetal endocrine function,
    103-110
  height, 161, 163, 171
  hormone deficiency, 106
  hyperthyroidism, 271
  rubella, 221
  starvation, 205, 206, 210, 215,
    219
    effect on fertility, 220
  syphilis, 271
  weight, 129, 161, 163, 170, 171,
    267
  x-ray exposure, 275
Maximum likelihood method, 230

McBride report, 186
  Australia, 186
  reduction deformities, 186
Medical-obstetrical risk, 139, 141,
  144, 149, 150
Meningitis, 220
Meningocele (true), 69, 76
Mercury, 196
Metabolic manipulation, 330-335
  dietary restriction, 330, 331-334
  metabolic inhibitors, 330, 334,
    335
  product replacement, 335
  surgical bypass procedures, 334
Metabolism of drugs, 122
Metachromasia, 309
Methotrexate, 196
Methylmalonic acid, 357, 359-361
Methylmalonic acidemia, 295,
  357-363
  in utero treatment of, 362
  prenatal treatment with Vitamin
    B, 357-363
Mineral deficiencies, 59
Mitral insufficiency, 234
Mitral valve atresia, 232, 233
Monitoring, 122, 129, 185, 190,
  196
"Monstrosity", 5, 7
  cyclopian, 5
Mortality, 3, 5, 11, 26, 27, 119
  data, 3, 5
  differential, 104
  fetal, 119, 124, 130
  infant, 5, 124-129, 140, 147,
    148, 150, 158
    in Canada, 125, 126
    in Chile, 125, 126
    in England and Wales,
      119-126
    in Japan, 126
    in New York City, 140, 141,

387

A 6
B 7
C 8
D 9
E 0
F 1
G 2
H 3
I 4
J 5